Resolving Ethical Dilemmas

A GUIDE FOR CLINICIANS

FIFTH EDITION

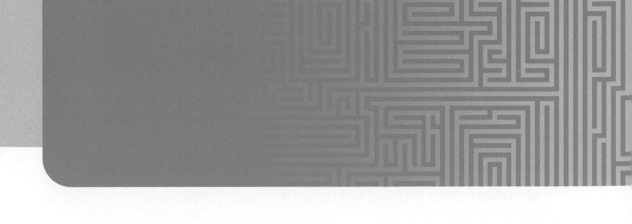

Resolving Ethical Dilemmas

A GUIDE FOR CLINICIANS

FIFTH EDITION

Bernard Lo, MD, FACP

President
The Greenwall Foundation
New York, New York
Professor Emeritus of Medicine
Director Emeritus, Program in Medical Ethics
University of California, San Francisco
San Francisco, California

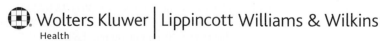

Wolters Kluwer | Lippincott Williams & Wilkins
Health

Philadelphia • Baltimore • New York • London
Buenos Aires • Hong Kong • Sydney • Tokyo

Senior Acquisitions Editor: Sonya Seigafuse
Senior Product Manager: Kerry Barrett
Vendor Manager: Bridgett Dougherty
Senior Manufacturing Manager: Benjamin Rivera
Senior Marketing Manager: Kim Schonberger
Design Coordinator: Stephen Druding
Production Service: S4Carlisle Publishing Services

Printed in China

Library of Congress Cataloging-in-Publication Data
Lo, Bernard.
    Resolving ethical dilemmas : a guide for clinicians / Bernard Lo. — 5th ed.
        p. ; cm.
Includes bibliographical references and index.
ISBN 978-1-4511-7640-7
ISBN 1-4511-7640-6
I. Title.
[DNLM: 1. Ethics, Clinical—Case Reports. WB 60]
174.2—dc23

                                                2012030892

DISCLAIMER
Care has been taken to confirm the accuracy of the information presented and to describe generally accepted practices. However, the authors, editors, and publisher are not responsible for errors or omissions or for any consequences from application of the information in this book and make no warranty, expressed or implied, with respect to the currency, completeness, or accuracy of the contents of the publication. Application of the information in a particular situation remains the professional responsibility of the practitioner.

The authors, editors, and publisher have exerted every effort to ensure that drug selection and dosage set forth in this text are in accordance with current recommendations and practice at the time of publication. However, in view of ongoing research, changes in government regulations, and the constant flow of information relating to drug therapy and drug reactions, the reader is urged to check the package insert for each drug for any change in indications and dosage and for added warnings and precautions. This is particularly important when the recommended agent is a new or infrequently employed drug.

Some drugs and medical devices presented in the publication have Food and Drug Administration (FDA) clearance for limited use in restricted research settings. It is the responsibility of the health care provider to ascertain the FDA status of each drug or device planned for use in their clinical practice.

To purchase additional copies of this book, call our customer service department at **(800) 638-3030** or fax orders to **(301) 223-2320**. International customers should call **(301) 223-2300**.

Visit Lippincott Williams & Wilkins on the Internet: LWW.com. Lippincott Williams & Wilkins customer service representatives are available from 8:30 am to 6:00 pm, EST.

10 9 8 7 6 5 4

CONTENTS

Preface to the First Edition   vii
Preface to the Fifth Edition   ix

SECTION I   FUNDAMENTALS OF CLINICAL ETHICS

  1 An Approach to Ethical Dilemmas in Patient Care 3
  2 Overview of Ethical Guidelines 12
  3 Informed Consent 19
  4 Promoting the Patient's Best Interests 32
  5 Confidentiality 41
  6 Avoiding Deception and Nondisclosure. 52
  7 Keeping Promises 62

SECTION II   SHARED DECISION MAKING

  8 An Approach to Decisions About Clinical Interventions 69
  9 Futile Interventions 71
 10 Decision-Making Capacity 77
 11 Refusal of Treatment by Competent, Informed Patients 85
 12 Standards for Decisions When Patients Lack
     Decision-Making Capacity 90
 13 Surrogate Decision-Making. 104
 14 Persistent Disagreements Over Care 110

SECTION III   DECISIONS ABOUT
LIFE-SUSTAINING INTERVENTIONS

 15 Confusing Ethical Distinctions 121
 16 Ethics Consultations and Ethics Committees 130
 17 Do Not Attempt Resuscitation Orders 135
 18 Tube Feedings 143
 19 Physician-Assisted Suicide and Active Euthanasia 149
 20 The Persistent Vegetative State. 159
 21 Determination of Death 163
 22 Legal Rulings on Life-Sustaining Interventions 168

SECTION IV   THE DOCTOR–PATIENT RELATIONSHIP

23   Overview of the Doctor–Patient Relationship 177
24   Refusal to Care for Patients 181
25   Gifts From Patients to Physicians 189
26   Sexual Contact Between Physicians and Patients 194
27   Secret Information About Patients 200
28   Clinical Research 202

SECTION V   CONFLICTS OF INTEREST

29   Overview Conflicts of Interest 211
30   Bedside Rationing of Health Care 216
31   Incentives for Physicians to Increase Services 223
32   Measures to Control Health Care Costs 227
33   Gifts From Drug Companies 234
34   Disclosing Errors 239
35   Impaired Colleagues 247
36   Ethical Dilemmas Students and House Staff Face 252

SECTION VI   ETHICAL ISSUES IN CLINICAL SPECIALTIES

37   Ethical Issues in Pediatrics 263
38   Ethical Issues in Surgery 271
39   Ethical Issues in Obstetrics and Gynecology 278
40   Ethical Issues in Psychiatry 286

SECTION VII   CURRENT CONTROVERSIES

41   Ethical Issues in Organ Transplantation 295
42   Ethical Issues in Genomic Medicine 304
43   Ethical Issues in Public Health Emergencies 314
44   Ethical Issues in Cross-Cultural Care 323
45   Ethical Issues in Digital Health Information 332

Cases for Discussion   *339*
Index   *353*

PREFACE TO THE FIRST EDITION

As a resident, I was paged by the intensive care unit late one night. I recognized the patient, a 17-year-old boy who had undergone bone marrow transplantation for leukemia and now had chronic interstitial fibrosis. The shy, bright smile I remembered from a previous admission was gone. According to the chart, he had developed progressive respiratory failure. His thin, intubated body was squirming restlessly in the bed. The patient's father grabbed my hand and pointed to the ventilator, saying, "Stop, it's enough. He doesn't want this." I phoned the attending physician, an eminent hematologist, who said that the patient was expected to die in the next few days. I asked whether we should extubate the patient, as his father had requested, and sedate him. The hematologist said that the bone marrow transplant service wanted to continue intensive care; although he did not defend their decision, he deferred to it. We did agree on a Do Not Resuscitate (DNR) order. I gave some sedation to the patient and tried to comfort him and his family. The boy died just before I went off duty the next morning, more comfortable perhaps, but by no means peaceful. The father asked me, "Why didn't they stop? Why?" Later, the attending physician told me that after my phone call, he couldn't get back to sleep. He said that he wanted to call me back to tell me to extubate the patient.

Like this boy's father, I kept asking, "Why?" Why were we so insistent on imposing our medical technology on dying patients? Why were decisions driven by physicians' personalities, hospital politics, research priorities, or staffing problems rather than by what was best for the patient? Why were we comfortable withholding cardiopulmonary resuscitation (CPR), but uneasy administering high doses of narcotics to a patient with intractable ventilatory failure? Although we spent much time on rounds talking about the use of immunosuppressive agents, antibiotics, ventilators, and a vast array of treatments, why did we avoid discussing what to do when such interventions were no longer helpful or appropriate?

My interest in medical ethics, and ultimately this book, grew from such perplexing cases as this and from the illnesses of family members and friends. From visiting my favorite aunt, who had developed multi-infarct dementia, I learned how hard it is to say that life is no longer worth living. She had become almost immobile, dependent on others for all her needs, and would often moan and shout when moved. But she would smile when I held her hands or stroked her cheek. Although mute most of the day, she laughed when I showed her pictures of my son and would ask me, "How old?" We could spend an hour looking at the same pictures over and over, with her repeating the same questions. But even as her family and I despaired over her deteriorating condition, it was not yet time to let her go. Life was still a precious gift, not yet an intolerable burden.

As I began writing and speaking about medical ethics, I learned that many colleagues shared my concerns. At professional meetings, practitioners often tell me about cases whose ethical dilemmas still bother them. I have tried to keep in mind such physicians struggling to do what was right in difficult situations. This book features realistic cases that physicians can relate to their own experience. The goal of *Resolving Ethical Dilemmas* is to help clinicians resolve the mundane ethical issues in patient care, as well as the dilemmas that keep them awake at night. In some cases, there are persuasive reasons for a course of action, but in others the countervailing arguments are equally compelling. Yet even when the philosophic debate is closely balanced, physicians must act, choosing one plan of care or another.

This book grew in several ways beyond my initial work on decisions regarding life-sustaining interventions. First, over the years I realized that physicians need help with many ethical issues. Friends and colleagues often asked me why no one has written about impaired colleagues, about patients' requests to deceive insurance companies, and about the ethical problems in managed care. Second, as the AIDS epidemic ravaged San Francisco, we grappled with new ethical dilemmas, such as the duty to provide care, access to experimental therapies, and the fear of nosocomial HIV infection. Third, a personal calamity broadened the issues of this book. On October 20, 1991, a firestorm raged through the Oakland hills. Our house and more than 2,000 others burned to the ground in a few hours. My wife and I felt sad, angry, frustrated, and overwhelmed by the task of putting our lives back together. It was hard to make any choices, much less informed or rational ones. Gradually, I realized I was struggling with the same issues in this book as in life. Issues of autonomy, informed consent, and fiduciary responsibility took on increasing prominence. How can people make informed decisions when they are emotionally overwhelmed? Why must physicians act in their patients' best interests, even to their personal financial disadvantage, when insurance companies and other businesses have no such obligation?

Colleagues sometimes ask me why I work on such "depressing" topics. Although the issues are indeed somber, it is also a special privilege when patients and their families trust us with their grief, anger, and tranquility and show us how to endure turmoil and sorrow. An elderly patient who had hidden for months the severity of her bone cancer pain was delighted when I made a home visit, saying, "I am so glad I could show you my garden. Now you know why I want to die here, looking at my flowers." Another of my patients died from breast cancer and recurrent pleural effusions. She always cried and moaned as we tapped her effusions, even though she knew that her breathing would be easier. I wondered whether we were hurting her rather than helping her. After her death, I said to her son that it must have been hard for him to care for her. He replied softly, "Doc, it made me a better man." As physicians, we see the worst and the best of people. At times, they are helpless and angry and make foolish decisions. But when confronting problems that are too large for them, people often become heroes. Ultimately, I hope this book will help patients who struggle with such problems by guiding the physicians who care for them.

Bernard Lo

PREFACE TO THE FIFTH EDITION

I have made several important changes in the fifth edition to keep it up-to-date with the best thinking in medical ethics and the most recent clinical developments.

The cases now provide considerably more detail on how to resolve the dilemmas the cases pose. These expanded discussions present practical examples of how to think through and resolve difficult cases. For example, Chapter 15, Confusing Ethical Distinctions, presents a detailed analysis of allegations of euthanasia during Hurricane Katrina in 2005, with lessons to be learned.

As medicine changes, ethics must address new clinical situations. Physicians are increasingly using electronic medical records rather than paper records. Furthermore, e-mail and social media allow doctors new ways to communicate with patients. A new Chapter 45, Ethical Issues in Digital Health Information, analyzes new ethical dilemmas related to physician use of e-mail and social media, health information available to patients on the Internet, and electronic health records.

The passage of the Patient Protection and Affordable Care Act in 2010 and the legal challenges to it have focused national attention on health care reform and the need to control the rising costs of health care. The heavily revised Chapter 32, Measures to Control Health Care Costs, analyzes how cost containment efforts now are increasingly based on incentives to physicians and incentives to patients. These efforts, in turn, raise ethical concerns that physicians must address.

The limitations of advance directives have become more widely and explicitly recognized. The heavily revised Chapter 12, Standards for Decisions When Patients Lack Decision-Making Capacity, focuses on advance care planning—discussions with patients and families about the patient's goals, values, concerns, and fears. The emphasis is on ongoing discussions rather than completing a legal form. We discuss the increasingly used Physician Orders for Life-Sustaining Treatment (POLST), analyze their advantages and limitations, and discuss a case in which POLST orders did not resolve difficult dilemmas. In addition, Chapter 44 extensively discusses a new case in which a Chinese American patient declines to participate in advance care planning and suggests how the physician might discuss end-of-life decisions with the family.

Several other chapters include important new material.

Chapter 4, Promoting the Patient's Best Interests, includes a new discussion of the problems of opioid abuse and diversion the need to balance concerns about these problems with the need to treat pain effectively.

Chapter 20, The Persistent Vegetative State, discusses new studies showing that some patients diagnosed as being in PVS have evidence of willful brain activity on functional magnetic resonance imaging or electroencephalography although they are clinically unresponsive.

Chapter 21, Determination of Death, analyzes recent controversies over using cardiopulmonary criteria for death in organ donors and objections to the conceptual basis for brain death.

Chapter 31, Incentives for Physicians to Increase Services, discusses new empirical evidence on how fee-for-service reimbursement incentives have changed the care of oncology and renal dialysis patients.

Chapter 41, Ethical Issues in Organ Transplantation, includes a new discussion of paired donation from living donors.

Chapter 42, Ethical Issues in Genomic Medicine, discusses prenatal screening through the analysis of fetal DNA present in maternal serum.

Chapter 43, Ethical Issues in Public Health Emergencies, has a new section on crisis standards of care.

In addition, the references have been updated. Finally, numerous revisions have been made to improve the clarity and flow of ideas.

Fundamentals
of Clinical Ethics

An Approach to Ethical Dilemmas in Patient Care

This case is really bothering me. I haven't been able to stop worrying about it. I'm just not sure what the right thing to do is." Cases with ethical dilemmas can perplex physicians. Strong reasons for an action might be balanced by cogent countervailing arguments. Common sense, clinical experience, being a good person, and good intentions do not guarantee that physicians will respond appropriately. Ethical dilemmas often evoke powerful emotions and strong personal opinions; however, emotions and opinions alone are not a satisfactory way of resolving ethical dilemmas. The following cases illustrate the range of ethical issues in clinical medicine.

CASE 1.1   Decisions about life-sustaining interventions

Mrs. D, an elderly woman with severe dementia, develops pneumonia. Her daughter insists that hospitalization and administration of antibiotics would be pointless and that the patient would not want such "heroics." Her son, however, demands that her pneumonia be treated because he believes that life is sacred. Should the physician withhold or administer antibiotics? Who should be Mrs. D's surrogate when she cannot speak for herself? Furthermore, what are the reasons that the physician can give to justify the decision to the patient's children and to the other health care workers caring for the patient?

CASE 1.2   Confidentiality of human immunodeficiency virus (HIV) test results

A 32-year-old man with a positive test for HIV antibodies refuses to notify his wife. "If she finds out, it would destroy our marriage." Should the physician notify the wife despite the patient's objections? Although maintaining patient confidentiality is important, it seems cruel not to warn the wife that she is at risk for a fatal infection. What are the reasons that justify the physician's decision?

CASE 1.3   Physician certification of eligibility

A 67-year-old man with chronic obstructive lung disease has dyspnea after walking one block. He is on an optimal medical regimen of inhaled bronchodilators and corticosteroids. His resting arterial O_2 level is 65 mm Hg, and it does not decrease with exercise. This exceeds the level that qualifies for Medicare coverage of home oxygen. The patient pleads, "Can't you just write that the oxygen level is 58? I need to do something about this breathing."

In such cases, physicians cannot avoid difficult decisions. This chapter describes how clinical ethics can help physicians deal with such dilemmas and presents approaches to resolving them. Specific ethical problems are discussed in detail in subsequent chapters.

WHAT IS CLINICAL ETHICS?

We use the term *clinical* to limit our topics to the doctor–patient encounter in the office or at the hospital bedside, when a physician is caring for an individual patient. Such patient care is the essence of a physician's work. Although the focus is primarily on the doctor's interaction with the patient, the physician's relationships with the family, other health care workers, and medical institutions, such as insurance companies, may also be pertinent.

We use the term *ethics* to refer to judgments about what is right or wrong and worthy of praise or blame; however, we refer to moral judgments about right and wrong, not biotechnical or clinical judgments about the most effective or safest test or treatment. Thus, in Case 1.1 the biotechnical issue is, which antibiotic would be most effective for community-acquired pneumonia? There may be medical uncertainty or controversy, for example, because of emerging patterns of antibiotic resistance. These biotechnical questions can often be resolved by referring to the medical literature or clinical experience. The clinical ethics question is whether to administer or withhold antibiotics.

We also distinguish clinical ethics from several other closely related fields that are beyond the scope of this book. *Health policy* refers to public policies that set the context in which physicians deliver care to patients. It includes health insurance, access to care for the uninsured, allocation of scarce resources, public health policies, and state laws regarding end-of-life care and confidentiality.

Bioethics refers to broader philosophical questions raised by biomedical advances, for example, whether genetically modified crops or germ-line gene therapy is acceptable.

HOW DOES CLINICAL ETHICS DIFFER FROM PROFESSIONAL ETHICS?

Many physicians seek ethical guidance from professional codes and the oaths that they took as students at white coat ceremonies and at graduation. New members of the profession pledge to the public and to their patients that they will be guided by the principles and values in the oath or code. Although professional oaths are important, they have several shortcomings (1). First, they are unilateral declarations by groups of physicians, without any input from patients or the public. Codes of ethics and professional oaths do not acknowledge that society has granted the medical profession autonomy to set standards for training and certification and, therefore, in exchange, may insist on certain expectations. Second, the content of professional codes has been criticized. The Hippocratic tradition is highly paternalistic, granting patients little role in making decisions. For instance, it does not require physicians to disclose information to patients, be truthful, or allow them to make informed choices. Third, oaths and codes articulate general precepts but are too brief to resolve specific dilemmas. Furthermore, the principles embodied in codes may be in conflict in a particular case, leaving the physician in a quandary about how to act. This book provides physicians the tools to interpret broad principles (such as those contained in professional codes) as they relate to specific situations and how to act when ethical principles conflict or do not apply.

HOW DOES CLINICAL ETHICS DIFFER FROM LAW?

Statutes, regulations, and court decisions also guide what physicians may or may not do. On many issues, the law reflects an ethical consensus in society. Moreover, appellate courts give reasons for decisions and, therefore, provide an analysis of pertinent issues. Hence, physicians should be familiar with what the law requires regarding issues in clinical ethics. However, the law may not provide definitive answers to ethical dilemmas.

First, the law, particularly criminal law, sets only a minimally acceptable standard of conduct. It identifies acts that are so *wrong* that physicians will be held legally liable for committing them. In contrast, ethics may focus on the *right* or the best decision in a situation. In Case 1.3, the Medicare criteria for coverage of home oxygen are clear: an arterial oxygen level of under 60 mm Hg. Giving false information to obtain Medicare coverage is considered fraud, a criminal violation. Physicians, like all citizens, should follow the law. However, professional ethics requires physicians to go beyond their legal duties, to act with compassion and respect, and to respond to the patient's distress. The law cannot compel such aspirations. Second, the law explicitly grants physicians discretion in some situations. In Case 1.1, most states allow physicians to determine when a patient lacks decision-making capacity and, thus, when a surrogate should make decisions with the physician (*see* Chapter 13). In Case 1.2, some states give physicians discretion whether or not to override confidentiality to protect partners of HIV-infected persons. In these circumstances, physicians must turn to ethical and clinical considerations, not legal ones. Third, the law might provide no clear guide to action on certain topics. For example, the law provides scant explicit guidance on the issue of disclosing genetic information to relatives when the patient objects to disclosure (*see* Chapter 42). Finally, law and ethics might differ. Abortion is currently legal throughout the United States, but remains controversial ethically. Conversely, people might consider some actions that are prohibited by law to be ethical. In a few states, the courts have rejected family decision making for incompetent patients who have not provided written advance directives or very specific oral directives. Ethically, however, the consensus is to respect surrogate decision making by concerned family members (*see* Chapter 12). In this situation, most physicians feel uncomfortable simply following the letter of the law.

SOURCES OF MORAL GUIDANCE

DISTINGUISHING MORALITY AND ETHICS

The terms "morality" and "ethics" are often used interchangeably to refer to standards of right and wrong behavior. It is helpful to draw some distinctions. Moral choices ultimately rest on values or beliefs that cannot be proved but are simply accepted. Morality usually refers to conduct that conforms "to the accepted customs or conventions of a people (2)." Children usually learn from parents and religious leaders what their culture or group regards as correct and might accept it without deliberation. Ultimately, such fundamental moral beliefs are part of a person's character. Yet ordinary moral rules, which usually provide an adequate guide for daily conduct, fail to provide clear direction in many clinical situations, as we have seen.

In contrast to morality, ethics connotes deliberation and explicit arguments to justify particular actions. Ethics also refers to a branch of philosophy that deals with the "principles governing ideal human character (2)." To philosophers, ethics focuses on the reasons *why* an action is considered right or wrong. It asks people to justify their positions and beliefs by rational arguments that can persuade others.

PERSONAL MORAL VALUES

Physicians, like all people, draw on many sources of moral guidance, including parental and family values, cultural traditions, and religious beliefs. However, additional guidance in clinical ethics is needed.

First, these personal moral values might not address important issues in clinical ethics. Often, doctors face an ethical dilemma for the first time during their training and clinical practice. Laypeople have little experience with such topics as life-sustaining treatment or surrogate decision making. In addition, personal moral values might offer conflicting advice on a particular situation. For instance, moral precepts to respect the sanctity of life can be used in Case 1.1 to justify both continuing and withholding antibiotics.

Second, physicians have role-specific ethical obligations that go beyond their obligations as good citizens and good persons. Doctors have special duties to maintain confidentiality, as in Case 1.2, and to avoid misrepresentation when certifying a patient's medical condition, as in Case 1.3. Personal moral values do not address these special professional roles.

Third, the physician's moral values might differ from those of the patient or other health care workers. The United States is increasingly diverse in terms of cultural heritage and religious beliefs. In such a pluralistic society, physicians cannot assume that other people directly involved in a case share their moral beliefs. Thus, physicians need to persuade other health care workers, patients, and family members of their plans to resolve ethical dilemmas in patient care, using reasons that do not depend on a particular religious or cultural perspective.

CLAIMS OF CONSCIENCE

Sometimes people explain their actions as a matter of conscience (3); to act otherwise would make them feel ashamed or guilty or violate their sense of integrity or deeply held values (2). Conscience involves self-reflection and judgment about whether an action is right or wrong. For example, in Case 1.2, a physician might declare, "I couldn't live with myself if I didn't notify his wife."

Deeply held claims of conscience are generally honored. It would be dehumanizing to compel people to act in ways that violate their sense of integrity and responsibility. Respecting claims of conscience, even though one disagrees with the decision or action, fosters moral reflection and striving to act with integrity. Claims of conscience, however, often do not resolve a dispute. There may be countervailing interests and ethical principles in play. Appeals to conscience do not end discussions; to persuade others to accept such claims, it is often necessary to provide reasons and arguments. Chapter 14 discusses physician insistence on interventions, and Chapter 24 discusses refusals to provide services, based on objections based on conscience.

CLAIMS OF RIGHTS

To explain their positions on ethical issues, people often appeal to rights, such as a "right to die" or a "right to health care." To philosophers, rights are justified claims that a person can make on others or on society (2). The language of rights is widespread in US culture, yet appeals to rights are often controversial. Other people might deny that the right exists or assert conflicting rights. For example, in Case 1.2, even if the seropositive patient has a right to confidentiality, the wife might have a countervailing right to know that she is at risk for a fatal infectious disease. Although claims of rights are often used to end debates, asserting a right should open a new discussion: whether there are persuasive arguments that support the claim of rights.

HOW CAN CLINICAL ETHICS HELP PHYSICIANS?

Certain situations commonly recur in clinical practice. Physicians learn to recognize individual cases as examples of syndromes, such as "angina" or "hyponatremia (4)." Placing cases into categories allows physicians to organize relevant data and draw on experiences with similar cases. For each type of case, the physician learns to gather additional information, to anticipate associated problems or complications, and to develop an approach. The more categories of cases physicians study, the better prepared they are for clinical practice.

Clinical ethics can help physicians identify, understand, and resolve common ethical issues in patient care. By studying paradigmatic "teaching cases," physicians can gain vicarious experience in identifying and resolving ethical dilemmas (5, 6). Doctors can learn how to interpret ethical guidelines in particular situations, how to identify features of a case that distinguish it from other apparently similar cases, and how to know when exceptions to guidelines are justified.

IDENTIFY ETHICAL ISSUES

By studying realistic cases that illustrate common ethical problems, physicians may better recognize the ethical issues in their own cases. In some cases, physicians might have only a vague uneasiness that important ethical issues are at stake. In other situations, health care workers might be perplexed about difficult decisions but fail to identify problems as specifically ethical in nature, as opposed to issues of clinical management or interpersonal conflict.

UNDERSTAND AREAS OF ETHICAL CONSENSUS AND CONTROVERSY

On many ethical issues, physicians, philosophers, and the courts agree on what should be done (7, 8). Such agreement is often possible even when people disagree on the reasons for their actions (9). For example, it is well established that trustworthy advance directives should be respected and that certain exceptions to confidentiality of medical information are ethically and legally appropriate. Subsequent chapters point out areas of widespread ethical agreement and areas of ongoing controversy.

Clinical ethics can identify actions that are clearly right or wrong and that are controversial. Philosophers distinguish among actions that are obligatory, permissible, and prohibited. In Case 1.3, there are strong reasons why physicians should not misrepresent the patient's condition to insurers (*see* Chapter 6). Some actions are optional or ethically *permissible,* but not required. The arguments for and against them may be so evenly balanced that reasonable people may disagree. Alternatively, it may be praiseworthy for the physician to perform them, but the physician should not be faulted for not doing so. For instance, it would be commendable for a busy physician in Case 1.3 to devote considerable time to explaining to the patient why he cannot fulfill his request. The physician should not be blamed, however, if she gave her recommendation with a brief explanation of her reasoning and referred the patient for more information on home oxygen to the website of the Global Initiative for Chronic Obstructive Lung Disease.

AN APPROACH TO ETHICAL DILEMMAS IN CLINICAL MEDICINE

A systematic approach to ethical problems helps ensure that no important considerations are overlooked and that similar cases are resolved consistently (Table 1-1). In any particular case, an experienced physician may need to modify the general approach.

WHAT IS THE PROBLEM OR DILEMMA?

As a first step, it is helpful to state the problem or dilemma in straightforward terms. In Case 1.2, should the wife be notified that she is at risk for HIV? In Case 1.3, should the physician report a false value for the patient's oxygen?

TABLE 1-1	An Approach to Ethical Dilemmas in Clinical Medicine

In plain terms, what is the problem or dilemma?

What are the medical facts and issues?

What are the concerns, values, and preferences of the physicians?

What are the concerns, values, and preferences of the patient?

What are the ethical issues?

What ethical guidelines are at stake?

What practical considerations need to be addressed?

WHAT ARE THE MEDICAL FACTS AND ISSUES?

Sound ethical decision making requires accurate medical facts and clinical judgment. The physician needs to clarify the patient's diagnosis and prognosis, the options for care, and the benefits and burdens of each alternative. Health outcomes need to be specified and characterized in quantitative terms insofar as possible. Furthermore, the strength of the medical evidence needs to be assessed. Uncertainty and disagreement over the medical facts are common. Often they can be resolved by going to the medical literature or by having the various specialty services or physicians caring for the patient meet face to face.

WHAT ARE THE PATIENT'S CONCERNS, VALUES, AND PREFERENCES?

Informed consent and shared decision making require the physician to understand the patient's perspective. A good first step is to ask open-ended questions about the patient's understanding of the clinical situation: "What is your understanding of your medical situation?" or "What have the doctors told you about your illness?" Any misunderstandings should be discussed and corrected.

Physicians should elicit the patient's or surrogate's concerns, hopes, and fears: "As you think about your medical situation, what concerns you the most?" Addressing the patient's concerns demonstrates caring, strengthens the doctor–patient relationship, and makes patients and surrogates more open to the physician's recommendations. Next, the physician needs to understand the patient's preferences regarding specific decisions that need to be made.

If the patient lacks decision-making capacity, an appropriate surrogate needs to be identified, generally a family member (*see* Chapter 13).

WHAT ARE THE CLINICIANS' CONCERNS, VALUES, AND PREFERENCES?

Physicians have expertise regarding diagnosis, prognosis, options for care, and their risks and benefits. They also have their own values and preferences. In Case 1.2, a physician might have a strong personal commitment to avoiding divorce or to women's rights. The physician's personal beliefs may differ from those of the patient or family. Physicians must identify their own values and distinguish medical expertise from value judgments, where the patient's values and preferences must be taken into account, and generally should be decisive.

Physicians commonly have different attitudes, preferences, and values regarding uncertainty, risk, and views of the doctor–patient relationship. They need to acknowledge that other health care workers may have different values and preferences. One way to assess such differences is to ask questions such as the following: Do the different clinical services on the case agree on the patient's prognosis and on recommendations for treatment? Would other attending physicians make different recommendations?

WHAT ARE THE ETHICAL ISSUES OR QUESTIONS?

It is generally fruitful to frame the ethical issues and questions in specific terms, rather than as broad ethical concepts, such as autonomy and beneficence. In Case 1.1, the questions might be as follows: When a patient has lost decision-making capacity, how should disputes between the daughter and son be resolved? Should antibiotics for pneumonia be considered heroic care in this context? With this framing, the physician can then address issues of selection of surrogate-makers and distinctions between ordinary and heroic care.

The importance of specificity can be illustrated by comparing how physicians pose medical issues. In a case of diabetic ketoacidosis, it is not useful to frame the issue as "homeostasis," although that is a fundamental unifying concept in this situation. For clinical management, it is much more useful to identify specific problems, such as volume replacement, hyperglycemia, potassium disorders, acidosis, and precipitating events. Posing medical issues in such specific terms facilitates clinical decisions and management. Each specific medical issue triggers considerations that the physician should take into account. For example, identifying serum potassium as an issue emphasizes that the potassium level should be elevated in the face of acidosis and suggests the magnitude of total body potassium loss and the rate of replacement.

WHAT ETHICAL GUIDELINES ARE AT STAKE, AND HOW CAN THE DILEMMA BE RESOLVED?

Once identified, specific ethical issues suggest ethical guidelines to be taken into account and an approach to resolving the issues. Subsequent chapters analyze how to resolve these specific ethical issues. The guidelines need to be more specific than "respect for persons," "beneficence," and so on, which are too abstract and general to guide the physician's decisions and actions.

In Case 1.2, maintaining patient confidentiality conflicts with preventing harm to another person. Ethical analysis helps the physician understand when it is appropriate to override confidentiality (*see* Chapter 5). There are several options for notifying the wife that she is at risk, each with advantages and disadvantages.

In Case 1.3, physicians have an ethical obligation to avoid misrepresentation (*see* Chapter 6) and to allocate scarce medical resources fairly (*see* Chapter 30).

Although physicians should learn an approach to each common ethical issue, difficult cases cannot be resolved by mechanically applying rules. Physicians must interpret guidelines in the particular circumstances of a case. Furthermore, guidelines may conflict or be accorded different weight in various circumstances. Physicians also need to think through the reasons supporting their plan, so that they can explain them to others in a persuasive manner.

WHAT PRACTICAL CONSIDERATIONS NEED TO BE ADDRESSED?

What Is the Plan for Communication?

The physician should consider how to discuss the ethical issues with other health care workers, patients, and surrogates. Team meetings can clarify the clinical situation and provide additional information about the patient's or surrogate's views. Health care workers from different clinical, personal, and cultural backgrounds can frequently point out hidden assumptions and value judgments, call attention to neglected issues, and suggest fresh alternatives. Health care workers caring for the patient should agree on a plan for care, or else clarify the points of disagreement and how they will be resolved.

A series of family meetings is usually required (10). Chapter 14 suggests how physicians can negotiate an ethically acceptable resolution when surrogates of a patient disagree. Often the key is to listen to the patient's and family's needs, concerns, and values. Patients or families might hear mixed messages from different clinicians, so family conferences that include key consulting services enhance consistent communication.

Physicians need to try to reach a decision that is acceptable to them, the patient or surrogate, and other health care providers caring for the patient. Decisions also need to be consistent with the ethical guidelines discussed in later chapters.

What Psychosocial Issues Complicate the Case?

Emotions, misunderstandings, interpersonal conflicts, and time pressures often complicate ethical dilemmas. Although analysis of ethical issues is essential, few dilemmas in clinical ethics are resolved solely by philosophical arguments. Indeed, many ethical dilemmas are settled by addressing psychosocial issues rather than through philosophical debate. Showing respect, concern, and compassion builds patient and family trust and makes them more likely to carefully consider the physician's recommendations.

When Should Physicians Seek Assistance?

In difficult cases, the physician may seek assistance from the hospital ethics committee or an ethics consultant (*see* Chapter 16). A second opinion from another physician not directly involved in the case might also be helpful. A chaplain, social worker, or nurse who has good rapport with the patient or family can help address their concerns or facilitate discussions.

What Are the Legal Constraints?

Physicians need to understand the legal risk of the course of action they have determined to be ethically appropriate; however, decisions should not be based primarily on defensive medicine. Ethics and law may differ. In many situations, the law is ambiguous or silent. In Case 1.2, states vary on whether they require physicians to notify public health officials of persons who are HIV-infected or whether they permit such notification. Physicians can minimize legal risk by documenting in the medical record the reasons that justify the plan for care.

CASE 1.1   *Continued*

The physician can follow the recommendations in Table 1.1.

What is the problem or dilemma? *Should antibiotics be administered, and who should decide?*
What are the medical facts and issues? *How likely is it that Mrs. D will be discharged from the hospital, return to her own home, and regain her former functional status if she receives antibiotics?*
What are the patient's concerns, values, and preferences? *Has Mrs. D indicated what is important to her and what she is concerned about? Has she indicated preferences for hospitalization and medical care in such a situation?*
What are the clinician's concerns, values, and preferences? *A physician might believe that she should provide effective, low-risk treatments that prolong life.*
What are the ethical issues or questions? *When a patient has lost decision-making capacity, how should disputes between the daughter and son about medical treatment be resolved? Should antibiotics for pneumonia be considered heroic care in this context?*
What ethical guidelines are at stake, and how can they be resolved? *Surrogates should base decisions on what the patient would want, not what they would decide for themselves (see Chapter 13). There are guidelines to evaluate what weight to give the patient's previous statements about end-of-life care (see Chapter 12). The doctor should orient the son and daughter to thinking about what Mrs. D would want and to obtain more information on what the patient previously said about her medical condition and life-sustaining treatments.*
What practical considerations need to be addressed? *Some states do not explicitly authorize surrogate decision making by family members who have not been designated as proxies by the patient, even though this is standard clinical practice and ethically sound.*

SUMMARY

1. Reading about ethical issues, thinking about them, and discussing them with colleagues can help physicians resolve ethical dilemmas.
2. As with any clinical problem, following a systematic approach helps ensure that all pertinent considerations are taken into account.
3. Physicians should gather information about the medical situation and the patient's values and preferences, identify the ethical guidelines at stake, and address practical considerations.

REFERENCES

1. Veatch RM. Assessing Pellegrino's reconstruction of medical morality. *Am J Bioeth.* 2006;6:72–75.
2. *Webster's New Dictionary of Synonyms.* Springfield, MA: Merriam-Webster Inc.; 1984:547.
3. Curlin FA, Lawrence RE, Chin MH, et al. Religion, conscience, and controversial clinical practices. *N Engl J Med.* 2007;356:593–600.
4. Kassirer JP. Diagnostic reasoning. *Ann Intern Med.* 1989;110:893–900.
5. Lo B, Jonsen AR. Ethical dilemmas and the clinician. *Ann Intern Med.* 1980;92:116–117.
6. Lo B, Quill T, Tulsky J. Discussing palliative care with patients. *Ann Intern Med.* 1999;130:744–749.
7. Meisel A. *The Right to Die.* 2nd ed. New York, NY: John Wiley & Sons; 1995.
8. Beauchamp TL, Childress JF. *Principles of Biomedical Ethics.* 6th ed. New York, NY: Oxford University Press; 2008.
9. Jonsen AR, Toulmin S. *The Abuse of Casuistry: A History of Moral Reasoning.* Berkeley, CA: University of California Press; 1988.
10. Lautrette A, Ciroldi M, Ksibi H, et al. End-of-life family conferences: rooted in the evidence. *Crit Care Med.* 2006;34:S364–S372.

Overview of Ethical Guidelines

E thical dilemmas arise in clinical medicine because there are often sound reasons for conflicting courses of action. In resolving dilemmas, physicians need to refer to general ethical guidelines to inform their choices and justify their decisions. This chapter provides an overview of guidelines in clinical ethics. Subsequent chapters discuss them in detail and apply them to specific cases.

RESPECT FOR PERSONS

Treating patients with respect entails several ethical obligations. First, physicians must respect the medical decisions of persons who are autonomous (1). The term *autonomy* literally means "self-rule." Autonomous people act intentionally, are informed, and are free from interference and control by others. People should be allowed to shape their lives in accordance with their core values and free from unwanted bodily intrusion or touching. The concept of autonomy includes the ideas of self-determination, independence, and freedom. Doctors should promote patient autonomy, for example, by disclosing information and helping patients deliberate.

With regard to health care, autonomy justifies the doctrine of informed consent (*see* Chapter 3). Informed consent has several specific aspects. Informed, competent patients may refuse unwanted medical interventions, such as surgery and invasive procedures, and may choose among medically feasible alternatives. Important clinical choices need not involve a major bodily invasion, for instance, choices whether to have an electrocardiogram or choices among several drugs for a condition. Competent, informed patients have the right to make choices that conflict with the wishes of family members or the recommendations of their physicians.

A person's autonomy is not absolute and may be justifiably restricted for several reasons. If a person is incapable of making informed decisions, trying to respect his or her autonomy might be less important than acting in his or her best interests. Autonomy might also be constrained by the needs of other individuals or society at large. A person is not free to act in ways that violate other people's autonomy, harm others, or impose unfair claims on society's resources.

A second meaning of respect for persons concerns patients who are not autonomous because their decision-making capacity is impaired by illness or medication. Physicians should still treat them as persons with individual characteristics, preferences, and values. Decisions should respect their preferences and values, so far as they are known. In addition, all patients, whether autonomous or not, should be treated with attention, dignity, and compassion.

Third, respect for persons requires physicians to avoid misrepresentation, maintain confidentiality, and keep promises. There are additional reasons for these other guidelines, as we will discuss.

MAINTAIN CONFIDENTIALITY

Maintaining the confidentiality of medical information respects patient privacy. It also encourages people to seek treatment and to discuss their problems frankly. In addition, confidentiality protects patients from harms that might occur if information about psychiatric illness, sexual preference, or alcohol or drug use were widely disseminated. Patients and the public expect physicians to keep medical information confidential. However, maintaining confidentiality is not an absolute duty. In some situations, physicians need to override confidentiality to protect third parties from harm (*see* Chapter 5).

AVOID DECEPTION AND NONDISCLOSURE

Truth telling—avoiding lies—is a cornerstone of social interaction. If people cannot depend on others to tell the truth, no one will make agreements or contracts. Physicians might mislead patients without technically lying, for example, by giving partial information that is literally true but intended to mislead. Deception violates the autonomy of people who are deceived because it causes them to make decisions on the basis of false premises. To cover these broader issues, this book uses the term "deception" rather than "lying." In addition, physicians sometimes withhold information about their diagnosis or prognosis from patients. Doctors may do so to protect patients from bad news. However, patients cannot make informed decisions about their medical care if they do not receive all pertinent information about their condition.

KEEP PROMISES

Promises generate expectations in other people, who, in turn, modify their plans on the assumption that promises will be kept. The very concept of promises is undermined if people are free to break them. It is unfair for someone to expect others to honor their promises, but to break his or her own. Keeping promises also enhances trust in both the individual physician and the medical profession. Furthermore, promises relieve patients' anxiety about the future by providing reassurance that doctors will not abandon them.

ACT IN THE BEST INTERESTS OF PATIENTS

The guideline of *nonmaleficence*, or "do no harm," forbids physicians from providing ineffective therapies or from acting selfishly or maliciously (2, 3). This oft-cited precept, however, provides only limited guidance, because many beneficial interventions also entail serious risks and side effects. Literally doing no harm would preclude risky treatments such as surgery and cancer chemotherapy.

The guideline of *beneficence* requires physicians to provide a net benefit to patients: the benefits of an intervention must outweigh the burdens and be proportionate (*see* Chapter 4). Because patients do not possess medical expertise and might be vulnerable because of illnesses, they rely on physicians to provide sound advice and to promote their well-being. Physicians encourage such trust. For these reasons, physicians have a fiduciary duty to act in the best interests of their patients.

UNWISE DECISIONS BY PATIENTS

Acting in patients' best interests might conflict with respecting their informed choices, as when patients' refusals of care might thwart their own goals or cause them serious harm. Simply accepting such refusals, in the name of respecting autonomy, would be highly problematic. Physicians should listen to patients, educate them, and try to persuade them to accept beneficial treatment, or negotiate a mutually acceptable compromise. If disagreements persist, the patient's informed choices and judgment of his best interests should prevail.

PATIENTS WHO LACK DECISION-MAKING CAPACITY

The choices and preferences of many patients who lack decision-making capacity are unknown or unclear. In this situation, respecting autonomy is not pertinent. Instead, physicians should be guided by the patient's best interests (*see* Chapter 4).

CONFLICTS OF INTEREST

Physicians should act in the patient's best interests rather than in their own self-interest when conflicts of interest occur (*see* Chapters 29–36). Patients trust their physicians to act on their behalf and feel betrayed if that trust is abused. When considering whether or not a conflict of interest exists, physicians should consider how patients, the public, and colleagues would react if they knew about the situation. Even the appearance of a conflict of interest might damage trust in the individual physician and in the profession.

ALLOCATE RESOURCES JUSTLY

The term *justice* is used in a general sense to mean fairness—that is, people should get what they deserve. People who are similar in ethically relevant respects should be treated similarly, and people who differ in ethically significant ways should be treated differently. Otherwise, decisions would be arbitrary and biased. To make this formal statement of justice operational, the physician would need to specify what counts as an ethically relevant distinction and what it means to treat people similarly.

In health care settings, "justice" also refers to the allocation of health care resources. Allocation decisions are unavoidable because resources are limited and could be spent on other social goods, such as education or the environment, instead of on health care. Ideally, allocation decisions should be made as public policy and set by legislatures or government officials, according to appropriate procedures. Physicians should participate in public debates about allocation and help set policies. In general, however, rationing medical care at the bedside should be avoided because it might be inconsistent, discriminatory, and ineffective. At the bedside, physicians usually should act as patient advocates within constraints set by society and sound clinical practice (*see* Chapter 30). In some cases, however, two patients might compete for the same limited resources, such as physician time or a bed in intensive care. When this occurs, physicians should ration their time and resources according to patients' medical needs and the probability and degree of benefit.

THE USE OF ETHICAL GUIDELINES

Having summarized guidelines for clinical ethics, we next discuss how physicians should use them in specific cases. This book uses the term *guidelines* to connote that ethical generalizations cannot be mechanically or rigidly applied but need to be used with discretion and judgment in the circumstances of a particular case. Guidelines are derived from decisions made in previous cases and from moral theories (4, 5). In turn, guidelines shape decisions in similar cases in the future. Guidelines might be difficult to apply in new cases for several reasons.

GUIDELINES NEED TO BE INTERPRETED IN THE CONTEXT OF SPECIFIC CASES

The meaning or force of a guideline might not be clear in a particular case. Uncertainty and case-by-case variation are inherent in clinical medicine. Furthermore, patients have different priorities and goals for care. A crucial issue is whether the case to be decided can be distinguished in ethically meaningful ways from previous cases to which the guideline was applied. Unforeseen or novel cases might point out the shortcomings of an existing guideline and suggest that it needs to be modified or an exception made.

EXCEPTIONS TO GUIDELINES MIGHT BE APPROPRIATE

Guidelines are not absolute. A particular case might have distinctive features that justify making an exception to a guideline (4). To ensure fairness, physicians who make an exception to a guideline should justify their decisions. The justification should apply not only to the specific case under consideration, but also to all similar cases faced by other physicians. Guidelines are stronger than rules of thumb that provide advice but are not binding. Many philosophers regard ethical guidelines as *prima facie* binding: they should be followed unless they conflict with stronger obligations or guidelines or unless there are compelling reasons to make an exception (5). The burden of argument is on those who claim that an exception to the guideline is warranted. Furthermore, when *prima facie* guidelines are overridden, they are not simply ignored. People often experience regret or even remorse that guidelines are being broken. Thus, people should minimize the extent to which *prima facie* guidelines are violated and mitigate the adverse consequences of doing so.

DIFFERENT GUIDELINES MIGHT CONFLICT

In many situations, following one ethical guideline would require the physician to compromise another guideline. Respecting a patient's refusal of treatment might clash with acting in the patient's best interests. Maintaining confidentiality might conflict with protecting third parties from harm. Allocating resources equitably might conflict with doing what is best for an individual patient. The practice of medicine would be much easier if there were a fixed hierarchy of ethical guidelines; for example, if patient autonomy always took priority over beneficence. Life is not so simple, however. In some clinical situations, respecting a patient's wishes should be paramount, whereas in others, a patient's best interests should prevail. Physicians need to understand why an ethical guideline should take priority in one situation but not in others.

The ability to make prudent decisions in specific situations has been described as *discernment* or *practical wisdom*. Discernment involves an understanding of how ethical guidelines are relevant in a variety of situations and to the particular case at hand (6).

PRINCIPLES, RULES, AND DUTIES

This book uses the term *guidelines* to refer to ethical generalizations that guide action because other terms, such as principles, rules, and duties, have undesirable connotations. According to the dictionary, *principle* connotes a "basis for reasoning or a guide for conduct or procedure." However, many philosophers use the term in a more restricted sense, to refer only to a comprehensive ethical theory that explains how to resolve conflicts among different precepts (7). A unified theory would also presumably provide clear, specific rules for action and a justification of those rules.

Philosophers have devoted considerable effort to developing comprehensive ethical theories. The two main types of ethical theory are consequentialist and deontologic. *Consequentialist* theories judge the rightness or wrongness of actions or guidelines by their consequences. Utilitarianism, the most prominent consequentialist theory, considers actions and rules appropriate when the overall benefits to all parties outweigh the overall harms. For instance, a utilitarian would consider it justified to tell a lie, breach confidentiality, or break a promise if, on the whole, the benefits of doing so outweigh the harms. In contrast, *deontologic* theories claim that the rightness or wrongness of an action depends on more factors than the consequences of an action. To a deontologist, actions such as telling a lie, breaching confidentiality, and breaking promises are inherently wrong. They would be morally suspect even if they produced no harmful consequences or led to beneficial ones.

Comprehensive theories of clinical ethics, however, are problematic (7). Utilitarian theories are flawed because they condone seemingly harmful actions that are not detected. For example, utilitarians might condone breaking a promise when no one else knows it is broken. Furthermore, acts that maximize the benefits for society as a whole may be considered acceptable even though they impose grave harms on individual persons. In a utilitarian analysis, harms to individuals might be outweighed by a sufficiently large benefit to society. Such an inequitable distribution of benefits and harms, however, might be unfair.

Deontologic theories can be criticized because they cannot provide a satisfactory account of which principles or rules take priority over others in cases of conflict. For example, deontologic theories would have difficulty determining whether beneficence or confidentiality would prevail when a patient with HIV infection refuses to notify his wife that she is at risk.

Detailed and lucid expositions of ethical theories and their critiques are available (7). Many writers, myself included, believe that a comprehensive and consistent theory of clinical ethics cannot be developed. This book avoids reference to ethical theories and to the term *principle* not only because of these conceptual problems, but also because ethical theories and principles are too abstract to guide physicians in specific cases.

The term *rule* is used in ethics to refer to generalizations that are narrower in scope than principles. The term is helpful because it focuses on individual conduct in specific situations, rather than on abstract generalizations; however, rules are generally regarded as binding, often prohibiting certain behaviors. In common language, "rule" might imply restrictions on individual conduct to maintain order in the group or for the sake of a goal. We speak of rules for a game or for an institution. The implication might be that rules can be applied in a straightforward manner, as when disputes in a game are settled by referring to the rules. In this sense, rules may be arbitrarily imposed to establish clear expectations for everyone. For example, rules for visiting hours may be established in a hospital to provide clear guidance for conduct, without any claim that one choice of hours is superior to another. The term "rule" is misleading in clinical ethics, because exceptions need to be made and because guidelines are not arbitrary conventions, but reflect deeply held values.

Finally, this book avoids the term *duty*, which might connote legal and ethical obligations. Ethical obligations, however, differ from legal duties imposed by legislation, regulations, or court rulings, as Chapter 22 discusses.

OTHER APPROACHES TO ETHICS

Because ethical theories and principles often do not help people resolve conflicts, other approaches to clinical ethics have been suggested (7).

CASUISTRY

Instead of constructing or relying on theories, some writers focus on how to resolve specific cases (4, 8, 9). According to these writers, people resolve dilemmas in everyday life by "looking at the concrete details of particular cases (8)." In this view, moral rules are not absolute; they merely create presumptions that may be rebutted, depending on the particular circumstances. The strategy is to compare a given case with clear-cut, paradigmatic cases. The key issue is whether the given case so closely resembles a paradigmatic case that it should be resolved in a similar manner or whether it can be distinguished and, therefore, treated differently. In some cases, the application of ethical maxims will be clear-cut. In more difficult cases, it might be unclear whether a guideline applies or different guidelines might provide conflicting advice. Proponents of case-based ethics emphasize the need for what Aristotle called practical wisdom, the ability to make appropriate decisions given the particular circumstances of the case. In educational terms, casuistry teaches by case analyses, starting with paradigmatic cases in which principles clearly apply and moving to complex, ambiguous cases over which reasonable people may disagree.

A case-based approach to clinical ethics takes into account the complexity of real-life decisions and offers readers a vicarious experience in resolving ethical problems (10). Dilemmas in clinical ethics generally present as specific decisions in patient care, not as clashes of abstract philosophical principles. This book emphasizes how to approach difficult cases and how to weigh different considerations in reaching a decision.

However, case-based analyses face a serious challenge: to provide a convincing basis for weighing some factors more heavily than others in reaching a decision. Indeed, casuistry runs the risk of ad hoc reasoning and inconsistent decisions. To avoid such pitfalls, this book will continually refer back to the ethical guidelines described in this chapter and explain why particular factors will be decisive in some situations, while different considerations will weigh most heavily in other circumstances.

ETHIC OF CARING

Some feminist writers argue that principles and rules provide an incomplete and inadequate conception of ethics (11). In this perspective, rule-based morality gives insufficient attention to maintaining or restoring relationships among individuals and avoiding interpersonal conflicts. In this view, responding to the needs and welfare of specific individuals might be more important than acting in accord with abstract standards. For example, when family members make decisions for an incompetent patient, traditional ethics might undervalue the need for the family members to get along with one another and live with the consequences of their decisions (12). In some situations, it might be more important to prevent serious family disputes than to follow the patient's prior directives. Such caring and responsiveness is often claimed to be a typically "feminine" orientation, as contrasted with a "masculine" orientation toward rules and principles. However, empirical studies do not support the hypothesis of gender-related orientations to ethics (13).

The emphasis on caring and on the well-being of others is welcome in medicine and other helping professions. Caring is essential in the doctor–patient relationship, and in clinical practice sympathy and compassion might be more important than following ethical guidelines mechanically. It is also important, however, to move beyond a sensitivity to these issues to a detailed description of exactly how caring should impact decisions in specific clinical situations. Furthermore, attending to the welfare of others might conflict with other important ethical imperatives, such as respecting the patient's autonomy.

VIRTUE ETHICS

Some writers point out that merely following guidelines might lead to a thin view of ethics. Physicians might perform the right actions but lack the spirit that should animate the medical profession. Virtue ethics emphasizes that the physician's characteristics are ultimately more important than the doctor's specific actions and their congruence with ethical principles (14). In this perspective, the essential questions are as follows: Is the doctor a good physician and good person? In one such view, the virtues of a good physician include fidelity, compassion, fortitude, temperance, integrity, and self-effacement (14).

Virtue ethics is helpful because it emphasizes the importance of such qualities as compassion, dedication, and altruism in physicians. Furthermore, in some complicated or unique situations, the physician's integrity might be a crucial factor in resolving dilemmas. Virtue ethics also has serious limitations because it lacks specificity on what the doctor should do in particular circumstances. A virtuous person might still commit wrong actions. Also, virtues might conflict with each other. In a given case, some people may believe that following a general guideline demonstrates the physician's integrity, while others believe that it would be compassionate to make an exception to the guideline.

SUMMARY

1. Ethical guidelines include showing respect for persons, avoiding deception, maintaining confidentiality, keeping promises, acting in the best interests of patients, and allocating resources justly.
2. These guidelines need to be applied to particular cases with discretion and judgment.

REFERENCES

1. Beauchamp TL, Childress JF. *Principles of Biomedical Ethics.* 5th ed. New York, NY: Oxford University Press; 2001:63–69.
2. Jonsen AR. Do no harm. *Ann Intern Med.* 1978;88:827–832.
3. Brewin TB. Primum non nocere? *Lancet.* 1994;344:1487–1488.
4. Sunnstein CR. *Legal Reasoning and Political Conflict.* New York, NY: Oxford University Press; 1996.

5. Beauchamp TL, Childress JF. *Principles of Biomedical Ethics*. 5th ed. New York, NY: Oxford University Press; 2001:19–23.
6. Beauchamp TL, Childress JF. *Principles of Biomedical Ethics*. 5th ed. New York, NY: Oxford University Press; 2001:34.
7. Beauchamp TL, Childress JF. *Principles of Biomedical Ethics*. 5th ed. New York, NY: Oxford University Press; 2001:337–377.
8. Jonsen AR, Toulmin S. *The Abuse of Casuistry: A History of Moral Reasoning*. Berkeley, CA: University of California Press; 1988.
9. Strong C. Critiques of casuistry and why they are mistaken. *Theor Med Bioeth*. 1999;20:395–411.
10. Lo B, Jonsen AR. Ethical dilemmas and the clinician. *Ann Intern Med*. 1980;92:116–117.
11. Gilligan C, Ward JV, Taylor JM, eds. *Mapping the Moral Domain: A Contribution of Women's Thinking to Psychological Theory and Education*. Cambridge, MA: Harvard University Press; 1988.
12. Alpers A, Lo B. Avoiding family feuds: responding to surrogates' demands for life-sustaining treatment. *J Law Med Ethics*. 1999;27:74–80.
13. Bebeau MJ, Brabeck MM. Ethical sensitivity and moral reasoning among men and women in the professions. In: Brabeck MM, ed. *Who Cares? Theory, Research, and Educational Implications of the Ethic of Care*. New York, NY: Praeger; 1989:144–163.
14. Pellegrino ED, Thomasma DG. *The Virtues in Medical Practice*. New York, NY: Oxford University Press; 1993.

ANNOTATED BIBLIOGRAPHY

1. Beauchamp TL, Childress JF. *Principles of Biomedical Ethics*. 6th ed. New York, NY: Oxford University Press; 2008. Comprehensive and lucid presentation of the philosophical foundations of biomedical ethics. Excellent references for further reading in the philosophical literature.
2. Pellegrino ED. Toward a reconstruction of medical morality. *Am J Bioeth*. 2006;6:65–71. Argues that the core of medical ethics is a healing relationship based on the patient's vulnerability and the physician's promise to help.
3. Jonsen AR, Toulmin S. *The Abuse of Casuistry: A History of Moral Reasoning*. Berkeley, CA: University of California Press; 1988. Offers a cogent rationale for a case-based approach to ethics and provides an overview of the accomplishments and downfall of casuistry.

3

Informed Consent

Although informed consent is legally required, many physicians are skeptical because patients can never understand medical situations as well as doctors and because they can usually persuade patients to follow their recommendations. In some situations, however, therapeutic options differ dramatically in terms of their side effects and impact on the patient, and no option is clearly superior. In these situations, there is no best approach, and the patient's values and preferences will be decisive. This chapter discusses the definition of informed consent, its justification, its requirements, and problems with informed consent. In some complex decisions, physicians should go beyond the minimum legal requirements of informed consent to promote shared decision making with patients.

CASE 3.1	Mastectomy or lumpectomy

Ms. B was a 58-year-old woman who was found to have a small breast cancer, stage T1N0M0. Her surgeon recommends mastectomy and informs her of the benefits and risks of the operation, including side effects such as lymphedema of the arm. The surgeon says that a less extensive operation may not remove all the tumor. Ms. B's daughter searched the Internet for information about breast cancer and learned that her mother's cancer could also be effectively treated with lumpectomy plus radiation therapy, which would avoid disfiguration and lymphedema.

Evidence-based practice guidelines recommend breast-conserving surgery for early breast cancer. Survival and disease-free survival are similar for mastectomy and for lumpectomy plus radiation. The percentage of women who receive breast-conserving surgery, however, varies strikingly by geographical region, and many women may not participate in decisions regarding surgery to the extent they wish (1). Before a mastectomy, the legal duty of informed consent requires surgeons to disclose the nature of the operation, its risks, and the alternatives. Case 3.1 illustrates, however, that a narrow vision of informed consent, while meeting legal standards, may result in suboptimal patient care decisions.

WHAT IS INFORMED CONSENT?

Discussions about informed consent are often confusing because people use this term in different senses.

AGREEMENT WITH THE PHYSICIAN'S RECOMMENDATIONS

Patients usually agree with physicians' recommendations, particularly in acute illness or injury, when the goals of care are clear, one option is superior, the benefits are great, and the risks are small. For example, a patient who suffers a wrist fracture needs a cast. A patient with a severe exacerbation of asthma that has not responded to inhaled bronchodilators needs systemic corticosteroids. In such situations, informed consent seems tantamount to obtaining the patient's agreement to the proposed intervention because there are no medically sound alternatives. Physicians often speak of "consenting the patient," implying that it is a foregone conclusion that the patient will agree, and indeed almost all patients do agree.

RIGHT TO REFUSE INTERVENTIONS

Patients have an ethical and legal right to be free of unwanted medical interventions and bodily invasions. Many early court cases associated with consent involved patients who had undergone surgery or invasive procedures and suffered serious adverse effects. The patients claimed that they would not have agreed to the intervention had they been told about these risks. Legally, competent patients must be informed of the risks of the proposed care and have the right to reject their physicians' recommendations. This right to refuse also extends to noninvasive care, such as diagnostic tests and medications.

CHOICE AMONG ALTERNATIVES

More broadly, patients should have the positive right to choose among medically feasible options, in addition to the negative right to refuse unwanted interventions. For instance, Case 3.1 involves a choice between two different types of surgery. This case also illustrates that patients or families may obtain medical information from sources other than the physician and may consider options that the physician has not mentioned.

SHARED DECISION MAKING

A still more comprehensive view is shared decision making by the physician and the patient (2). Both parties play essential roles in clinical decisions. The physician has medical knowledge and judgment. Patients know their values and preferences, for example, what risks and side effects are acceptable. Shared decision making is a back-and-forth process. The physician can also help educate patients, correct misunderstandings, help them deliberate, make recommendations, and to try to persuade them to accept the recommendations (2, 3).

Shared decision making is a continuum (4). The physician may simply explain the medical options or may also make a recommendation based on the patient's goals and values. Or the patient and physician may be equal partners and deliberate together. In informed dissent, the patient may reject the physician's plan or agree tacitly. Finally, the physician may decide about predominately technical issues, keeping in mind that patients or surrogates may have preferences regarding apparently value-neutral aspects of care or want to be involved in them. Patients may have different preferences for decision-making procedures for different decisions or at different times.

REASONS FOR INFORMED CONSENT AND SHARED DECISION MAKING

Several ethical and pragmatic reasons justify a broader conception of informed consent (5).

RESPECT PATIENT SELF-DETERMINATION

People want to make decisions about their bodies and health care in accordance with their values and goals. One court declared, "Every human being of adult years and sound mind has a right to determine what shall be done with his own body (6)."

Patient choice should be promoted because in most clinical settings, different goals and approaches are possible, outcomes are uncertain, and an intervention might cause both benefit and harm (7). Individuals place different values on health and the risk of medical interventions. Some patients are wary about the side effects of treatment, while others want to try risky therapies that have a higher probability of achieving desirable outcomes. Most women choose lumpectomy because it is less disfiguring and has fewer side effects. For some older women, however, conservation of the breast may be unimportant and returning for 6 weeks of radiation therapy may be burdensome. Physicians might not accurately predict patients' preferences. Doctors and patients often disagree on treatment preferences (8). For example, patients with newly diagnosed cancer are more likely than physicians, nurses, and the general public to prefer intensive chemotherapy with little chance of cure.

ENHANCE THE PATIENT'S WELL-BEING

The goal of medical care is to enhance patient well-being, which can be judged only in terms of the patient's goals and values. The patient's values are particularly important if various treatment approaches have very different characteristics or complications and involve trade-offs between short-term and long-term outcomes, if one option carries a small chance of a serious complication, if the patient has strong aversions toward risk or certain outcomes, or if there is uncertainty and disagreement among physicians (9). The choice between mastectomy and lumpectomy/radiation in Case 3.1 has many of these characteristics. In addition, participation in decisions might have other beneficial consequences for patients, such as increased sense of control, self-efficacy, and adherence to plans for care.

REQUIREMENTS FOR INFORMED CONSENT

Ethically and legally, informed consent requires discussions of pertinent information, obtaining the patient's agreement to the plan of care, and freedom from coercion (5).

INFORMATION TO DISCUSS WITH PATIENTS

Physicians need to discuss with patients information that is relevant to the decision at hand (Table 3-1). Most court decisions and legal commentaries use the term *disclose*, and, when summarizing legal doctrine, this book also uses this term. In general, however, we prefer the term *discuss* to emphasize that a dialog with the patient is preferable to a monolog by the physician.

Patients must be told the *nature* of the intervention, the expected *benefits*, the *risks*, and the likely *consequences*. Risks that are common knowledge, already known to the patient, of trivial impact, or very infrequent do not need to be discussed. For instance, patients do not need to be told the risks of venipuncture. For invasive interventions, courts have ruled that physicians need to discuss rare but serious risks, such as death or stroke.

Patients also need to understand the *alternatives* to the proposed test or treatment and their risks, benefits, and consequences. In particular, alternatives that are recommended in the medical literature and by evidence-based consensus guidelines need to be offered, even if the physician personally disagrees. The alternative of no intervention needs to be discussed. If a patient declines the recommended intervention, the physician needs to explain the adverse consequences of the refusal. In a case where a woman refused a Pap smear, the court ruled that the physician needed to discuss how the test could diagnose cancer at an early stage and avert death through early treatment (10).

The extent of disclosure will depend on the clinical context. For conditions such as appendicitis or fracture, where there is only one realistic option and it is highly effective, relatively safe, and

TABLE 3-1	Information to Discuss with Patients
The nature of the test or treatment	
The benefits, risks, and consequences of the intervention	
The alternatives and their benefits, risks, and consequences	

strongly recommended, a detailed discussion of alternatives offers little benefit to patients (11). However, the physician still needs to tell the patient the nature of the treatment, the risks, and the consequences, such as the course of convalescence.

Physicians must take the initiative in discussing information rather than wait for patients to ask questions. Patients might be uncomfortable asking questions or not even know what questions to ask. Discussions about the proposed test or treatment and the alternatives should be conducted by the attending physician or by the physician performing the intervention.

It is controversial whether physicians need to inform patients of alternatives for care that they do not believe are medically indicated. Obviously, physicians do not need to mention treatments that have no scientific rationale, would provide no medical benefit, or are known to be ineffective or harmful. However, physicians should inform patients of alternatives that other reasonable physicians would recommend, particularly if there is strong evidence of effectiveness and safety.

CASE 3.1   *Continued*

Ms. B's surgeon needs to discuss alternatives to the mastectomy he is recommending. Because lumpectomy plus radiation therapy has fewer complications and equivalent long-term outcomes, it needs to be offered. Physicians' recommendations should be supported by published evidence and evidence-based guidelines. Even if Ms. B's surgeon believed that mastectomy was the best approach, he still should inform her about the option of lumpectomy plus radiation therapy and tell her that it is recommended in evidence-based guidelines. He can then explain why he thinks mastectomy is better for her. The surgeon should not expect Ms. B or her daughter to take the lead in asking about alternatives to mastectomy. From the patient's perspective, the Internet may be an invaluable source of information about cancer treatments. The National Cancer Institute, the American Cancer Society and medical school websites offer reliable information.

Some kinds of information that the law does not require be disclosed may still be ethically desirable to disclose, as the following case illustrates (12).

CASE 3.2   **Disclosure of prognostic information**

Mr. A was a 50-year-old man who, after resection of a carcinoma of the pancreas, was recommended to have adjuvant chemo- and radiation therapy. He had indicated to his oncologist that he wished "to be told the truth about his condition." The doctor told him that the therapy was unproven, that most patients with pancreatic cancer die of the disease, and that there was a serious risk of recurrence. He died a year later, and his family sued, claiming that had he been told outcomes data, he would have declined chemo- and radiation therapy and put his business affairs in order. At the time, adjuvant chemo- and radiation therapy were unproven. The California Supreme Court ruled that physicians did not need to give patients statistical data on outcomes. "Statistical morbidity values derived from the experience of population groups are inherently unreliable and offer little assurance regarding the fate of the individual patient."
Based on Arato v. Avedon, 858 P.2d 598 (Cal. 1993)

After resection for pancreatic cancer, the 5-year survival rate is about 20% for patients with clear surgical margins and negative nodes. Quantitative information may be material to patients' decisions, notwithstanding the court's ruling. Physicians can explain why an individual patient might be expected to do better or worse than average. Even if not legally required, it is ethically desirable for physicians to provide such information to patients.

Other information may also be ethically desirable to discuss, although not legally required. The hospital's and surgeon's *experience* might be pertinent to a patient's decision, because increased volume is associated with significantly better outcomes for some operations and surgeons have a "learning curve" for new procedures. For example, the mortality for pancreatic resection is over 12% higher in low-volume hospitals than in high-volume hospitals (13). Similarly, patients might find it pertinent to know the *outcomes* of a surgical procedure at a given institution or by a particular surgeon, not outcomes reported in the literature. Some states make such surgeon- and hospital-specific, risk-adjusted outcome data for coronary artery bypass surgery publicly available (14). For cardiology procedures, it was recommended that patients receive information about clinician and institutional outcomes, with benchmark comparisons, or, at a minimum, information about experience and procedure volumes (15). Although some courts have ruled that physician-specific experience needs to be disclosed for some operations, other courts have not (16). The majority of surgical patients regard it as essential to their decision to have surgery knowing the surgeon's experience with a highly innovative procedures (17). Another issue that many patients might find pertinent is the *role of trainees* in their care, particularly with invasive or surgical procedures, as Chapter 36 discusses.

CASE 3.2   *Continued*

Although the courts do not require physicians to offer to present outcomes statistics to patients, there are good ethical reasons to do so. Although it is true to statistics cannot predict what will happen in a particular case, they do provide estimates of the likelihood of outcomes. Physicians can always discuss with patients the features of the individual case that make it likely that their prognosis is better or worse than the numbers in the literature.

Public health experts and evidence-based guidelines are now advocating that patients calculate individualized probabilities of outcomes to help them guide decisions about their care. The Framingham cardiac risk index and the World Health Organization fracture risk tool are available online for patients to use to guide their decisions regarding treatment of cardiac risk factors or treatment for osteoporosis.

This case illustrates how ethical standards for informed consent may be higher than legal requirements.

PATIENT AGREEMENT WITH THE TREATMENT PLAN

Patients must agree with the intended plan of care. For major interventions, such as surgery, obtaining explicit written authorization is standard. Written consent signals to the patient that the decision is important. In ambulatory care, oral agreement to the plan of care is usual because the risks are lower and because patients can choose to discontinue medications (18, 19).

AGREEMENT SHOULD BE VOLUNTARY

Coercion and manipulation undermine free choices by patients. Coercion involves threats that are intended to control patients' behavior and that patients find irresistible (20). An example is a threat to discharge a patient from the hospital if he does not agree with the recommended care. Manipulation of information might also thwart informed decisions. For example, physicians might misrepresent the patient's condition or the nature of the proposed intervention. Coercion and manipulation contrast with persuasion, which is an attempt to convince the patient to act in a certain way by providing rational arguments and accurate data (20). Persuasion respects patient autonomy and, indeed, enhances it by improving the patient's understanding of the situation.

Certain constraints on patients' choices are not coercive (21). The patient's prognosis might be so grim that all alternatives are undesirable and the patient has no "real choice." Warnings by the physician about the outcomes of choices or about the natural history of the illness are also not coercive because the physician makes no threat to bring about undesirable outcomes. Indeed, physicians would be ethically remiss if they did not point out to patients the consequences of unwise choices.

If patients lack the capacity to make informed decisions (*see* Chapter 10), advance directives or appropriate surrogates should guide decisions (*see* Chapters 12 and 13).

PROBLEMS WITH INFORMED CONSENT

Physicians need to understand common problems with informed consent so that they can take steps to minimize them.

PATIENTS DO NOT UNDERSTAND MEDICAL INFORMATION

Patients often do not recall information they have discussed with physicians, even basic information about the proposed treatment. Patients considering knee/hip replacement and lower back surgery have poor knowledge about the surgery. Fewer than 50% of patients could answer basic questions about the procedure (22). For back surgery, only 14% of patients knew how many will not improve after surgery and only 33% knew how many will experience complications of surgery. Furthermore, patients facing common medical decisions cannot accurately assess how well informed they are (23).

PHYSICIANS DO NOT PROVIDE KEY INFORMATION

In audiotaped office visits, orthopedic surgeons discussed the nature of the decision to be made in 92% of cases, alternatives in 62%, and risks and benefits in 59%. They rarely discussed the patient's role in decision making (14%) or assessed the patient's understanding (12%) (24). For outpatient decisions involving a new medication or change in dose, physicians described the decision in of 75% cases but checked patient preferences in only 27% of cases. For complex decisions such as PSA screening or counseling regarding surgery, physicians discussed alternatives in only 30% of cases and pros and cons in only 26% (25). Furthermore, doctors often use technical jargon that is incomprehensible to laypeople, and informed consent forms are usually difficult to read and understand.

SOME PATIENTS DO NOT WANT TO MAKE DECISIONS

Some patients might not want to make decisions, but instead defer to physicians or family members.

CASE 3.3	Reluctance to make a decision

Mr. T was an 88-year-old man with severe chronic obstructive pulmonary disease (COPD), coronary artery disease, and peptic ulcer disease. He developed an adenocarcinoma of the lung, which could be treated with surgery or radiation therapy. His physician was reluctant to recommend surgery because of the patient's increased operative risk. In addition, his COPD was so severe that he might be dyspneic after a pneumonectomy. When his doctor discussed alternatives for treatment, Mr. T said, "Do what you think is best. You're the doctor."

Like Mr. T, about 25% to 50% of Americans prefer to leave medical decisions to their physicians, depending on the physicians (26). Women, more educated, and healthier people are more likely to prefer an active role in decision making. Furthermore, persons from cultures where informed consent is not as important as in the United States may defer to physicians.

PATIENTS MIGHT NOT WANT TO MAKE DECISIONS INDIVIDUALLY

In some cultures, patients might be expected to involve their families in medical decisions rather than make decisions as individuals. Women might traditionally be expected to defer decisions to their husbands or fathers. Clearly, physicians need to allow patients to involve others in their medical decisions if they choose to do so, recognizing that with a culture individuals vary in their preferences for decision making.

Although patients might not use all disclosed information, it is nonetheless important that physicians give them pertinent information. A patient who decided to pursue a course of medical care upon first hearing about it might reconsider upon learning more information.

PATIENTS CANNOT ANTICIPATE THEIR FUTURE REACTIONS

People cannot accurately predict how future situations will affect their preferences (27). Healthy patients underestimate the quality of life that patients with illness or disability report. When people imagine what it would be like to have a severe illness or disability, they overlook the many activities they might still be able to enjoy and do not appreciate how patients adapt to their circumstances (28). The concern is that people will make important decisions based on transient feelings or inaccurate perceptions of how they will feel in future states of illness.

PATIENTS MAKE DECISIONS THAT CONTRADICT THEIR BEST INTERESTS

Some physicians fear that information about risks might cause patients to refuse medically beneficial interventions. Empirical studies do not support this concern. In an older study of 104 refusals of inpatient treatment, none resulted from disclosure of information but 14 patients refused care because of inadequate information about tests or information (29).

LEGAL ASPECTS OF INFORMED CONSENT

Court rulings have shaped the doctrine of informed consent, with particular focus on what information must be disclosed to patients.

MALPRACTICE

Physicians who do not obtain informed consent might be found liable in civil suits for battery or negligence (5). *Battery*, the harmful or offensive touching of another person, includes surgery without the patient's consent or surgery beyond the scope of patient consent. For instance, a physician might be liable for performing a mastectomy on a patient who had consented to only a biopsy, even if the intervention was medically appropriate, skillfully performed, and beneficial. This battery model, however, fits medicine poorly. Many cases do not involve physical touching of the patient, for example making a diagnosis or prescribing drugs. In addition, battery requires that the physician intended to provide care without the patient's consent. Most cases of malpractice, however, are unintentional.

The modern approach to malpractice, which has supplanted the battery model, is to hold physicians liable for *negligence*: the physician breached a duty to the patient, the patient suffered harm, and the breach of duty caused the harm. The patient needs to prove that the physician failed to disclose a risk that should have been disclosed, that the patient would not have consented had the risk been discussed, and that the risk occurred and caused harm. A crucial issue in malpractice law, therefore, is what risks should be discussed.

STANDARDS FOR DISCLOSURE

Full or complete disclosure of all information that physicians know about a particular condition is impossible. Thus, the issue is not *whether* physicians should limit the amount and types of information they discuss with patients, but rather *what* information to discuss or omit.

Courts have used several standards to determine what information to disclose to patients (5). About half of the states have adopted a *professional standard*: The physician must disclose what a reasonable physician of ordinary skill would disclose in the same or similar circumstances. This is equivalent to providing the information that colleagues customarily provide. The professional standard has been criticized because it is based on what physicians customarily discuss, not on what information patients need and because it may impede improvements in clinical care (30). In Case 3.1, a physician would not be liable for failing to inform a patient of breast-conserving surgery if surgeons in the area had not adopted it, even if there is rigorous evidence favoring it.

Other states have adopted a patient-oriented standard for disclosure: Physicians should disclose what a *reasonable patient* in the same or similar situation would find material to the medical decision; that is, it would influence the decision. Generally, this standard requires more disclosure than the professional standard and is more consistent with the goal of promoting patient decision making and choices. However, this standard has been criticized because it does not take into account how patients vary in their preferences regarding what information is relevant (30).

Some patients might desire more information than the standard "reasonable" patient. For example, a carpenter might be particularly concerned that a new medication might impair his or her dexterity or alertness. In clinical practice, as a practical matter, physicians need to answer direct questions from patients to maintain the doctor–patient relationship. A few states have adopted a subjective standard for disclosure: The physician must provide information that the *individual patient* would find pertinent to the decision. This subjective standard for disclosure is problematic in malpractice litigation. If a rare, undisclosed complication occurs, the patient might claim that he would not have consented to the intervention if the physician had mentioned that particular risk. In hindsight, it might be difficult to decide whether this assertion is plausible.

In some states, laws specify that certain risks need to be disclosed—for example, "brain damage" or "loss of function of any organ or limb (5)."

CONSENT FORMS

The consent form documents that the patient agreed to treatment. In some states, a signed consent form provides a legal presumption of valid consent. A signed consent form, however, is not equivalent to informed consent because the discussion of the risks, benefits, alternatives, and consequences might be inadequate (5). Physicians should document in the progress notes that the indications, risks, benefits, and alternatives were discussed and that the patient agreed to the care.

LAWS RESTRICTING PHYSICIAN DISCUSSIONS WITH PATIENTS

A few states have passed laws that forbid or mandate what physicians may say to patients. Florida prohibits physicians from asking about firearms in the home, although an exception is allowed if the physician believes in good faith that it is relevant to the safety of the patient or others (31). Supporters argued that the law protected the privacy of gun owners and prevented doctors from harassing and discriminating against them. Critics charged that this law is an unconstitutional restriction on the free speech of physicians and undermines efforts to reduce the public health risk of injuries and deaths caused by firearms. South Dakota mandates specific language that physicians must if a woman requests an abortion. The physician must tell the woman that abortion ends the life of a "whole, separate, unique, living human being" with whom she has a Constitutionally protected relationship. The physician must also say that depression and suicide are risks of abortion, although there is no credible scientific evidence that this is the case (32). Backers of the law say that it assures that women have information needed to make an informed decision. Critics object that the law violates a physician's First Amendment right to be free of government-mandated ideologic speech. Moreover, critics charge that the law compels physicians to give false and misleading to patients (32).

EXCEPTIONS TO INFORMED CONSENT

Several exceptions to informed consent illustrate how acting in the patient's best interests might supersede patient self-determination. These exceptions need to be carefully limited so that they do not undermine informed consent.

LACK OF DECISION-MAKING CAPACITY

When patients lack decision-making capacity, an appropriate surrogate should give permission or refusal, following the patient's previously stated preferences or his or her best interests (*see* Chapter 4).

EMERGENCIES

In an emergency, delaying treatment to obtain informed consent might jeopardize the patient's health or life. Courts have recognized a doctrine of *implied consent*: Because reasonable persons would consent to treatment in such emergency circumstances, physicians may presume that the patient in question also would consent. Few people would object to treating life-threatening emergencies, such as an impending airway obstruction in anaphylaxis, without the patient's explicit consent. It is often possible to abbreviate the process of disclosure and consent in an urgent situation, rather than dispense with it altogether. In addition, the process of informed consent can often be initiated while the treatment is being started.

The emergency exception should not be used when informed consent is feasible or if it is known that a particular patient does not want the treatment. For example, terminally ill patients might have indicated that they do not want cardiopulmonary resuscitation.

Some physicians claim that consent is implied when a patient seeks care from a hospital or signs a general consent form upon admission. The implication is that informed consent for specific tests or treatments is unnecessary. However, this use of "implied consent" is unacceptable, because it allows physicians to administer any type of care they choose. When patients come to a hospital, they do not give physicians *carte blanche*. Most patients would probably agree to certain interventions, such as diagnostic testing, but would want to base further decisions on new information.

THERAPEUTIC PRIVILEGE

Physicians may withhold information when disclosure would severely harm the patient or undermine informed decision making by the patient. For example, a patient might be depressed and have a history of previous suicide attempts in response to serious medical diagnoses. Telling such a patient that he has cancer might provoke another suicide attempt. The concept of therapeutic privilege, however, needs to be circumscribed (33). The possibility that the patient will feel sad does not justify withholding a serious diagnosis. Also the physician may not "remain silent simply because divulgence might prompt the patient to forego therapy the physician feels the patient really needs (34)."

WAIVER

Patients such as Mr. T in Case 3.3 might not want to participate in making decisions about their care. Ethically and legally, patients' requests to waive the right of informed consent should be respected. Self-determination would be undermined if patients were forced to participate in decision making against their wishes. Shared decision making entitles patients to participate actively in health care decisions, but does not require them to do so (21). To be ethically valid, a waiver of informed consent must itself be informed. Patients must appreciate that they have the right to receive information and to make decisions about their care. Patients might later decide to participate more actively in decisions.

PROMOTING SHARED DECISION MAKING

The process of shared decision making generally requires multiple discussions between the physician and patient (Table 3-2) (32).

TABLE 3-2	Promoting Shared Decision Making

Encourage the patient to play an active role in decisions.
> Elicit the patient's perspective about the illness.
> Build a partnership with the patient.

Ensure that patients are informed.
> Provide comprehensible information.
> Try to frame issues without bias.
> Interpret the alternatives in light of the patient's goals.
> Check that the patients have understood information.

Protect the patient's best interests.
> Help the patient deliberate.
> Make a recommendation.

Try to persuade patients.

ENCOURAGE THE PATIENT TO PLAY AN ACTIVE ROLE

Physicians can encourage patient involvement in decisions, even with patients like Mr. T in Case 3.3, who defer to their judgment.

Elicit the Patient's Perspective About the Illness

Physicians can elicit the patient's concerns, expectations, and values regarding medical care through open-ended questions, such as:

- "As you think about the next few years, what is most important to you?"
- "What concerns you the most about your health?"

Build a Partnership With the Patient

Physicians can acknowledge that the decision is complex and difficult (35). Moreover, doctors can affirm their dedication to working for the patient's well-being: "We'll work together to make the best decisions for you."

ENSURE THAT PATIENTS ARE INFORMED

Provide Comprehensible Information

To enhance patient understanding, physicians should use simple language and avoid medical jargon. Decision aids, such as interactive CDs or computer programs, increase patients' knowledge about their condition and the options and reduce their sense of conflict over decisions (36). For patients like Ms. B in Case 3.1, decision aids increase the use of breast-conserving surgery by about 25% (1). Decision aids also have the advantage of not requiring additional face-to-face time between physicians and patients. Talking to other patients who have experienced an intervention such as mastectomy or colectomy can help patients appreciate how they can adapt.

Try to Frame Issues Without Bias

People are more likely to accept a treatment if the outcomes are phrased in terms of survival, rather than in terms of death (37). Lung cancer patients are more likely to prefer surgery to radiation therapy if outcomes are framed as the probability of living rather than the probability of dying (38). Moreover, surgery is more attractive when survival data are presented as the average number of years lived rather than as the probability of surviving a given time period.

Physicians also need to consider how to discuss rare but serious risks, such as anaphylactic reactions to radiographic contrast material (39). Patients might infer incorrectly that a risk is significant because the physician has mentioned it. Physicians can put the risk in context: "I believe that this is a very small risk, compared with the information we would gain from the test."

Check That Patients Have Understood Information

Disclosure by the physician is not equivalent to comprehension by the patient. It is helpful to ask patients to repeat the information in their own words and to invite them to ask questions (40). This repeat back technique improves patient comprehension, while maintaining patient satisfaction, reducing anxiety slightly and adding only 4 minutes to an ambulatory visit (41, 42).

PROMOTE THE PATIENT'S BEST INTERESTS

The guideline of beneficence requires physicians to help patients make decisions that are in their best interests (*see* Chapter 4). In addition to providing information, physicians should help patients deliberate about their choices in complex situations.

Help Patients Deliberate

Some situations are close calls or toss-ups: various options may have similar net health outcomes, but strikingly different consequences for the patient. In deciding whether to start coumadin for atrial fibrillation, patients differ in how they balance the risk of serious bleeding against the risk of an embolic complication of the disease (43, 44). The patient's goals and values should be decisive. The physician can help the patient clarify whether to try to prevent a complication or to accept the natural course of illness rather than severe adverse effects of interventions.

Make a Recommendation

Physicians should not merely list the alternatives and leave it to the patient to decide (45, 46). Patients commonly ask physicians what they would do. Physicians need to clarify what exactly the patient is asking (47). If the patient is asking if he is making the right choice, the physician needs to be supportive and compassionate. If the patient wants to know what the physician would do, it is helpful for physicians to describe the process of decision making they would use, including talking with relatives, friends, and religious leaders. If the patient still wants to know what the physician would do, it is appropriate to offer a recommendation based on the patient's values and goals, acknowledging that may differ from the physician's.

Try to Persuade Patients

Physicians should also try to dissuade patients from choices that are clearly contrary to their best interests, as judged by their own values (3). Chapter 4 discusses this issue in depth.

| CASE 3.3 | *Continued* |

Mr. T's doctor said, "I'd be glad to tell you what I think is best for you. But first I need to understand what is important to you." When the physician asked Mr. T what was most important to him over the next few years, he replied that he wanted to care for his sister, who had stomach cancer. The physician explained that he would be unable to care for his sister while recuperating from surgery and also that he might die from the operation. Given Mr. T's priorities, his doctor recommended radiation therapy. Mr. T tolerated radiation well and cared for his sister during her terminal illness. He had several more years of good health before he developed hemoptysis from spread of his lung cancer. He ultimately died an inpatient hospice.

SUMMARY

1. Shared decision making respects patient self-determination.
2. For patients to make informed choices, physicians must discuss with them the alternatives for care and the benefits, risks, and consequences of each alternative.
3. Physicians need to encourage patients to play an active role in decision making and to ensure that patients are informed.

REFERENCES

1. Waljee JF, Rogers MA, Alderman AK. Decision aids and breast cancer: do they influence choice for surgery and knowledge of treatment options? *J Clin Oncol.* 2007;25:1067–1073.
2. Murray E, Charles C, Gafni A. Shared decision-making in primary care: tailoring the Charles et al. model to fit the context of general practice. *Patient Educ Couns.* 2006;62:205–211.
3. Emanuel EJ, Emanuel LL. Four models of the physician-patient relationship. *JAMA.* 1992;267:2221–2226.
4. Kon AA. The shared decision-making continuum. *JAMA.* 2010;304:903–904.
5. Berg JW, Lidz CW, Appelbaum PS. *Informed Consent: Legal Theory and Clinical Practice.* 2nd ed. New York, NY: Oxford University Press; 2001.
6. Schloendorff v. Society of New York Hospitals. 211 N.Y. 125,105 N.E. 92 (1914).
7. Shultz MM. From informed consent to patient choice: a new protected interest. *Yale Law J.* 1985;95:219–299.
8. Montgomery AA, Fahey T. How do patients' treatment preferences compare with those of clinicians? *Qual Health Care.* 2001;10(suppl 1):i39–i43.
9. Kassirer JP. Incorporating patient preferences into medical decisions. *N Engl J Med.* 1994;330:1895–1896.
10. Truman v. Thomas. 27 Cal. 3d 285, 165 Cal. Rptr. 308, 611 P.2d 902 (Cal. 1980).
11. Whitney SN, McGuire AL, McCullough LB. A typology of shared decision making, informed consent, and simple consent. *Ann Intern Med.* 2004;140:54–59.
12. Annas GJ. Informed consent, cancer, and truth in prognosis. *N Engl J Med.* 1994;330:223–225.
13. Birkmeyer JD, Siewers AE, Finlayson EV, et al. Hospital volume and surgical mortality in the United States. *N Engl J Med.* 2002;346:1128–1137.
14. Steinbrook R. Public report cards—cardiac surgery and beyond. *N Engl J Med.* 2006;355:1847–1849.
15. Krumholz HM. Informed consent to promote patient-centered care. *JAMA.* 2010;303:1190–1191.
16. Howard v. University. 172 N.J. 537; 800 A.2d 73 (N.J. 2002).
17. Lee Char SJ, Hills NK, Lo B, et al. What do patients want to know before an innovative surgical procedure? In press.
18. Braddock CH, Fihn SD, Levinson W, et al. How doctors and patients discuss routine clinical decisions: informed decision making in the outpatient setting. *J Gen Intern Med.* 1997;12:339–345.
19. Diem SJ. How and when should physicians discuss clinical decisions with patients? *J Gen Intern Med.* 1997;12:397–398.
20. Faden RR, Beauchamp TL. *A History and Theory of Informed Consent.* New York, NY: Oxford University Press; 1986.
21. Brock DW. *Life and Death.* New York, NY: Cambridge University Press; 1993.
22. Fagerlin A, Sepucha KR, Couper MP, et al. Patients' knowledge about 9 common health conditions: the DECISIONS survey. *Med Decis Making.* 2010;30:35S–52S.
23. Sepucha KR, Fagerlin A, Couper MP, et al. How does feeling informed relate to being informed? The DECISIONS survey. *Med Decis Making.* 2010;30:77S–84S.
24. Braddock C III, Hudak PL, Feldman JJ, et al. Surgery is certainly one good option: quality and time-efficiency of informed decision-making in surgery. *J Bone Joint Surg Am.* 2008;90:1830–1838.
25. Braddock CH III, Edwards KA, Hasenberg NM, et al. Informed decision making in outpatient practice: time to get back to basics. *JAMA.* 1999;282:2313–2320.
26. Levinson W, Kao A, Kuby A, et al. Not all patients want to participate in decision making. A national study of public preferences. *J Gen Intern Med.* 2005;20:531–535.
27. Halpern J, Arnold RM. Affective forecasting: an unrecognized challenge in making serious health decisions. *J Gen Intern Med.* 2008;23:1708–1712.
28. Ubel PA, Loewenstein G, Schwarz N, et al. Misimagining the unimaginable: the disability paradox and health care decision making. *Health Psychol.* 2005;24:S57–S62.
29. Appelbaum PS, Roth LH. Patients who refuse treatment in medical hospitals. *JAMA.* 1983;250:1296–1301.
30. King JS, Moulton BW. Rethinking informed consent: the case for shared medical decision-making. *Am J Law Med.* 2006;32:429–501.
31. Murtagh L, Miller M. Censorship of the patient–physician relationship: a new Florida law. *JAMA.* 2011;306:1131–1132.

32. Curfman GD, Morrissey S, Greene MF, et al. Physicians and the First Amendment. *N Engl J Med.* 2008;359:2484–2485.

33. Sirotin N, Lo B. The end of therapeutic privilege? *J Clin Ethics.* 2006;17:312–316.

34. Canterbury v. Spence. 464 F.2d 772 (D.C. Cir. 1972).

35. Epstein RM, Alper BS, Quill TE. Communicating evidence for participatory decision making. *JAMA.* 2004;291:2359–2366.

36. Fowler FJ Jr, Levin CA, Sepucha KR. Informing and involving patients to improve the quality of medical decisions. *Health Aff (Millwood).* 2011;30:699–706.

37. McNeil BJ, Weichselbaum R, Pauker SG. Speech and survival: tradeoffs between quality and quantity of life in laryngeal cancer. *N Engl J Med.* 1981;305:982–987.

38. McNeil BJ, Weichselbaum R, Pauker SG. Fallacy of the five-year survival in lung cancer. *N Engl J Med.* 1978;299:307–401.

39. Brody H. *The Healer's Power.* New Haven, CT: Yale University Press; 1992.

40. Gaster B, Edwards K, Trinidad SB, et al. Patient-centered discussions about prostate cancer screening: a real-world approach. *Ann Intern Med.* 2010;153:661–665.

41. Fink AS, Prochazka AV, Henderson WG, et al. Enhancement of surgical informed consent by addition of repeat back: a multicenter, randomized controlled clinical trial. *Ann Surg.* 2010;252:27–36.

42. Schenker Y, Fernandez A, Sudore R, et al. Interventions to improve patient comprehension in informed consent for medical and surgical procedures: a systematic review. *Med Decis Making.* 2011;31:151–173.

43. Protheroe J, Fahey T, Montgomery AA, et al. The impact of patients' preferences on the treatment of atrial fibrillation: observational study of patient based decision analysis. *BMJ.* 2000;320:1380–1384.

44. Devereaux PJ, Anderson DR, Gardner MJ, et al. Differences between perspectives of physicians and patients on anticoagulation in patients with atrial fibrillation: observational study. *BMJ.* 2001;323:1218–1222.

45. Quill TE, Brody H. Physician recommendations and patient autonomy: finding a balance physician power and patient choice. *Ann Intern Med.* 1996;125:763–769.

46. Ubel PA. What should I do, doc?: some psychologic benefits of physician recommendations. *Arch Intern Med.* 2002;162:977–980.

47. Kon AA. Answering the question: "Doctor, if this were your child, what would you do?". *Pediatrics* 2006;118:393-397.

ANNOTATED BIBLIOGRAPHY

1. Berg JW, Lidz CW, Appelbaum PS. *Informed Consent: Legal Theory and Clinical Practice.* 2nd ed. New York, NY: Oxford University Press; 2001.
   Comprehensive and lucid book, covering ethical, legal, and practical aspects of informed consent. Stresses the need for dialogue between doctors and patients.

2. Mlller FG, Wertheimer A. *The Ethics of Consent.* New York, NY: Oxford University Press; 2010.
   Interdisciplinary analyses of consent in many situations, including clinical medicine and research.

3. Whitney SN, McGuire AL, McCullough LB. A typology of shared decision making, informed consent, and simple consent. *Ann Intern Med.* 2004;140:54–59.
   Argues that detailed informed consent is not required when there is only one medically feasible option; however, shared decision making is important whenever several options exist.

4. Murray E, Charles C, Gafni A. Shared decision-making in primary care: Tailoring the Charles et al. model to fit the context of general practice. *Patient Educ Couns.* 2006;62:205–211.
   Conceptual framework for shared decision making, with an emphasis on outpatient care and chronic illness.

5. Epstein RM, Alper BS, Quill TE. Communicating evidence for participatory decision making. *JAMA.* 2004;291:2359–2366.
   Suggests how physicians can communicate information to patients in ways that enhance shared decision making.

6. Kon AA. The shared decision-making continuum. *JAMA.* 2010;304:903–904.
   Suggests how physicians can give recommendations while not imposing their values on patients.

Promoting the Patient's Best Interests

Patients may reject the recommendations of their physicians, refusing beneficial interventions or insisting on interventions that are not indicated. In such cases, physicians are torn between respecting patient autonomy and acting in the patients' best interests. If physicians simply accept unwise patient decisions in the name of respecting patient autonomy, their role seems morally constricted. This chapter discusses how physicians can protect the well-being of patients, while avoiding the pitfalls of paternalism. Chapter 12 addresses how to assess the best interests of a person who lacks decision-making capacity.

PATIENT REFUSAL OF BENEFICIAL INTERVENTIONS

The following case illustrates how patients may refuse beneficial interventions.

CASE 4.1 **Refusal of surgery for critical aortic stenosis**

Mrs. N is a 76-year-old widow with aortic stenosis. For several years she has been refusing further evaluation, saying that she would not want surgery. After an episode of near-syncope, she agrees to echocardiography, mostly to humor her primary care physician. Critical aortic outflow obstruction is found. Her physician strongly recommends valve replacement. The risks of surgery are unacceptable to her, particularly the risk of prolonged hospitalization or neurologic or cognitive impairment after surgery. Having lived a full life, she says she welcomes a sudden death rather than a prolonged decline. In the past, she has been reluctant to visit physicians, undergo tests, or take medications. She leads an active life, writing a resource book for senior citizens, leading several volunteer organizations, and enjoying concerts.

Mrs. N's physicians believe that her refusal conflicts with her best interests. With valve replacement, she is likely to live longer and avoid debilitating symptoms, such as chest pain and dyspnea. Refusal of surgery might result in what she fears most: progressive decline and loss of independence.

How can physicians respond to Mrs. N's refusal? On the one hand, it would be disrespectful and impractical to override her refusal and operate without her consent. On the other hand, accepting her refusal without further discussion might result in severe disability that she would not want. What attempts by physicians to persuade Mrs. N to agree to surgery are warranted? To address these issues, physicians need to understand the ethical guidelines of doing no harm and acting in their patients' best interests.

DOING NO HARM TO PATIENTS

The ethical guideline of nonmaleficence requires people to refrain from inflicting harm on others. Prohibiting harmful actions is the core of morality. For instance, the Ten Commandments prohibit killing, lying, and stealing. Avoiding harm is generally considered a more stringent ethical obligation than providing benefit.

The widely quoted maxim "Do no harm" has several distinct meanings (1). First, physicians should not provide interventions that are known to be ineffective. Second, physicians should not act maliciously, as by providing substandard care because they dislike the patient's ethnic background or political views. Third, doctors should also act with due care and diligence. Fourth, the maxim sometimes is cited as "Above all, do no harm," or, more impressively in Latin, *Primum non nocere.* If physicians cannot benefit patients, they should at least not harm them or make the situation worse. Fifth, when benefits and burdens are evenly balanced, physicians should err on the side of not intervening.

The precept "do no harm" provides only limited guidance. Many medical interventions, such as the aortic valve replacement mentioned in Case 4.1, offer both great benefits and high risks and adverse effects. Doing no harm would literally preclude such interventions, yet many patients with serious illness may accept substantial risks to gain medical benefits. Furthermore, as we next discuss, merely doing no harm seems a limited view of the physician's role.

PROMOTING THE PATIENT'S BEST INTERESTS

The ethical guideline of beneficence requires physicians to promote patients' "important and legitimate interests (2)." This guideline arises from the nature of the doctor–patient relationship and of medical professionalism.

THE FIDUCIARY NATURE OF THE DOCTOR–PATIENT RELATIONSHIP

Physicians have special responsibilities to act for the well-being of patients because patients are often impaired in significant ways by their illness. Furthermore, the stakes are high; poor decisions might place patients' health or lives at risk.

Reasons for the Fiduciary Relationship

Patients are vulnerable.   Because illness often undermines patients' independence and judgment, people might be less able to look after their own interests when they are sick.

Physicians have expertise that patients lack.   Physicians have expert knowledge, as well as the experience and judgment to apply it to the patient's individual circumstances.

Patients rely on their physicians.   Even in the Internet era, it is often difficult for patients to obtain information and individualized advice except from physicians. Often, they have no previous experience in making medical decisions. With serious illnesses, patients might have little time to seek second opinions. It is hard for laypeople to determine whether a physician's advice is sound or to evaluate a physician's skills. Hence, patients commonly rely on the advice of their physicians.

Definition of a Fiduciary Relationship

Legally, relationships between professionals and clients are characterized as fiduciary. The term *fiduciary* is derived from the Latin word *fidere*, to trust. Fiduciaries must act in the best interests of their patients or client, subordinating their self-interest. Fiduciaries are held to higher standards than business people, who use their knowledge and skill for their own self-interest, rather than for the benefit of their customers. Ordinary business relationships are characterized by the phrase *caveat emptor*, "let the buyer beware," not by trust and reliance. Some financial incentives challenge the fiduciary nature of the doctor–patient relationship, as Chapter 34 discusses.

THE NATURE OF PROFESSIONALISM

In professional codes of ethics, physicians promise to serve the best interests of patients. Literally, physicians "profess" to use their skills to heal and comfort the sick, encouraging patients to rely on them and promising to act in a fiduciary manner (3). In return for physicians acting for the good of their patients, society allows physicians to regulate themselves by, for example, selecting applicants for medical schools and postgraduate training, establishing standards for certification, and disciplining practitioners.

Professionalism is a core competency for students and residents and is regularly assessed during training. It may refer to several different things. First, it may be a set of core values that physicians should follow, such as primacy of patient welfare, respect for patient autonomy, and honesty (4). Second, professionalism may refer to attitudes, beliefs, and skills that foster these core values, such as the ability to solve challenges to these core values and a willingness to engage in reflection, deliberation, and discussions with peers (5). Third, it may refer to observed behaviors, particularly in training settings. When faculty evaluate students' professionalism, however, they do not agree with other, and their own evaluations are inconsistent across different cases. Furthermore, the same behavior (such as lying) might be considered professional by one faculty member and unprofessional by another (6). This inconsistency may result from the importance of context and motivation in judging people's behaviors. Finally, patterns of unprofessional actions may predict future undesirable behavior. Ratings during training that a student was irresponsible or had diminished capacity for self-improvement are significantly associated with a higher risk for subsequent disciplinary actions by state licensing boards (7). The relationship between professionalism and clinical ethics (as discussed in this book) merits clarification. As we use the term, ethics helps physicians specify values and principles, decide what to do when these are in conflict, and articulate persuasive reasons for their decisions and actions.

PROBLEMS WITH BEST INTERESTS

The idea that physicians should act in the best interests of patients is indisputable. In any given case, however, determining what actions are in the patient's best interests might be controversial.

DISAGREEMENTS OVER WHAT IS BEST FOR A PATIENT

People may disagree over the goals of care or the assessment of the benefits and burdens of an intervention. In Case 4.1, the physicians' goal is to increase the patient's likelihood of survival; however, the patient's goal is to avoid physical and mental decline. Furthermore, the physicians and patients may weigh the risks and benefits of surgery differently. Physicians tend to focus on the prospect of long-term survival, while Mrs. N. is more concerned about the short-term risks of surgery and her quality of life (8).

QUALITY OF LIFE

The term *quality of life* is used in many ways. Factors that might be considered include the following:

- The symptoms of the illness and the side effects of treatment
- The patient's functional ability to perform activities of daily life, such as walking, shopping, and preparing meals
- The patient's subjective experiences of happiness, pleasure, pain, and suffering
- The patient's independence, privacy, and dignity

Competent patients usually consider their quality of life, as well as the duration of life, when making health care decisions. In some situations, a patient with a serious illness may decide that his or her quality of life is so poor that interventions are unacceptably burdensome. The principle of respect for persons requires respecting judgments about quality of life made by patients who are competent and informed. More controversy exists if other persons are making the judgments.

Quality of Life Judgments by Others Might Be Problematic

Quality of life judgments by others often differ sharply from patient's own assessment. Persons with chronic illness, such as coronary artery disease and chronic obstructive lung disease, rate their quality of life higher than do their physicians or other healthy persons (9). Similarly, elderly patients who have survived a hospitalization in the intensive care unit view their quality of life higher than their family members do. Such discrepancies are not surprising. Many patients learn to cope with chronic illness over time, develop support systems, and continue to find substantial pleasure in life. Furthermore, quality of life might improve substantially if in-home assistance or adaptive devices are provided. In addition, assessments of quality of life made by others might be discriminatory if they are based on the patient's economic value to society or social worth.

Some people reject all quality of life considerations because they will lead to discrimination against people with disabilities. Proponents of a "right to life" may believe that biologic life should be prolonged, regardless of prognosis or quality of life, a position often based on religious beliefs about the sacredness of life. However, it is disrespectful for people to impose their view of quality of life on a patient who does not agree. Moreover, interventions that may prolong life also have burdens that should be taken into account.

These disagreements illustrate how determinations of quality of life by others are problematic unless they are based on the patient's own judgments.

MEDICAL PATERNALISM

Historically, beneficence rather than respect for persons was the dominant ethical principle for physicians. Doctors made decisions for the patient on the basis of what they believed was the patient's best interest. This approach to decision making has been termed *medical paternalism*, analogous to how parents make decisions for their children. Deferring to the physician's recommendations is reasonable in many acute illnesses or emergencies: when cure is possible, when the benefits of therapy far outweigh the risks, and when treatment must be started promptly.

Definition of Paternalism

Paternalism is intentionally overriding a person's known preferences or actions to benefit that person. Philosophers distinguish two types of paternalism. In weak or soft paternalism, the patient's decisions are not informed or are not voluntary. If a patient's autonomy is impaired or in doubt, it is appropriate for physicians to intervene, at least temporarily. The justification is that patients should be protected from harming themselves through nonautonomous decisions and actions. Intervening to determine whether a patient is competent and informed is a minimal imposition on patient autonomy, compared with the possible harms of allowing an incompetent patient to act unwisely.

In strong or hard paternalism, a patient's autonomous choices are overridden. An example is withholding a diagnosis or a test result requested by a patient because the physician believes the information will greatly upset the patient. When writing about paternalism, philosophers generally mean strong or hard paternalism. Strong or hard paternalism has been sharply criticized, as we discuss in the next section.

Problems With Medical Paternalism

Critics of (strong) paternalism raise several objections (2). First, value judgments are unavoidable in clinical medicine, and patients, not physicians, should make them. Physicians can define the burdens and benefits of an intervention, but in Case 4.1 only Mrs. N can decide whether the surgical risk and side effects are worth the chance for long-term survival and relief of her symptoms.

Second, the belief that patients cannot make wise medical decisions is a self-fulfilling prophecy. If patients are not informed, they will not be able to make meaningful choices. If they are empowered to make decisions, most patients ask questions, seek information, and take responsibility for difficult choices.

Third, physicians might seek to override a patient's wishes because of their own psychological and emotional reactions to the case. Some physicians are affronted and angry if patients reject their recommendations.

CASE 4.1 *Continued*

Mrs. N's physician wanted to be sure that her refusal of aortic valve replacement was informed. He explained the situation as a dilemma: without valve replacement she might have a sudden death, but she might also have progressive disability from congestive heart failure or angina. Valve replacement offered the prospect of avoiding such disability, but with a trade-off of major risks and recuperation. He reassured her that the decision was hers to make. She agreed to speak with a cardiologist, cardiac surgeon, and several elderly patients who had undergone the procedure. Her physician also encouraged her to bring a friend (she had no close living relatives) to these meetings. Afterwards, she still declined surgery because of the operative risks.

Several years later, transcather aortic valve replacement became available. However, her blood vessels were to narrow to allow the procedure. Two more years later, when a keyhole approach to aortic valve replacement became available, she declined because her quality of life was unacceptable because of memory loss and severe osteoarthris.

PATIENT REQUESTS FOR INTERVENTIONS

Patients might insist on medical interventions that physicians consider far more harmful than beneficial, frustrating and angering physicians. Such disagreements are often framed as conflicting rights: Patients claim the right to decide about their medical care, while the physician asserts a countervailing right to follow her professional judgment. However, framing the issues in this way generally leads to stalemate. A more fruitful approach is to examine the benefits and burdens for the patient.

INTERVENTIONS OUTSIDE APPROPRIATE MEDICAL PRACTICE

CASE 4.2 **Request to monitor side effects of a performance-enhancing drug**

A 22-year-old college swimmer is taking oral anabolic steroids, which she obtains through friends at the gym where she lifts weights. She is aware of the long-term side effects but plans to use the drugs only for the next year while she is competing. Some of her competitors are using steroids, and she cannot remain competitive unless she takes them also. She asks her physician to monitor her for side effects, but not to prescribe the drugs.

In this case, the patient is using drugs for enhancement, not for the treatment or prevention of illness. Many physicians believe that enhancement of normal function is not an appropriate goal of medicine. In this case, the medical risks might be serious. There are additional reasons that the physician might decline this request. Using performance-enhancing drugs is unfair to other competitors and violates rules governing athletic competitions (10). Even though this patient is not asking the physician to prescribe the steroids, the physician might believe that monitoring for side effects condones the practice.

From another perspective, however, the physician can frame the request as preventing harm to the patient. Patients commonly use other substances that might harm their health, such as cigarettes, alcohol, and illicit injection drugs, which they obtain without prescription, and physicians continue to follow patients who use such substances, monitor them for adverse effects, and treat complications, while still urging them to stop. Indeed, by maintaining a supportive doctor–patient relationship, physicians might be better positioned to persuade patients to stop taking harmful substances.

INTERVENTIONS WHOSE BENEFIT CAN BE ASSESSED ONLY BY THE PATIENT

CASE 4.3   Request for controlled drug for pain

Mr. R, a 56-year-old man, has been disabled by chronic back pain for 10 years. Extensive evaluations, including a magnetic resonance (MR) scan, have been negative. Exercises and physical therapy have provided only minor improvement. After changing health insurance plans, the patient visits a new physician and requests a refill of a prescription for eight 160-mg tablets of oxycodone (Oxycontin) daily. He says that he has not changed the dosage in several years. His new physician does not prescribe opioids at this strength and dosage for chronic pain. She wants to wean the patient off opioids and to help him live an active life despite the pain. The patient refuses a referral to a pain clinic. "I know that Oxycontin works. Nothing else helps me."

Pain is undertreated by physicians and causes substantial suffering. The fact that pain can be assessed only through the patient's self-report should not lead physicians to downplay the importance of treating it effectively. However, the evidence that opioids are effective in chronic noncancer pain is weak (11). Some physicians are uncomfortable prescribing opioids, particularly when the dosage seems high, only on the basis of the subjective patient reports. In this case the risks of opioids are significant. Oxycodone has been abused, diverted to illegal sales, and implicated in outbreaks of opioid abuse.

The ethical guideline of respecting patient autonomy and the legal doctrine of informed consent gives patients the *negative* right to refuse unwanted treatments (*see* Chapter 3). This patient, however, claims the *positive* right to receive a specific drug. Some countries allow patients to buy many drugs, including antibiotics, without a physician's prescription. In the United States, however, only physicians are licensed to order tests or prescribe medications. Prescriptions for opioids, such as oxycodone, require special physician registration numbers from the Drug Enforcement Agency and special prescription forms. The federal government has announced new regulations to better balance making opioids available to patients in need with preventing the public health harms of opioid abuse and diversion. These new policies include required education for physicians prescribing opioids, financial incentives to physicians to check state Prescription Drug Monitoring Programs databases for prescriptions from multiple providers, and security standards for electronic prescribing of controlled substances.

CASE 4.3   *Continued*

Mr. R's physician offered to provide opioids only as part of a comprehensive plan of pain management that included referral to physical therapy, a pain specialist, and behavioral medicine for other approaches to managing the pain, regularly scheduled visits for re-evaluation and refills, and no refills by other physicians (including emergency room or urgent care physicians). She acknowledged that only he could assess the severity of pain. A contract with these conditions, signed by Mr. R and physician, was placed in the medical record.

INTERVENTION WITH SMALL BENEFIT

CASE 4.4   Request for an expensive, low-yield test

Ms. D, a 41-year-old bus driver, has episodes of crampy abdominal pain, episodes of diar-rhea, and some constipation. One year ago, after an evaluation that included colonoscopy, she was diagnosed with irritable bowel syndrome (IBS). Dietary manipulations and increased dietary fiber have been ineffective. On the advice of a friend, she asks her doctor to order an abdominal magnetic resonance imaging (MRI) scan because when the cramps are severe she fears something serious has been missed. She also says that "if doctors could only find out what is causing this, they would be able to do something about it." She refuses to discuss psychosocial issues about her illness or to try antidepressants that inhibit serotonin reuptake, saying that "my problems aren't in my head."

The physician's goal in Case 4.4 is to help Ms. D cope with a chronic medical condition and live an active life despite her symptoms. However, Ms. D's goals are relief of her symptoms and reassurance that her condition is not dangerous. Having different goals for care, Ms. D and her physician disagree on the benefits and burdens of a MRI scan.

To Ms. D, a scan has little medical risk and potentially great benefit. She believes that a negative scan would provide reassurance. In the unlikely event that the scan is abnormal, her course of care would be dramatically changed. In contrast, from the physician's perspective, a negative scan result is unlikely to lead to reassurance. Patients who seek "just another test" for reassurance often request further tests in a fruitless quest for a definitive diagnosis. Articles on IBS advise against additional diagnostic tests if a thorough initial work-up is negative and the clinical course is typical (12). In other situations, the medical risks of the requested intervention might be substantial. If the patient in Case 4.5 had requested exploratory surgery for reassurance or to establish a definitive diagnosis, the physicians should certainly demur.

ALLOCATING RESOURCES FAIRLY

Given the soaring cost of health care, physicians have a duty to allocate health care resources fairly and cannot ignore the costs of patient requests. Expensive, low-yield high-technology procedures, such as the MRI scans noted in Case 4.4, drive up the cost of medical care. In addition, MRI scans commonly reveal incidental findings that require further costly and sometimes risky evaluation, but ultimately prove to be clinically insignificant.

However, cost should not be the main reason for refusing patient requests. Under the current health care system, physicians have no explicit societal mandate to limit care to control costs. In managed care systems, potential conflicts of interest make it problematic to limit highly beneficial care on the basis of cost (*see* Chapter 32).

The primary consideration should be the benefits and risks to the patient, rather than costs. If the intervention's medical risks outweigh any benefits for the patient, the patient's request can be refused without reference to costs. Patients who have financial incentives to control costs—through substantial copayments—are less likely to request such interventions. Thus, when patients and physicians both have financial incentives for cost-effective medicine, situations like Case 4.4 are easier to resolve.

Cost might determine how much time and effort physicians should spend on trying to dissuade the patient. The physician should spend more time trying to discourage an expensive MRI scan than in discouraging inexpensive tests. If Ms. D with IBS in Case 4.4 wanted a simple blood count that offered little benefit, few physicians would strongly object.

> **CASE 4.4** **Continued**
>
> *Ms. D's physician acknowledged her concerns and frustrations about a serious illness regarding a chronic illness. Rather than ordering a MRI scan, the physician recommeneded referral to a gastroenterologist to help develop a comprehensive approach, possibility including new medications. The doctor explained how the digestive system responds physiologically to stress and anxiety. The physician also explained the problem of incidental findings on MRI scans and reviewed recommendations for screening for cervical, breast, and colon cancer. She recommended that regular visits regardless of symptoms could provide reassurance that there was "nothing serious."*

REACHING AGREEMENT ON BEST INTERESTS

The cases in this chapter illustrate how the patient's choices may conflict with what the physician's view of the patient's best interests. Through continued discussions with patients, physicians can promote the best interests of patients while respecting patients' ultimate power to decide (Table 4-1). Chapter 14 gives detailed recommendations for such discussions. Physicians should recommend what they believe is best for the patient from the perspective of the patient's values and preferences. In shared decision making, physicians should not merely present patients with a list of alternatives and leave them to decide.

Physicians also should try to dissuade patients from unwise decisions. Persuasion respects patients and fosters their autonomy. Persuasion might include talking to the patient about the decision on several occasions and asking the patient to talk to family members, friends, other physicians, or other patients who have had the intervention. The goal is to negotiate a mutually acceptable plan for care, while respecting the patient's right to refuse unwanted interventions. Persuasion needs to be distinguished from deception and threats, which are wrong because they undermine the patient's autonomy. Persuasion must also be distinguished from badgering the patient. Continual attempts to convince patients to change their minds are disrespectful and might also be counterproductive.

TABLE 4-1 **Promoting the Patient's Best Interests**
Understand the patient's perspective.
Address misunderstandings and concerns.
Try to persuade the patient.
Negotiate a mutually acceptable plan of care.
Ultimately let the patient decide.

SUMMARY

1. Physicians need to respect patient autonomy and act in the patient's best interests simultaneously.
2. Doctors have a fiduciary obligation to act for the well-being of patients as patients would define it.
3. Physicians can satisfy the ethical guidelines of beneficence and autonomy by understanding the patient's perspective, by trying to persuade patients, respecting the power to refuse unwanted interventions, and by negotiating a mutually acceptable plan.

REFERENCES

1. Brewin T. Primum non nocere? *Lancet.* 1994;344:1487–1488.
2. Beauchamp TL, Childress JF. *Principles of Biomedical Ethics.* 6th ed. New York, NY: Oxford University Press; 2009:197–237.
3. Pellegrino ED, Thomasma DG. *For the Patient's Good: The Restoration of Beneficence in Health Care.* New York, NY: Oxford University Press; 1988.
4. ABIM Foundation, American Board of Internal Medicine, ACP-ASIM Foundation, et al. Medical professionalism in the new millennium: a physician charter. *Ann Intern Med.* 2002;136:243–246.
5. Lesser CS, Lucey CR, Egener B, et al. A behavioral and systems view of professionalism. *JAMA.* 2010;304: 2732–2737.
6. Ginsburg S, Regehr G, Lingard L. Basing the evaluation of professionalism on observable behaviors: a cautionary tale. *Acad Med.* 2004;79:S1–S4.
7. Papadakis MA, Teherani A, Banach MA, et al. Disciplinary action by medical boards and prior behavior in medical school. *N Engl J Med.* 2005;353:2673–2682.
8. McNeil BJ, Weichselbaum R, Pauker SG. Fallacy of the five-year survival in lung cancer. *N Engl J Med.* 1978;299:307–401.
9. Ubel PA, Loewenstein G, Schwarz N, et al. Misimagining the unimaginable: the disability paradox and health care decision making. *Health Psychol.* 2005;24:S57–S62.
10. Murray TH. Making sense of fairness in sports. *Hastings Cent Rep.* 2010;40:13–15.
11. Manchikanti L, Ailinani H, Koyyalagunta D, et al. A systematic review of randomized trials of long-term opioid management for chronic non-cancer pain. *Pain Physician.* 2011;14:91–121.
12. Longstreth GF. Irritable bowel syndrome: diagnosis in the managed care era. *Dig Dis Sci.* 1997;42:1105–1111.

ANNOTATED BIBLIOGRAPHY

1. Beauchamp TL, Childress JF. *Principles of Biomedical Ethics.* 6th ed. New York, NY: Oxford University Press; 2009:197–237.
   In-depth discussion of the ethical principle of beneficence.
2. Pellegrino ED, Thomasma DG. *For the Patient's Good: The Restoration of Beneficence in Health Care.* New York, NY: Oxford University Press; 1988.
   Comprehensive exposition of the importance of beneficence in the doctor–patient relationship.
3. Ubel PA, Loewenstein G, Schwarz N, et al. Misimagining the unimaginable: The disability paradox and health care decision making. *Health Psychol.* 2005;24:S57–S62.
   People who are living with chronic illness and disability report their quality of life to be higher than what healthy people predict they would experience under the circumstances. Thus patient assessments of their quality of life may differ from how others judge it.

CHAPTER 5

Confidentiality

P atients reveal to physicians sensitive personal information about their medical and emotional problems, alcohol and drug use, and sexual activities. The presumption is that physicians should keep patient information confidential unless the patient gives permission to disclose it; however, exceptions to confidentiality might be warranted to prevent serious harm to third parties or to the patient (Table 5-1). The HIV epidemic, the development of computerized medical records, and the explosion of genetic information have sharpened controversies over confidentiality. In 2003, the federal government issued health privacy regulations, commonly known as HIPAA regulations, because the Health Insurance Portability and Accountability Act mandated them.

The terms privacy, confidentiality, and security should be distinguished (1). Privacy refers to patients' interest in controlling information about themselves, access to their bodies, and freedom to make decisions about their health care. In particular, patients may choose what information about themselves they disclose to their physicians. They may regard some information as too intimate or sensitive to disclose or simply not relevant to the issue at hand. Privacy may also refer to whether information collected for one purpose may be used for another purpose, for example whether information collected for patient care may be used for research or quality improvement.

TABLE 5-1 Exceptions to Confidentiality
Exceptions to Protect Third Parties
Reporting to public officials
Infectious diseases
Impaired drivers
Injuries caused by weapons or crimes
Partner notification by public health officials
Warnings by physicians to persons at risk
Violence by psychiatric patients
Infectious diseases
Exceptions to Protect Patients
Child abuse
Elder abuse
Domestic violence

There is no single concept of privacy that is universally accepted; instead, privacy may be viewed as a bundle of overlapping and related interests, which are also related to other interests such as liberty and autonomy.

Confidentiality refers to the further disclosure of information that the patient has provided to the physician. For example, after a patient has disclosed information to a physician, may that information be disclosed to the patient's family, insurance company, or to public health officials? The focus of confidentiality is on what the physician may reveal to third parties, rather than what the patient chooses to disclose to the physician. In everyday conversation, the distinction between privacy and confidentiality is blurred.

Security refers to the procedural and technical measures to prevent inappropriate access, use, and disclosure of personal information in health records. In this era of electronic health records, increased security is an important means to prevent breaches of confidentiality that may affect thousands of patients. Current security standards include training of physicians and staff regarding privacy and confidentiality, basing access to a patient's health record on need to know, logins, passwords, time-outs, audit trails, and encryption of personal health information transmitted to remote computers and mobile devices.

THE IMPORTANCE OF CONFIDENTIALITY IN MEDICINE

REASONS FOR CONFIDENTIALITY

Keeping medical information confidential shows respect for patients (2), who expect physicians to maintain confidentiality. Maintaining confidentiality also has beneficial consequences for patients and for the doctor–patient relationship. It encourages people to seek medical care and discuss sensitive issues candidly. In turn, treatment for these conditions benefits both the individual patient and public health. Furthermore, confidentiality prevents harmful consequences to patients, such as stigmatization and discrimination. Patients might fear that employers will gain access to their health information and discriminate against them.

Respect for confidentiality is a strong tradition in medicine, dating back to the Hippocratic Oath. The legal system may also hold physicians liable for unwarranted disclosure of medical information.

DIFFICULTIES MAINTAINING CONFIDENTIALITY

Maintaining confidentiality is increasingly difficult in modern medicine. Many people have access to medical records, including the attending physician, house staff, students, consultants, nurses, social workers, pharmacists, billing staff, medical records personnel, insurance company employees, and quality-of-care reviewers. Computerized medical records, which improve access to medical information, also allow more serious breaches of confidentiality. Confidentiality can be violated at any computer station, making available extensive data on many patients. Fax and e-mail also present opportunities for confidentiality to be broken.

Many breaches of confidentiality, however, result from health care workers' indiscretions. Caregivers might discuss patients by name in hospital elevators or cafeterias (3). Although many physicians take such discussions for granted, patients object to such breaches of confidentiality.

WAIVERS OF CONFIDENTIALITY

Patients commonly authorize disclosure of information about their condition, for example, to other physicians, insurers, employers, or benefits programs such as disability or workers' compensation (4). Patients might not appreciate that signing a general release allows the insurance company to further disseminate the information without restriction. Insurance companies generally place patients' diagnoses in a computerized database that is accessible to other insurance companies or to employers without further permission from the patient.

COUNTERVAILING ETHICAL GUIDELINES

Although confidentiality is important, it is not an absolute value. In some situations, overriding confidentiality might be justified in order to provide important benefits to patients or to prevent serious harm to third parties. Access to information might be needed to improve the quality of care or protect the public health. These exceptions require careful justification, because not every instance of benefit to patients or prevention of harm to others warrants the disclosure of identifiable medical information without the patient's permission.

FEDERAL HEALTH PRIVACY REGULATIONS

The privacy regulations require health care providers—both individual health care workers and institutions—to obtain patient authorization to use or disclose individually identifiable health information, with certain broad exceptions (5). Providers must make reasonable efforts to use and disclose only the minimum identifiable information that is needed to accomplish the intended purpose. In addition, health care providers must take reasonable safeguards against prohibited or incidental use or disclosure of personal health information and maintain "reasonable and appropriate" safeguards to prevent violations of the privacy regulations.

Patients must receive written notice of their privacy rights and the organization's privacy practices. They may inspect and copy their medical records and request that corrections be made. They may request to receive information by alternative means and locations (such as not leaving messages on an answering machine) and to obtain a list of disclosures of their information. Health care providers must develop privacy policies and procedures and train all staff about the privacy regulations. The regulations also address how individually identifiable health information may be used or disclosed for research and marketing and by business associates of the health care provider. The HIPAA regulations apply to virtually all health care providers. Because the regulations set criminal penalties for intentional violations, many risk managers interpret them conservatively. These federal regulations establish a minimum level of protection; state laws and organizational policies may be stricter.

HIPAA regulations are not intended to impede access to individual patient information needed for high quality and efficient patient care. No patient authorization is needed to use or disclose identifiable information for treatment, payment, and operations, including quality improvement, quality assurance, and education. Furthermore, HIPAA permits required disclosures of identifiable information to public health officials, health oversight agencies, and as required by law or a court. The "minimum necessary" restriction does not apply to treatment or to disclosures required by law.

Good patient care requires communication among various health care providers. In the course of care, incidental disclosure of information and breaches of confidentiality might occur. Physicians should take reasonable precautions to prevent inappropriate disclosures, but should not forego communications that might be essential in patient care (6). For example, physicians may communicate with other providers by e-mail or fax without explicit patient authorization, but should take such precautions as using secure e-mail systems and keeping fax machines in areas where other patients cannot access them. Furthermore, physicians may discuss patients at the nursing station, provided that they keep their voices down and pause when someone such as a patient or visitor approaches.

DISCLOSING THE PATIENT'S CONDITION TO OTHERS

Disclosing patient information to family members, friends, or the press might raise ethical issues.

DISCLOSURE TO RELATIVES AND FRIENDS

Relatives and friends often ask about the patient's condition. Generally patients want the physician to talk to their family, and usually physicians do not even ask the patient's permission to do so. In some cases, however, the patient might not want the information disclosed.

> **CASE 5.1**   **Estrangement from relatives**
>
> *Ms. D, a 32-year-old woman, is admitted to the hospital after a serious automobile accident. She is disoriented and confused. Her sister requests that Ms. D's husband not be given any information. Ms. D has previously told the physician about her hostile divorce proceedings, and this is well documented in the electronic health record at the hospital. The husband learns that she is hospitalized and inquires about her condition.*

The HIPAA privacy regulations establish a reasonable approach to this issue. Health care providers need to notify patients that relatives will be informed unless the patient requests that they not be. In ethical terms, the physician can presume that patients would want their relatives notified. The reasons are that generally the patient would want them told, that they might provide valuable information, that they have the patient's best interests in mind, and that their assistance might be needed with decision making or discharge planning. However, this presumption can be reversed in Cases like 5.1. Physicians may provide information about a patient's condition and treatment to family members and other people involved in the patient's care, provided that the patient does not object. Often, such communication is needed to help monitor the patient's condition, administer medications, or arrange follow-up care.

> **CASE 5.1**   *Continued*
>
> *If the inpatient physician knows about the contentious divorce proceedings between Ms. D and her husband, he should regard them as estranged and not give the husband information about Ms. D's condition, instead referring him to her sister. In a hospitalist system, such social history may not be transmitted to the covering physician or nursing staff. How much should physicians who do not know the patient question the presumption that they may tell family members about the patient's condition? It would be reasonable to expect the admitting physician to review information in the electronic record. However, screening family members to ask if they are estranged would be disrespectful for the vast majority of family members who care about the patient and might lead to mistrust between them and the medical team.*

INFORMATION ABOUT PUBLIC FIGURES

The press might seek information about patients who are public figures or celebrities. The public and the news media might have legitimate reasons to know medical information about a public figure. For instance, a political candidate's health is an important concern to voters (7). However, famous people have a right to confidentiality, like all patients. The physician and hospital should ask the patient or appropriate surrogate what information, if any, should be released.

OMITTING SENSITIVE INFORMATION FROM MEDICAL RECORDS

Patients who are concerned about breaches of confidentiality sometimes ask physicians to omit sensitive information from their medical records.

> **CASE 5.2**   **Omission of information from the medical record**
>
> *Mr. N, "a 41-year-old nurse," is in excellent health, has a routine checkup at the hospital where he works. He asks his physician not to write in the medical record that was severely depressed several years ago. Mr. N knows that many people in the hospital might see his record, and he does not want colleagues to know his psychiatric history. He also fears that he will have difficulty changing jobs if his history is known.*

Physicians might fear that omitting medical information from patient records might compromise the quality of care. Important clinical information might not be available in an emergency. In addition, documentation of the patient's current condition and treatment might be required for insurance payment or authorization for services. Furthermore, it might not be feasible to exclude information from an electronic medical record. Even if a diagnosis is omitted from the record, it might be inferred from the patient's laboratory tests or medications.

The purpose of the medical record is to enhance patient well-being and quality of care. Generally, patients are the best judge of their best interests. Some patients might regard breaches of confidentiality as more threatening than the risk of suboptimal care resulting from incomplete medical records. Thus, a patient's informed preferences to exclude sensitive information from the medical record should be respected if feasible. Many psychiatrists, for example, keep their detailed psychotherapy notes separate from the rest of the patient's medical record.

CASE 5.2   *Continued*

Mr. N's concerns are understandable because depression might be considered stigmatizing. Many electronic health records allow patients to limit access to some information only to persons providing direct care. The Americans with Disabilities Act restricts access by potential employers to a worker's health records and basing hiring and promotion decisions on medical conditions that do not affect job performance. Mr. N's physician should explain how the prior history can be useful to other doctors providing care. If Mr. N persists in his request, the physician should try to accommodate it, preferably with a note in the medical record alerting other treating physicians to contact her for additional history not in the record. However, electronic ordering of medications cannot be omitted from an electronic medical record.

OVERRIDING CONFIDENTIALITY TO PROTECT THIRD PARTIES

Overriding patient confidentiality might prevent serious harm to third parties, as the following case illustrates. HIPAA expressly permits these exceptions to confidentiality, which are often required by state law.

CASE 5.3   Risk of HIV transmission

Mr. H, a 28-year-old accountant, reveals to his physician that he had a positive test for HIV antibodies at an anonymous testing center. He asks his physician not to disclose the test results to anyone, because he is concerned about losing his job and health insurance. Mr. H's physician encourages him to notify his wife so that she can be tested and treated if necessary. After several discussions, Mr. H continues to refuse to notify his wife or allow others to do so. He declares, "If she finds out, it would destroy our marriage." Should the physician notify the wife despite the patient's objections?

The ethical guideline of nonmaleficence requires both patients and physicians to avoid harming other people and to prevent harm to others. Infected persons have a moral duty not to harm others and to notify persons whom they have placed at risk. This duty is particularly strong when trust is expected, as in marriage. The common law may also impose on infected persons a legal duty to notify persons whom they place at risk. In Case 5.3, the patient abrogates this responsibility. In addition, physicians may override confidentiality to prevent serious harm to third parties in some circumstances, as we discuss next.

JUSTIFICATIONS FOR OVERRIDING CONFIDENTIALITY

The balance between preventing harm to third parties and protecting confidentiality is ultimately set by society through statutes, public health regulations, and court decisions. Setting this balance as public policy allows all points of view to be represented and is preferable to decisions by the individual physicians in their offices or at the bedside. Laws on confidentiality vary from state to state. In general, exceptions to confidentiality are warranted when all the following conditions are met (Table 5-2) (2):

- The potential harm to identifiable third parties is serious.
- The likelihood of harm is high.
- There is no less invasive alternative means for warning or protecting those at risk.
- Breaching confidentiality allows the person at risk to take steps to prevent harm.
- Harm to the patient resulting from the breach of confidentiality is minimized and acceptable. Disclosure should be limited to information essential for the intended purpose, and only those persons with a need to know should receive information.

In these circumstances, the overall harm to the third parties at risk is judged to be greater than the harm to the index case resulting from overriding confidentiality.

Confidentiality can be overridden in several ways: reporting to public officials, partner notification by public health officials, and direct warnings to third parties at risk.

WARNINGS TO PATIENTS

As a first step, physicians need to explain to patients how their condition might put others at risk and to advise how the patient should protect those at risk. For instance, doctors need to explain how to avoid transmitting a contagious disease. Similarly, they should warn patients about driving if they are taking medications that might impair their alertness. Physicians should also explain if public health officials will reserve results from clinical laboratory and if contact tracing will be carried out.

REPORTING TO PUBLIC OFFICIALS

In certain situations, physicians are legally required to break confidentiality and to report the name of a patient to appropriate public officials (Table 5-1).

Infectious Diseases

Physicians, clinical laboratories, and hospitals are required by law to report to public health officials the names of patients with specified infectious diseases, such as tuberculosis, gonorrhea, and enteric pathogens. Such reporting allows accurate outbreak investigations, surveillance, and public health planning and facilitates partner notification.

HIV Infection

In certain conditions, stigma and discrimination are greater than in other illnesses. Early in the HIV epidemic, HIV testing received special protection, including pretest counseling and written

TABLE 5-2   Situations in Which Overriding Confidentiality Is Warranted
The potential harm to third parties is serious.
The likelihood of harm is high.
No alternative for warning or protecting those at risk exists.
Breaching confidentiality will prevent harm.
Harm to the patient is minimized and acceptable.

informed consent (8). Alternative test sites were established in which people could be tested for HIV antibodies anonymously. Furthermore, although AIDS cases had to be reported, HIV infection was not reportable in many states.

As highly active antiretroviral therapy became available and overt discrimination decreased, HIV infection has been treated like other infectious diseases, with reporting of persons with HIV infection by name to public health officials (9). Because prognosis has improved dramatically with highly active antiretroviral therapy, there is a stronger rationale for partner notification. Also, reporting only AIDS cases gives an inaccurate picture of the epidemic, compromises public health planning, and leads to inequitable distribution of funding based on caseload. Moreover, HIV viral load and CD4 counts are reported in some states, to better link testing with treatment (10). Anonymous testing, however, is still permitted.

Impaired Drivers

Many states require physicians to report to the department of motor vehicles persons with specified medical conditions that impair their ability to drive safely. Such conditions include epilepsy, syncope, dementia, sleep apnea, and other conditions that impair consciousness (11). Even if the underlying condition is treated, the patient might not be able to drive safely. For example, after placement of an implantable cardiac defibrillator, about 10% of patients experience syncope or near-syncope associated with defibrillation in the first year (12). The physician's role is not to stop the patient from driving or to decide whether the patient should be permitted to drive. Such determinations are properly made by the department of motor vehicles. The physician only informs officials of persons who warrant evaluation. Reporting is particularly important for patients who drive commercially and present greater risks because they spend more hours on the road, drive heavy vehicles, and might be responsible for passengers.

Reporting of patients with seizures is particularly controversial (13). The physician has knowledge of seizures only through patient reports. Mandatory reporting may lead some patients to withhold from physicians information on breakthrough seizures, precluding adjustments of medications to improve control of the seizures.

Injuries Caused by Weapons or Crimes

Almost all states require physicians to report injuries involving a deadly weapon or criminal act (14). The rationale is to protect the public from further violence.

PARTNER NOTIFICATION BY PUBLIC HEALTH OFFICIALS

In partner notification, persons at risk for an infectious disease are warned that they have been exposed. More partners are notified when public health officials carry out the notification than when patients do it themselves. In the AIDS epidemic, the term *partner notification* has replaced the traditional term *contact tracing* (15). During partner notification, partners should be told only that they have been exposed. Although the identity of the index case is not revealed, partners can often infer it.

Many contagious diseases, such as tuberculosis, are spread through aerosolized particles and can be transmitted by casual contact. Casual contacts might be located without the cooperation of the index case, as by going to the index case's workplace. In contrast, for blood-borne and sexually transmitted diseases such as HIV, sexual or injection partners can be identified only with the infected person's cooperation, and for all practical purposes partner notification must be voluntary (15). If patients do not wish to cooperate, they can deny that they have partners or give inaccurate names and addresses. Any perception that partner notification programs are punitive or disrespectful to index cases might further reduce cooperation.

WARNINGS BY PHYSICIANS TO PERSONS AT RISK

In addition to notifying public officials, physicians might have a legal duty or the legal option to directly warn identifiable persons whom a patient places at risk (Table 5-1).

Violence by Psychiatric Patients

Physicians have a legal responsibility to override confidentiality to protect persons who are potential targets of violence by psychiatric patients (*see* Chapter 42). The landmark Tarasoff ruling declared, "Protective privilege ends where public peril begins (16)." Although many physicians believe that the law requires them to *warn* the persons who are potential targets, in fact, the law requires a broader duty to *protect* the person who is a potential target from harm (17). This duty to protect might require more intensive therapy, voluntary or involuntary hospitalization, convincing the patient to give up weapons, or notifying the police.

Infectious Diseases

Courts might require physicians to warn patients with infectious diseases to take precautions to prevent their infectious disease from afflicting others (18). In addition, some courts require physicians to notify identified persons whom their infected patients place at risk. Generally, physicians can fulfill this duty by notifying public health officials.

PHYSICIAN JUDGMENT

Although society has set legal requirements for public health reporting, physicians might still face dilemmas in Case 5.3. Some jurisdictions explicitly give physicians discretion on partner notification in some situations. For example, in California, physicians are *permitted* but not *required* to notify partners of HIV-infected patients (or notify public health officials). Physicians who decide to notify cannot be held liable in civil or criminal proceedings. Doctors should notify the patient of their intent to notify, so that the patient has the opportunity to notify himself. When notifying a partner, the name of the index case should not be disclosed.

Sound medical ethics might require notification even though the law does not.

CASE 5.3   *Continued*

Mr. H promises to use condoms but refuses to notify his wife. In one study, more than 60% of physicians were willing to allow a patient with gonorrhea to tell his wife that he had nonspecific urethritis (19). This strategy, however, is ethically problematic in the case of HIV infection, because HIV is an incurable but preventable and treatable infection. Unless notified, the wife would not be aware of her risk or the need for testing and prevention or treatment. Women may object that male physicians unfairly favor the man's interests over the woman's well-being and autonomy.

The physician should try to persuade Mr. H to agree to partner notification. She also can try to elicit Mr. B's concerns and address them. It is unlikely his wife will not eventually learn his diagnosis, and failure to disclose now will likely undermine the marriage. In the long run, telling his wife is in Mr. B's self-interest. Physicians should offer Mr. H's choices about how notification is done. For instance, he may prefer that a public health official notify his wife rather than his physician.

OVERRIDING CONFIDENTIALITY TO PROTECT PATIENTS

In several situations, physicians are required to override confidentiality to protect the patient rather than third parties (Table 5-1). In these situations, the ethical justification for intervening is that patients might not be able to protect themselves. The HIPAA privacy regulations allow physicians to comply with state requirements for such reporting.

CHILD ABUSE

All states require health care workers to report suspected child abuse or neglect to child protective services agencies (20). The parents' privacy is overridden to protect vulnerable children from an imminent risk of serious harm. More than 1,000 children die of neglect and abuse each year; most are under the age of 5. Health care workers might be the only people outside the family to have close contact with preschool children. State laws vary regarding the types of situations that must be reported and the kinds of persons who must report. In some states, only helping professionals, such as health care workers, school personnel, child care providers, law enforcement workers, and mental health professionals, must report; in other states, any person who suspects abuse or neglect has a mandatory duty to report.

A report should be triggered if there is reasonable belief or suspicion of abuse and neglect that justifies fuller investigation. Definitive proof is not needed (21). To encourage reporting, most states grant legal immunity when reporting is done in good faith. Intervention might enable parents to obtain enough assistance and support to prevent further abuse. In extreme cases, the child might be removed from parental custody. In evaluating possible child abuse, pediatricians should treat parents with respect, keeping in mind that most parents are trying their best to deal with the challenges of childrearing.

ELDER ABUSE

Most states require health care workers to report cases of elder abuse to adult protective services (22). The goal is to identify persons who are incapable of seeking assistance on their own and to offer them help. Elderly persons who are dependent on their caretakers might be unwilling or unable to complain about physical or psychological abuse or neglect. Patients might not be aware of available in-home supportive services or might feel intimidated by caretakers. They might fear that if they complain, they will be worse off, perhaps placed in a nursing home. Most abusers of elderly persons are family members who are overwhelmed by caring for a frail elderly person. Thus, reporting and intervention might provide resources that allow the elderly person to continue to live safely at home. Elderly persons who are truly capable of making informed decisions and are free from coercion are at liberty to decline offered assistance.

Specific laws for reporting elder abuse vary from state to state. Generally, reasonable suspicion of abuse is sufficient to trigger reporting. Health care workers typically must report abuse only when they obtain information about a patient in their professional roles. Thus, although physicians as private citizens *may* report an elderly neighbor whom they suspect is abused, they are not *required* to do so. Health care workers receive legal immunity when they report suspected abuse in good faith.

DOMESTIC VIOLENCE

Domestic violence or intimate partner violence is physical, sexual, or psychological assault against intimate partners. The vast majority of people who are assaulted are women. Some states require health care workers to report suspected domestic violence or abuse, while most states require reporting of injuries caused by a deadly weapon or illegal act (14). Persons who are assaulted often are unable to take steps on their own to escape further violence. Although reporting is intended to protect the person assaulted and to hold perpetrators of violence accountable, it might be ineffective or even counterproductive (14). Mandatory reporting might put victims at risk of retaliation from their assailants. The police and courts often respond poorly to reports of abuse. In one study, 44% of victims of domestic violence opposed mandatory reporting, preferring instead that physicians notify authorities only with the approval of the victim rather than in every case. Thus, physicians might face conflicting obligations: a legal mandate to report and the patient's desire not to report the abuse. Physicians should provide emotional support, ask about safety, and refer patients to a shelter, legal and social services, and counseling. Particular concerns about an increased risk of violence should be communicated to the police when making a report (14). Whenever possible, physicians should promote the abused person's autonomy—for example, respecting a request to delay reporting until the person can find shelter.

SUMMARY

1. Physicians should maintain confidentiality unless there are compelling reasons to override it.
2. In some situations, the law provides clear guidance for physicians about confidentiality; however, the law might be silent about other situations, or it might defer to the judgment of physicians.
3. Even if public health reporting is required by law, it is respectful to tell patients that reporting will occur, obtain their agreement if possible, and take steps to address their concerns and minimize harm to them.

REFERENCES

1. Allen A. *Privacy and Medicine. In Stanford Encyclopedia of Philosophy*. http://plato.stanford.edu/entries/privacy-medicine/. Accessed August 22, 2011.
2. Beauchamp TL, Childress JF. *Principles of Biomedical Ethics*. 6th ed. New York, NY: Oxford University Press; 2009:302–310.
3. Ubel PA, Zell MM, Miller DJ, et al. Elevator talk: observational study of inappropriate comments in a public space. *Am J Med*. 1995;99:190–194.
4. Rothstein MA, Talbott MK. Compelled disclosure of health information: protecting against the greatest potential threat to privacy. *JAMA*. 2006;295:2882–2885.
5. Department of Health and Human Services. 45 CFR Parts 160 and 164. *Standards for Privacy of Individually Identifiable Health Information*. http://www.hhs.gov/ocr/hipaa/finalreg.html. Accessed December 2, 2008.
6. Lo B, Dornbrand L, Dubler NN. From hippocrates to HIPAA: confidentiality, government regulations, and professional judgment. *JAMA*. 2005;293:1766–1771.
7. Annas GJ. The health of the president and presidential candidates: the public's right to know. *N Engl J Med*. 1995;333:945–949.
8. Bayer R, Fairchild AL. Changing the paradigm for HIV testing—the end of exceptionalism. *N Engl J Med*. 2006;355:647–649.
9. Fairchild AL, Gable L, Gostin LO, et al. Public goods, private data: HIV and the history, ethics, and uses of identifiable public health information. *Public Health Rep*. 2007;122(suppl 1):7–15.
10. Fairchild AL, Bayer R. HIV surveillance, public health, and clinical medicine—will the walls come tumbling down? *N Engl J Med*. 2011;365:685–687.
11. Gupta M. Mandatory reporting laws and the emergency physician. *Ann Emerg Med*. 2007;49:369–376.
12. Epstein AE, Baessler CA, Curtis AB, et al. Addendum to "Personal and public safety issues related to arrhythmias that may affect consciousness: implications for regulation and physician recommendations: a medical/scientific statement from the American Heart Association and the North American Society of Pacing and Electrophysiology": public safety issues in patients with implantable defibrillators: a scientific statement from the American Heart Association and the Heart Rhythm Society. *Circulation*. 2007;115:1170–1176.
13. Meador KJ. To drive or not to drive: roles of the physician, patient, and state. *Neurology*. 2007;68:1170–1171.
14. Hyman A, Schillinger D, Lo B. Laws mandating reporting of domestic violence: do they promote patient well-being? *JAMA*. 1995;273:1781–1787.
15. Bayer R, Toomey KE. HIV prevention and the two faces of partner notification. *Am J Public Health*. 1992;82:1158–1164.
16. Tarasoff v. Regents of the University of California. 551 P.2d 334 (Cal. 1976).
17. Anfang SA, Appelbaum PS. Twenty years after Tarasoff: reviewing the duty to protect. *Harv Rev Psychiatry*. 1996;4:67–76.
18. Gostin LO. *Public Health Law: Power, Duty, Restraint*. 2nd ed. Berkeley, CA: University of California Press; 2008:287–330.
19. Novack DH, Detering BJ, Arnold R, et al. Physicians' attitudes toward using deception to resolve difficult ethical problems. *JAMA*. 1989;261:2980–2985.
20. Dubowitz H, Bennett S. Physical abuse and neglect of children. *Lancet*. 2007;369:1891–1899.
21. Levi BH, Portwood SG. Reasonable suspicion of child abuse: finding a common language. *J Law Med Ethics*. 2011;39:62–69.
22. Mosqueda L, Dong X. Elder abuse and self-neglect: "I don't care anything about going to the doctor, to be honest..." *JAMA*. 2011;306:532–540.

ANNOTATED BIBLIOGRAPHY

1. Allen A. *Privacy and Medicine. In Stanford Encyclopedia of Philosophy.* http://plato.stanford.edu/entries/privacy-medicine/. Accessed August 22, 2011.
   Comprehensive, thoughtful review.
2. Lo B, Dornbrand L, Dubler NN. From hippocrates to HIPAA: confidentiality, government regulations, and professional judgment. *JAMA.* 2005;293:1766–1771.
   Analyzes the federal confidentiality regulations (also known as HIPAA regulations) and how physician judgment is still required to determine what risk of a breach of confidentiality is acceptable when disclosing information to other health care workers caring for a patient.
3. Hyman A, Schillinger D, Lo B. Laws mandating reporting of domestic violence: do they promote patient well-being? *JAMA.* 1995;273:1781–1787.
   Explains that recent laws mandating reporting of domestic violence may place physicians in a dilemma if reporting is likely to lead to retaliation by the perpetrator.
4. Gostin LO. *Public Health Law: Power, Duty, Restraint.* Berkeley, CA: University of California Press; 2000:85–109.
   Lucid discussion of overriding confidentiality to protect the public health.
5. Mosqueda L, Dong X. Elder abuse and self-neglect: "I don't care anything about going to the doctor, to be honest..." *JAMA.* 2011;306:532–540.
   Comprehensive review of elder abuse.

6

Avoiding Deception and Nondisclosure

Children are taught to tell the truth and avoid lies. In clinical medicine, however, the distinction between telling the truth and lying can seem simplistic. Even doctors who condemn outright lying might consider withholding a grave diagnosis from a patient, covertly administering needed medications to a psychotic patient, or exaggerating a patient's condition to secure that patient's insurance coverage. This chapter analyzes the ethical considerations regarding lying, deception, misrepresentation, and nondisclosure. Such actions might mislead either the patient or a third party, such as an insurance company or a disability agency.

DEFINITIONS

The following case illustrates some ways physicians might provide misleading information.

CASE 6.1	Family request not to tell the patient the diagnosis of cancer

Ms. Z, a 70-year-old Cantonese-speaking woman, with a change in bowel habits and weight loss is found to have a carcinoma of the colon. The daughter and son ask the physician not to tell their mother that she has cancer. They say that people in her generation are not told they have cancer and that if Ms. Z is told she will lose hope. A colleague suggests that you tell the patient that she has a "growth" that needs to be removed.

Physicians might provide misleading information in different ways. *Lying* refers to statements that the speaker knows are false or believes to be false and that are intended to mislead the listener. For example, the physician might tell the patient that the tests were normal.

Deception is broader than lying, and it includes all statements and actions that are intended to mislead the listener, whether or not they are literally true. An example would be telling the patient that she has a "growth," hoping that she will believe nothing is wrong. Other techniques used to mislead people include employing technical jargon, ambiguous statements, or misleading statistics; not answering a question; and omitting important qualifying information.

Misrepresentation is a still broader category, including unintentional, as well as intentional statements and actions. The statements might or might not be literally true. Unintentional misrepresentation might result from inexperience, poor interpersonal skills, or lack of diligence or knowledge. For instance, a physician might not tell Ms. Z she has cancer because the physician misread the biopsy report.

Nondisclosure means that the physician does not provide information about the diagnosis, prognosis, or plan of care. For example, a physician might not tell Ms. Z she has cancer unless the patient specifically asks.

Many writers on medical ethics use terms such as *truth-telling* or *veracity*. This book, however, avoids these terms because ethically difficult cases usually do not involve outright lies.

ETHICAL OBJECTIONS TO LYING

Traditional religious and moral codes forbid lying. The Old Testament, for example, exhorts people not to bear false witness. Lying and deception also show disrespect for others. Those who are lied to or deceived generally feel betrayed or manipulated, even if the liar has benevolent motives. Lying also undermines social trust because listeners cannot be confident that other statements by the person will be truthful. This loss of trust is particularly grave in medicine because trust is essential in a doctor–patient relationship. In addition to undermining the speaker's integrity, lying is further condemned because a single lie often requires continued deception.

Lying and deception are considered prima facie wrong; they are presumed to be inappropriate, and they require a justification (1, 2). Many people regard lying as more blameworthy than other types of deception (1). Some "white" lies, however, may be accepted as social customs that do not deceive anyone and might prevent people from feeling rejected.

The ethical issue is whether general prohibitions on lying also apply to deception and nondisclosure in situations like Case 6.1.

DECEPTION OR NONDISCLOSURE TO THE PATIENT

Traditional codes of medical ethics did not require physicians to be truthful or forthcoming to patients. The writings of Hippocrates urge physicians to conceal "most things from the patient while you are attending him." Until recently, many physicians in the United States either did not tell patients about serious diagnoses, such as cancer, or deceived them (3).

WITHHOLDING BAD NEWS FROM A PATIENT

Reasons for Deception or Nondisclosure

Deception and nondisclosure prevent serious harm to patients. Although many families fear that a patient might lose hope, refuse medically beneficial treatment, or become depressed after learning a serious diagnosis, this is rarely the case (4). Although sadness and anxiety might occur, major depression or suicide attempts are rare. Some patients, however, have active major depression or previously attempted suicide. In such cases, it would be justified to withhold the diagnosis while obtaining psychiatric consultation and assessing the likelihood of harm. In exceptional cases, the risk of harm might be so serious as to justify withholding the diagnosis until the patient's mental health improves. Another common example occurs in organ transplantation. A potential living donor may not want to donate but fears criticism or rejection from relatives. The donor evaluation team may say that he is not a suitable donor without specifying the reason.

Deception is culturally appropriate. In many cultures, patients traditionally are not told they have cancer or other serious illness. In one study, although 87% of European American patients and 89% of African American patients wanted to be told if they have cancer, only 65% of Mexican Americans and 47% of Korean Americans wanted to be told (5). Some cultures believe disclosure of a grave diagnosis causes patients to suffer, while withholding information gives serenity, security, and hope (6). Being direct and explicit might be considered insensitive and cruel. Families and physicians might try to protect the patient by taking on decision-making responsibility (7, 8). However, the crucial ethical issue is whether the individual patient wants to know the diagnosis, not what most people in their culture would want.

Deception may enhance patient autonomy. Some patients might not want to know their diagnoses. It would be autocratic to force them to receive information against their will, even in the name of promoting informed decisions.

Reasons Against Deception and Nondisclosure

Most patients want to know their diagnosis.   The vast majority of patients in the United States want to know if they have a serious diagnosis. In one survey, 94% of those asked said that they "would want to know everything" about their medical condition, "even if it is unfavorable" (9). Ninety-six percent wanted to know a diagnosis of cancer. In a recent study, 87% of relatives of patients on mechanical ventilation for 3 to 5 days wanted doctors to discuss prognosis, even if it was uncertain (10). The desire to be told a serious diagnosis is so strong in the United States that the majority of patients want radiologists to tell them of abnormal results at the time of the imaging study rather than waiting for their primary physician to do so (11, 12). Even among patients from cultures in which nondisclosure is traditional, many want to be informed of their diagnosis (5).

Patients need information for decisions.   For patients to make informed decisions, physicians need to disclose pertinent information (*see* Chapter 3). Under the doctrine of informed consent, doctors are expected to disclose such information without patients having to ask for it.

Disclosure has more beneficial than harmful consequences.   Disclosure of the diagnosis and prognosis can benefit patients. Patients are more likely to adhere to treatment if they understand the rationale. Many patients with a serious diagnosis already suspect it. Silence might lead them to imagine that the situation is worse than it actually is. Patients often feel relieved when their illnesses are diagnosed and they can focus on treatment options.

Deception and nondisclosure require more deception.   Deception and nondisclosure usually require additional, more elaborate deceptions. If a patient is not told the diagnosis of cancer, deception is needed to explain the reasons for surgery or other treatments.

Deception and nondisclosure might be impossible.   In the long run, it is unrealistic to keep patients from knowing their diagnoses. A nurse, house officer, or x-ray technician might disclose it. When patients belatedly find out their diagnoses, they generally feel angry and betrayed. Thus, the practical issue is not whether to tell the patient the diagnosis, but rather how to tell.

DECEIVING A PATIENT TO ADMINISTER NEEDED MEDICATIONS

The following case illustrates deception in the administration of medications (13).

CASE 6.2	Covert administration of medications

Mr. E, a 32-year-old man with bipolar disorder, discontinued his medications and developed mania. He formed a specific plan to murder his father and kill himself. Mr. E's sister persuaded him to come to the emergency department (ED), but he would not let anyone touch him or examine him and refused medications and admission. She said that previous violent confrontations with ED staff during periods of mania had caused physical and psychological injury. Mr. E's sister agreed to injecting haloperidol and lorazepam into a sealed juice container and gave him the juice. These events were documented in the medical record. Mr. E accepted the drink, and 45 minutes later was calm and cooperative and agreed to psychiatric hospitalization.

In Case 6.2, using deception to administer medications averted a risk of serious harm to a patient who lacks decision-making capacity, as well as to his father. Covert administration of medications in food is also common in the care of patients with dementia, who commonly refuse medications (13). Many caregivers feel they have no other alternative in patients who lack decision-making capacity to administer drugs to treat serious medical problems, such as diabetes or infection. There are reasons for and against such deception, in addition to the reasons previously discussed.

Additional Reasons in Favor of Deception

There are no less problematic alternatives to prevent serious harm. Covert administration of medications may be the least bad of a set of poor alternatives. In Case 6.2, other options, such as physical restraints or parenteral administration of medications over the patient's objections, are also ethically problematic because they violate the patient's autonomy and bodily integrity, seem inhumane, and might injure the patient and staff. The strongest case for deception is as a last resort, after attempts to persuade the patient to accept beneficial care have failed.

The medication would restore the patient's autonomy. In Case 6.2, untreated mania rendered Mr. E incapable of making an informed decision. Thus, although the deception violates his autonomy, its purpose is to restore his autonomy.

The patient's surrogate authorizes deception. Mr. E's sister agreed to the deception and to administer the medications that he needed. In trying to bring him to care, she acted in his best interests. As the surrogate of a patient who lacks decision-making capacity, she judges that it is better for him to receive needed care through deception than to remain in untreated mania.

Additional Reasons Against Deception

Slippery slopes. If allowed in one case, deception may become more widely used in other cases where the level of impairment is not as serious, when persuasion has not been vigorously attempted, or when adequate staffing and facilities are not available.

Long-term and indirect consequences. Abuses might occur if the practice of deception becomes widespread in the treatment of patients in psychiatric crisis or with dementia. Health care workers may not take time and effort to work with distressed patients (13).

RESOLVING DILEMMAS ABOUT MISREPRESENTATION AND NONDISCLOSURE TO PATIENTS

Physicians often can respond to dilemmas about informing patients of serious diagnoses without resorting to misrepresentation or nondisclosure (Table 6-1).

Anticipate Dilemmas Regarding Deception and Nondisclosure

Dilemmas regarding deception and nondisclosure can often be anticipated. When ordering a cancer test, physicians can ascertain whether the patient wishes to be informed of the results: "Many patients want to know their test results, while other patients want the doctor to tell a family member. I will do whatever you prefer. What do you want me to do?" After the physician has received the test results, inquiring about the patient's preferences for disclosure might reveal the diagnosis. Simply asking the question suggests that the results are abnormal because there is no reason to withhold normal results from the patient.

TABLE 6-1 Resolving Dilemmas About Deception and Nondisclosure to Patients
Anticipate dilemmas about disclosure.
Determine what the patient wants.
Elicit the family's concerns.
Focus on how to tell the diagnosis, not whether to tell.
If you are withholding information, then plan for future contingencies.

In bipolar disorder or schizophrenia, relapses and refusal of treatment while mentally incapacitated are common. Patients in remission can be asked whether they prefer covert administration or physical restraint if they need to be given medications to prevent grave harm.

Respect the Patient's Preferences

When a family requests that a patient not be told of a serious diagnosis, the physician should assess whether this is the patient's wish or the family's. Convincing evidence that the patient himself would not want to be told should be respected.

Address Concerns that Prompted the Request for Deception or Nondisclosure

The physician can often address these concerns without resorting to deception or nondisclosure.

Maintain Transparency and Accountability

Any decision to use deception or nondisclosure and its rationale should be documented in the medical record. Such documentation fosters accountability because the physician must explain her reasoning and others can review it.

Minimize the Amount of Deception and Its Adverse Consequences

If Ms. Z asks the physician directly what the test showed, there are strong arguments for responding forthrightly. The question indicates that the patient wants some information. Furthermore, patients realize that an evasive response is bad news, because physicians do not hesitate to tell patients normal results.

Long-term nondisclosure of cancer generally is not feasible. Physicians should not promise family members that the patient will not learn a serious diagnosis. Surgeons may decline to operate unless a competent patient gives informed consent. A nurse, an x-ray technician, or an clinic scheduler might inadvertently disclose the diagnosis. It is usually counterproductive to devise elaborate schemes to try to keep patients from knowing the diagnosis instead of helping them cope with the bad news.

CASE 6.1   Continued

The physician can elicit the family's concerns by asking, "What do you fear most about telling your mother she has cancer?" Also the physician can validate the family's feelings as the natural reactions of loving relatives and explain how bad news usually can be disclosed in supportive ways that help patients cope. Physicians should soften bad news by being compassionate, responding to the patient's concerns, offering empathy, and helping mobilize support (14, 15). Often the physician can persuade relatives that the patient should be told of the diagnosis.

If Ms. Z chooses not to know her diagnosis, the physician should leave open the possibility that she might change her mind. Physicians should regularly ask patients if they have questions or want to discuss anything else about their condition.

CASE 6.2   Continued

Mr. E's surrogate gave permission to use deception. Furthermore, if Mr. E had indicated previously that he would prefer covert medication over forced parenteral administration in this situation, ethical concerns about deception would also be resolved.

The physician should debrief the patient after he recovers from his psychiatric crisis and address the issue of trust explicitly. Such disclosure shows respect for the patient and offers an opportunity to plan for similar situations in the future.

DECEPTION OR NONDISCLOSURE TO THIRD PARTIES

Patients who seek benefits, such as insurance coverage, disability, and excused absences from work, often need physicians to give information about their condition to third parties (16). Physicians might consider using deception to help them gain such benefits. Although such deception might be motivated by a desire to help the patient, it is ethically problematic. Throughout this section, it is assumed that the patient has authorized disclosure to the third party.

REASONS SUPPORTING DECEPTION

Physicians might claim they are acting in the best interest of patients when using deception. In doing so, physicians might regard themselves as patient advocates, helping their patients gain medical and social benefits.

CASE 6.3	Insurance coverage

Mr. M, a 42-year-old accountant, presents with a 2-month history of lower back pain that has not responded to conservative therapy with rest, nonsteroidal anti-inflammatory agents, and exercises. There are no neurologic symptoms, and the physical examination is normal. His father had prostate cancer that presented as back pain, and he is concerned that he might have a serious disease causing his symptoms. Mr. M requests a magnetic resonance imaging (MRI).

Mr. M and his physician agree that an MRI scan would reassure him. His health insurance policy requires preauthorization for MRI studies, which are usually authorized only if there are neurologic findings or other findings suggesting a systemic disease. The physician considers putting on the requisition that Mr. M has numbness and weakness in his legs to obtain insurance authorization for the study, as diagnostic yield of imaging without neurologic symptoms is low.

In one survey, 39% of physicians reported that during the past year they had exaggerated the severity of a patient's condition, changed a patient's billing diagnosis, or reported signs and symptoms the patient did not have to help the patient get needed care (14). Such deception is more common if physicians believe that the care is necessary, the appeals process is burdensome, and the patient's condition is more serious (15). The physician might regard his actions as redressing a wrong rather than breaking an ethical guideline. Some doctors might state that the patient has numbness and tingling in his legs and rationalize it as literally true because most people have such symptoms at some time in their lives.

CASE 6.3	*Continued*

Mr. M's physician needs to consider other tests, such as plain films of the spine, which would reveal metastases and a PSA to rule out prostate cancer. The doctor needs to discuss the possibility of incidental findings and false positive results that will require additional tests and risks. Even if the benefits of deception for Mr. M seem to outweigh the harms, there are consequences for the doctor–patient relationship generally that need to be considered. Insurers consider such deception to be fraud and might bring legal charges (15).

In other situations, the harms of deception might seem very small, as in the following case.

CASE 6.4	Excuse from work

A patient asks a physician to sign a form excusing an absence from work. He says that he had a severe upper respiratory infection, from which he has now recovered. The physician did not see the patient while he was ill.

In Case 6.4, the physician might sign the form, even though the physician does not know whether the patient was actually sick. The doctor might consider the harm—inappropriate absenteeism—minor and better handled directly by the employer (17). It makes little sense for patients to visit physicians for all self-limited illnesses that keep them from work. Even if the worker was not sick, perhaps he had a good reason to stay home—to care for a sick child, for example. For these reasons, physicians commonly certify work absences even when they have not examined the patient during the illness.

REASONS NOT TO DECEIVE

Deception Undermines Trust in Physicians

Physicians dealing with a specific case might not appreciate the impact of a practice of deception in these situations. Lying and deception undermine social trust because people cannot trust that other statements are truthful. It is especially problematic for physicians to lie or intentionally deceive others because their relationship with patients and society depends on trust. If physicians are known to use deception in some situations to help patients, they might also use it in other situations for other purposes.

Third parties expect truthful information. Physicians have an obligation to avoid misrepresentation to patients because of the fiduciary nature of the doctor–patient relationship (*see* Chapter 4). Physicians should also avoid deceiving third parties, but for different reasons. The relationship between physicians and third parties is contractual rather than fiduciary. In contracts, both parties are required to avoid deception and deal fairly (18). Insurers commonly require physicians to affirm that the information provided is accurate and complete.

It is unrealistic to expect that such deception to third parties will not be discovered. Computers help insurers to identify questionable claims. Similarly, other physicians review applications for disability from Social Security and worker's physicians. Once misled, third parties will mistrust other information from physicians and might require additional documentation. Physicians, who already complain of bureaucratic intrusions on the practice of medicine, might then face additional paperwork.

The Harms of Deception Outweigh the Benefits

When indirect and long-term harms are taken into account, the overall harms of deception outweigh the benefits (19). Deception about a patient's condition indirectly harms other people. Giving disability parking permits to those who do not need them makes it more difficult for persons who are truly disabled to park. Deceptive claims for disability or insurance coverage force the others patients, employers, or the public to pay higher taxes or insurance premiums.

RESOLVING DILEMMAS ABOUT DECEPTION TO THIRD PARTIES

The following suggestions might help physicians deal with patients' requests to use deception to gain benefits (Table 6-2).

TABLE 6-2   Resolving Dilemmas About Deception to Third Parties
Consider whether an important health benefit is at stake.
Deception might not be necessary.
Exhaust other alternatives.
Involve patients who request deception.

Consider Whether an Important Health Benefit Is at Stake

Physicians need to ask in what sense they are helping the patient. In some cases, health care is not the issue.

CASE 6.5   Cancellation of travel plans

A healthy patient who has bought a vacation tour wishes to change his plans. He asks his physician to write a note saying that he is ill so he can obtain a refund.

In Case 6.5, the patient simply wants to break a business deal with the travel agency and avoid a financial penalty. Although physicians have a duty to provide beneficial medical care, they have no obligation to help patients gain financial advantages.

In other cases, physicians might want to help patients receive disability payments to obtain food, clothing, and shelter. Such necessities are essential for good health. Physicians have an obligation to provide truthful information that will help patients get social benefits to which they are entitled, but it is not at all clear that physicians should use deception to help certain patients get social benefits for which they do not qualify. Even if physicians believe that the current social system is unjust, deception in selective cases seems an inadequate way to address this unfairness.

Deception Might Not Be Necessary

The literal truth might resolve the dilemma. The strategy of using the literal truth is unethical if it is intended to deceive. However, employing the literal truth is appropriate if it is not deceptive and prevents harm to the patient (15). In Case 6.4, the physician was asked to certify an absence from work without having examined the patient during the illness. Some physicians simply write, "The patient reports that he was sick and unable to work" (17). This statement, which is true, shifts the dilemma back onto the patient and employer rather than having the physician take responsibility for secondhand information (16). Furthermore, this strategy obviates physician visits simply to obtain work excuses. The physician should also explain to the patient the substance of his note and the reasons for it.

Exhaust Other Alternatives

Physicians can often benefit patients without using deception. In Case 6.3, the physician has other options for reassuring the patient, as discussed below. Pursuing these alternatives requires the physician's effort, but exhausting them gives physicians a stronger ethical justification for using deception as a last resort.

Involve Patients Who Request Deception

Physicians often believe that they alone must decide how to respond to requests for deception. In fact, patients who make such requests have ethical responsibilities as well. If patients ask physicians to use deception on a disability application or an insurance bill, then physicians can frankly say that they feel caught between two ethical duties—to help the patient and to be truthful. Physicians can reflect the dilemma back to patients, saying, "If I mislead your insurer, how would my patients trust me not to mislead them in other situations?" Furthermore, the physician can point out the problems that will occur later if the insurer requests additional documentation.

DECEPTION WITH COLLEAGUES

Trainees sometimes use deception with colleagues. In one study, 19% of residents reported that they would fabricate a test result they had not checked if they were likely to be "ridiculed and reprimanded" for not checking it (20). In another scenario, 8% of residents said they would lie about checking for occult blood in a patient with anemia who had suffered a myocardial infarction. Furthermore, more than 40% of respondents reported that they had witnessed another resident lying to an attending physician or another resident during the past year (20).

Deception with other physicians is ethically troubling for several reasons. If a physician tells other physicians that a test result is normal, without actually checking the results, the patient might be harmed. If the result was actually abnormal, then needed treatment might be delayed or omitted. In addition, if physicians need to trust information from colleagues, they may feel they need to duplicate that doctor's work, which would waste effort and cause resentment.

As discussed in more detail in Chapter 36, it is understandable that trainees want to have a good reputation. Using deception to bolster one's reputation, however, cannot be condoned.

SUMMARY

1. There are strong ethical reasons for physicians to avoid deception and nondisclosure with patients.
2. Physicians should try to avoid deception about the patient's condition to third parties who have a right to such information.

REFERENCES

1. Sokol DK. Can deceiving patients be morally acceptable? *BMJ.* 2007;334:984–986.
2. Bok S. *Secrets: On Ethics of Concealment and Revelation.* New York, NY: Pantheon Books; 1982.
3. Novack DH, Plumer R, Smith RL, et al. Changes in physicians' attitudes toward telling the cancer patient. *JAMA.* 1979;241:897–900.
4. Appelbaum PS, Roth LH. Patients who refuse treatment in medical hospitals. *JAMA.* 1983;250:1296–1301.
5. Blackhall LJ, Murphy ST, Frank G, et al. Ethnicity and attitudes toward patient autonomy. *JAMA.* 1995;274:820–825.
6. Gordon DB, Paci E. Disclosure practices and cultural narratives: understanding concealment and silence around cancer in Tuscany, Italy. *Soc Sci Med.* 1997;46:1433–1452.
7. Surbone A. Truth telling to the patient. *JAMA.* 1992;268:1661–1662.
8. Surbone A. Telling the truth to patients with cancer: what is the truth? *Lancet Oncol.* 2006;7:944–950.
9. President's Commission for the Study of Ethical Problems in Medicine and Biomedical and Behavioral Research. *Making Health Care Decisions.* Washington, DC: U.S. Government Printing Office; 1982.
10. Evans LR, Boyd EA, Malvar G, et al. Surrogate decision-makers' perspectives on discussing prognosis in the face of uncertainty. *Am J Respir Crit Care Med.* 2009;179:48–53.
11. Raza S, Rosen MP, Chorny K, et al. Patient expectations and costs of immediate reporting of screening mammography: talk isn't cheap. *AJR Am J Roentgenol.* 2001;177:579–583.
12. Schreiber MH, Leonard M Jr, Rieniets CY. Disclosure of imaging findings to patients directly by radiologists: survey of patients' preferences. *AJR Am J Roentgenol.* 1995;165:467–469.
13. Treloar A, Philpot M, Beats B. Concealing medication in patients' food. *Lancet.* 2001;357:62–64.
14. Wynia MK, Cummins DS, VanGeest JB, et al. Physician manipulation of reimbursement rules for patients: between a rock and a hard place. *JAMA.* 2000;283:1858–1865.
15. Everett JP, Walters CA, Stottlmyer DL, et al. To lie or not to lie: resident physician attitudes about the use of deception in clinical practice. *J Med Ethics.* 2011;37:333–338.
16. Toon PD. Practice Pointer. "I need a note, doctor": dealing with requests for medical reports about patients. *BMJ.* 2009;338:b175.
17. Holleman WL, Holleman MC. School and work release evalutions. *JAMA.* 1988;260:3629–3634.
18. Farnsworth EA. *Contracts.* 2nd ed. Boston, MA: Little, Brown and Company; 1990:249–272.
19. Bok S. *Lying: Moral Choices in Public and Private Life.* New York, NY: Pantheon Books; 1978.
20. Green MJ, Farber NJ, Ubel PA, et al. Lying to each other: when internal medicine residents use deception with their colleagues. *Arch Intern Med.* 2000;160:2317–2323.

ANNOTATED BIBLIOGRAPHY

1. Everett JP, Walters CA, Stottlmyer DL, et al. To lie or not to lie: resident physician attitudes about the use of deception in clinical practice. *J Med Ethics.* 2011;37:333–338.
   Comprehensive discussion of different types of lies that doctors make.

2. Surbone A. Telling the truth to patients with cancer: What is the truth? *Lancet Oncol.* 2006;7:944–950.
   Points out that in most other cultures it is customary for families and physicians to shield patients from disturbing information about their diagnosis or prognosis.
3. Sokol DK. Can deceiving patients be morally acceptable? *BMJ.* 2007;334:984–986.
   Analysis of deception in clinical medicine.
4. Ross LF. What the medical excuse teaches us about the potential living donor as patient. *Am J Transplant.* 2010;10:731–736.
   Thoughtful analysis of providing true but misleading information to third parties, in the context of persons who do not want their family to know they do not wish to donate.

7

Keeping Promises

Keeping promises reduces uncertainty and promotes trust. Physicians, like all people, make promises and are sometimes tempted to break them. Although promises are regarded as binding, in retrospect, some promises might seem imprudent or mistaken. The following cases demonstrate that some promises can be kept only if important ethical guidelines are violated.

CASE 7.1 **Promise not to tell the patient that she has cancer**

Mrs. G, a 61-year-old Mexican American widow, is found to have cancer on a needle aspiration of a breast mass. Her primary care physicians agrees to a request from her daughter and son to tell her she has cancer because they fear that she would not be able to handle the bad news. They point out that it is not customary in Mexico to tell women of her age that they have cancer. After breast cancer is diagnosed, the physician refers Mrs. G to a surgeon. The surgeon believes that patients need to be involved in decisions regarding mastectomy or lumpectomy. In addition, Mrs. G asks a Spanish-speaking nurse, "Why do I need surgery? Do I have cancer?" The nurse does not want to deceive a patient who asks a direct question. The surgeon and nurse feel constrained by the primary physician's promise not to tell Mrs. G her diagnosis.

Case 7.1 illustrates that in some situations, keeping promises might be problematic. The surgeon and nurse believe that the primary physician's promise not to tell Mrs. G her diagnosis fails to respect her as a person. They question why they should violate their sense of moral integrity to keep someone else's promise.

CASE 7.2 **Promise to schedule tests**

Mr. H, a 54-year-old heavy smoker, is hospitalized for hemoptysis, weight loss, and angina pectoris. A chest x-ray shows a 2-cm proximal lung mass, with hilar adenopathy. A bronchoscopy is scheduled to obtain a biopsy. When the intern walks by his room, the patient shouts, "This is outrageous. I haven't had breakfast, I haven't had lunch. Now they say they don't know when the test will be done and that I might have to go through all this again tomorrow. If this is how the hospital is run, I'm leaving." The intern, eager to appease the patient and continue with his other work, promises the patient that the test will be done that afternoon. He tells the nurse to call the bronchoscopy suite to say that the procedure needs to be done that afternoon.

In Case 7.2, the intern makes a promise so Mr. H will cooperate with getting a needed test. However, the bronchoscopy schedule is not under his control. Even though the intern's motive is beneficent—to help the patient receive needed medical care—the means of achieving his goal is ethically problematic.

THE ETHICAL SIGNIFICANCE OF PROMISES

A promise is a commitment to act a certain way in the future, either to do something or to refrain from doing something. Promises generate expectations in others, who, in turn, modify their plans and actions on the assumption that promises will be kept (1). In everyday social interactions, people expect others to keep the ones they make. Promises might be exchanged for other promises, as in a business contract. For example, a merchant might promise to deliver goods in exchange for the promise of payment on delivery.

Keeping promises is desirable for several reasons. It results in beneficial consequences by making the future more predictable, relieving anxiety, and promoting trust. Indeed, the dictionary definition of "promise" is "that which causes hope, expectation, or assurance." Keeping promises is also important even if there are no short-term beneficial consequences. Promise-keeping is essential for harmonious social interactions. If promises are commonly broken, then people would be unwilling to rely on others to keep commitments.

Breaking promises may cause significant harm. The person to whom the promise was made may suffer a setback, such as inconvenience and monetary losses. It seems unfair to allow people to break promises that others have relied on (2). The very concept of promises is negated if people break them and gain an advantage but expect others to honor promises (2).

Promise-keeping is especially important for physicians. Because the doctor–patient relationship is based on trust, patients might feel betrayed if physicians break promises. Once betrayed, patients might be less likely to trust the individual physician or the medical profession. Promises by physicians might help patients cope with the uncertainty and fears inherent in being sick. In addition, promises establish mutual expectations that benefit both physicians and patients. For example, physicians promise confidentiality of medical information; in return, patients are more candid about discussing sensitive issues pertaining to their health. Thus, promises enhance the patient's well-being and facilitate the physician's work.

PROBLEMS WITH KEEPING PROMISES

None of us wants to keep all the promises we make. Some promises are made on the spur of the moment, under emotional stress, with inadequate information, or without proper deliberation (2). Foolish promises that put one at a great disadvantage are often retracted, particularly if they confer a gratuitous boon on the other person. People might excuse breaking such promises if the other person has taken no action in reliance on the promise and is no worse off than if the promise had never been made.

Clinical dilemmas occur when keeping promises would require actions that violate other ethical guidelines. In Case 7.1, the surgeon and nurse believe the initial promise not to tell the patient violates the guideline of respect for persons.

SUGGESTIONS FOR PHYSICIANS

DO NOT MAKE PROMISES LIGHTLY

A statement that the physician regards as kindly reassurance might be interpreted by the patient or family as a promise. Even if the physician does not think a promise is important, the patient may. Patients typically are more upset when physicians break promises than the physicians are.

ADDRESS THE CONCERNS UNDERLYING THE REQUEST FOR A PROMISE

If someone asks the physician to make an unrealistic promise, then the physician can elicit the underlying concerns and try to address them in other ways.

DO NOT PROMISE OUTCOMES THAT ARE OUT OF YOUR CONTROL

Physicians should not make promises that are beyond their power to keep. Given the complex organization of modern medicine, it is misleading to make promises about other physicians and nurses, who are autonomous agents with their own moral and professional values.

Because clinical outcomes are inherently uncertain, it is unrealistic to make a promise that guarantees a good outcome or the absence of complications after a procedure.

DO NOT VIOLATE ETHICAL GUIDELINES BECAUSE OF AN ILL-CONSIDERED PROMISE

Although promise-keeping is important, it is not an absolute duty. Other ethical guidelines are also important and might take priority in some situations. In some cases, breaking the promise might be the lesser of two evils. The strongest case for overriding the promise-keeping occurs when the following conditions are met:

- Keeping the promise would violate another important ethical guideline. In Case 7.1, keeping the promise would require deception by the physician and, thereby, compromise the patient's autonomy.
- The countervailing ethical considerations were not taken into account when the promise was made.
- The clinical and ethical situation has changed significantly since the promise was made.
- Someone else made the promise. Although a person's promise can bind his own future actions, it need not bind others.
- The promise was stated implicitly rather than explicitly.

CASE 7.1	*Continued*

When Mrs. G's children asked that she not be told she has cancer, the primary care physician should elicit the concerns underlying their request. The doctor should anticipate future problems if she is not told, including the possibilities that other health care workers may decide to disclose the diagnosis or the patient may ask someone directly what her diagnosis is. Another health care worker, like the surgeon in this case, may decide that she cannot provide care without offering to discuss Mrs. G's diagnosis with her. In her view, avoiding deception should prevail over keeping a promise made by a third party. Similarly, when asked by the patient if she has cancer, it would be disrespectful to deceive her rather than giving a direct and compassionate answer.

CASE 7.2	*Continued*

Physicians should not make promises about situations they cannot control. In the short run, it might seem easier to promise that the test will be done rather than to have the patient complain. However, making a promise that may not be kept will cause more problems in the long run. It might be better simply to listen and acknowledge that the patient has every right to be angry. Realistically, the doctor can promise to look into the matter and to do his best to get the procedure done as soon as possible, for instance, phoning the pulmonary consultant.

In summary, promises can allay patients' fears and uncertainty. It is important to keep promises because other people rely on them. Breaking promises undermines trust in the individual physician and in the medical profession, yet keeping promises is not an absolute ethical duty. Sometimes, respecting a promise might require the physician to violate other important ethical guidelines. In exceptional situations, breaking a promise might be justified as the lesser of two evils.

SUMMARY

1. Physicians should keep promises because other people rely on them.
2. In exceptional circumstances, breaking a promise might be justified as the lesser of two evils.

REFERENCES

1. Farnsworth EA. *Contracts*. 2nd ed. Boston, MA: Little, Brown and Company; 1990:39–110.
2. Fuller LL, Eisenberg MA. *Basic Contract Law*. 4th ed. St. Paul, MN: West Publishing Co.; 1981:1–8.

Shared Decision Making

An Approach to Decisions About Clinical Interventions

Medical interventions might allow accurate diagnosis and effective treatment, but they might also be applied when their benefit is questionable or when patients would not want them. Physicians, therefore, must try to avoid two types of errors: withholding potentially beneficial tests and therapies that the patient would want and imposing interventions that are not beneficial or not wanted.

This brief chapter presents an approach to decisions about clinical interventions. The general approach to ethical issues in Chapter 1 can be adapted to such decisions (Fig. 8-1). The key questions are as follows.

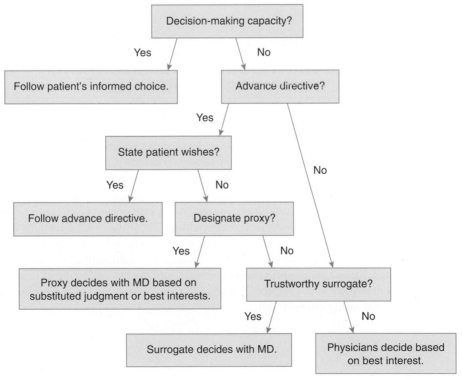

FIGURE 8-1. Flowchart for clinical decisions.

IS THE INTERVENTION FUTILE IN A STRICT SENSE?

Sound ethical judgments require accurate medical information. Physicians are under no obligation to provide interventions that are futile in a strict sense (*see* Chapter 9).

DOES THE PATIENT HAVE ADEQUATE DECISION-MAKING CAPACITY?

This is a crucial branch point in decision making. Chapter 10 discusses how to determine whether a patient lacks decision-making capacity.

IF THE PATIENT IS COMPETENT, THEN WHAT IS THE PATIENT'S INFORMED DECISION?

Competent, informed patients may refuse medical interventions (*see* Chapter 11). Patients frequently lack decision-making capacity when decisions about medical interventions must be made. If the patient lacks decision-making capacity, then two additional questions need to be posed.

IF THE PATIENT IS NOT COMPETENT, THEN HAS HE OR SHE GIVEN ADVANCE DIRECTIVES?

Clear and convincing advance directives should be respected (*see* Chapter 12). In the absence of such advance directives, decisions should be based on what the patient would want or what is in his or her best interests (*see* Chapter 12).

IF THE PATIENT HAS NOT CLEARLY INDICATED WHAT HE OR SHE WOULD WANT DONE IN THE SITUATION, THEN WHO SHOULD SERVE AS SURROGATE?

Generally, the surrogate should be a person designated by the patient or a close family member (*see* Chapter 13).

This book then considers disagreements between doctors and patients over medical interventions. Chapter 14 analyzes insistence by patients or surrogates on interventions that physicians regard as inappropriate. Chapter 15 discusses conclusions about life-sustaining interventions that are commonly drawn but that prove misleading on closer analysis. Chapter 16 discusses how ethics committees or ethics consultants can help physicians resolve ethical dilemmas.

Next, this book analyzes life-sustaining interventions in specific situations. Chapter 17 discusses Do Not Resuscitate (DNR) orders. Often, discussions about DNR orders are the first step in a comprehensive evaluation of the goals and plans for care. Chapters 18 through 21 discuss physician-assisted suicide, tube feedings, the persistent vegetative state, and the determination of death.

Legal issues are then presented. Chapter 22 analyzes landmark legal cases that have dramatized dilemmas about life-sustaining interventions.

9

Futile Interventions

P atients or surrogates sometimes request medical interventions that physicians consider irrational or pointless. The concept of futility seems an appealing way to resolve such disagreements. The term *futility* comes from a Latin word meaning "leaky" (1). In classical mythology, the gods condemned the daughters of Danaus to carry water in leaky buckets. No matter how hard they tried, they could never achieve their goal of transporting water. By analogy, futile medical interventions would serve no meaningful purpose, no matter how often they are repeated.

Physicians might claim that judgment of futility is a matter of professional expertise and that they may decide unilaterally to forego futile interventions rather than share decision making with patients or surrogates. Because the term futility gives decision-making power to physicians, however, it must be used with caution. The term is fraught with confusion, inconsistency, and controversy.

STRICT DEFINITIONS OF FUTILITY

Physicians use the term in different ways (2–4). In three strictly defined senses, medical futility justifies unilateral decisions by physicians to withhold or withdraw interventions (Table 9-1).

INTERVENTION HAS NO PATHOPHYSIOLOGIC RATIONALE

CASE 9.1	Antibiotics not active against organism

A 74-year-old woman has progressive septic shock with methicillin-resistant Staphylococcus aureus *(MRSA) infection despite treatment with appropriate antibiotics, fluids, and vasopressors. The patient's family requests an antibiotic that they learned about on the Internet. The patient's organism is resistant to this antibiotic.*

In this case, there is no pathophysiologic rationale for the antibiotic because the organisms causing this patient's illness are resistant. No clinical or physiologic benefit can be expected. Even if the family insists on the drug, there is no medical reason to administer it.

TABLE 9-1	When Is an Intervention Futile in a Strict Sense?

Intervention has no pathophysiologic rationale.

Cardiac arrest occurs after refractory progressive hypotension or hypoxemia.

The intervention has already failed in the patient.

CARDIAC ARREST OCCURS AFTER PROGRESSIVE REFRACTORY HYPOTENSION OR HYPOXEMIA

CASE 9.2	Progressive multiorgan failure

The patient in Case 9.1 is now comatose, on renal dialysis, and on a ventilator. Despite fluid replacement and increasing doses of vasopressors, her mean arterial pressure is below 60 mm Hg. Her physicians want to write an order not to resuscitate her in case of a cardiopulmonary arrest.

In Case 9.2, cardiopulmonary arrest occurs because of progressive hypotension despite maximal support of the patient's circulation and oxygenation. Effective circulation cannot be sustained in this patient despite all appropriate therapy. If her refractory hypotension progresses to cardiopulmonary arrest, cardiopulmonary resuscitation (CPR) could not restore effective circulation. Similarly, CPR would be ineffective if cardiac arrest occurs after progressive hypotexia that is refractory to treatment.

INTERVENTION HAS ALREADY FAILED IN THE PATIENT

CASE 9.3	No response to CPR

A 54-year-old man suffers a cardiac arrest in the emergency room. CPR and advanced cardiac support are initiated promptly. The initial rhythm is asystole. After 30 minutes, there has not been any return of spontaneous cardiac rhythm or circulation. All measures recommended in the American Heart Association guidelines have been attempted. His family insists that resuscitation be continued.

An adequate clinical attempt of CPR has failed to achieve the fundamental goal of restoring effective circulation and breathing. It is pointless to continue or repeat interventions that have already failed.

These three strict senses of "futility" are as plain as the root metaphor of carrying water in leaky buckets. Such interventions will not achieve the goals set by the patient, and all physicians would agree that the interventions are useless. The determination that an intervention is futile in these strict senses is based on objective data or judgments within the expertise of physicians. Physicians have no ethical duty to provide interventions that are futile in these strict senses; indeed, they generally have an ethical obligation *not* to provide them.

LOOSE DEFINITIONS OF FUTILITY

The term futility is also used in several looser senses that are confusing, involve contested value judgments, and do not justify unilateral decisions by physicians to withhold interventions (3, 5, 6). The phrase "not medically indicated" commonly is used in similar ways.

CASE 9.4	Recurrent aspiration pneumonia and severe dementia

A 74-year-old man with severe dementia is hospitalized for the third time in 6 months for aspiration pneumonia. At baseline, he sometimes recognizes his daughter and smiles when watching television or listening to music. The daughter, his only surviving relative, insists that he be treated with antibiotics. The resident exclaims, "Treating him is futile! His dementia is not going to improve, and it's inhumane to keep alive someone with such a poor quality of life." The resident also argues that a Do Not Attempt Resuscitation (DNAR) order should be written on the basis of futility because CPR is so unlikely to succeed.

THE LIKELIHOOD OF SUCCESS IS VERY SMALL

Some physicians contend that an intervention should be considered futile if the likelihood of success in a given situation is extremely small—for example, no success in the last 100 attempts or less than a 1% chance of success (7). There are problems, however, in setting a quantitative, probabilistic concept of futility. Why set the threshold at 1%? Some patients or families might consider a likelihood of success of 1% worth pursuing in some circumstances. However, some physicians might desire to make unilateral decisions to forego interventions whose likelihood of success is 2% or even 5%. Indeed, physicians commonly describe interventions as futile when the likelihood of success is far greater than 1% (8, 9).

NO WORTHWHILE GOALS OF CARE CAN BE ACHIEVED

Futility can be defined only in terms of the goals of care (4). Some ethicists contend that the proper goal of medicine is not simply to correct physiologic derangements. For these writers, it is inappropriate to prolong life if the patient will not regain consciousness or leave the intensive care unit (ICU) alive (1, 7).

Individual patients or the public, however, may have sharply different views. Some people regard life as precious even if the patient will not regain consciousness. Indeed, some states have public policies that favor prolonging life in patients who will not regain consciousness (10). Thus, physicians cannot define goals of care unilaterally, but should be guided by the patient's values.

THE PATIENT'S QUALITY OF LIFE IS UNACCEPTABLE

In some situations, some physicians might declare an intervention futile because they consider the patient's quality of life unacceptable, for example, if he is in a persistent vegetative state (PVS) (1). These physicians contend that sustaining biologic life is not an appropriate goal when the patient has no likelihood of regaining consciousness or interacting with other people. However, patients generally view their quality of life more favorably than family members or physicians. Quality of life needs to be assessed according to the goals and values of the patient and cannot be determined unilaterally by physicians.

PROSPECTIVE BENEFIT IS NOT WORTH THE RESOURCES REQUIRED

An intervention might be termed futile because the expected outcomes are not considered worth the effort and resources required. Allocation of resources, however, should be decided by society as a whole, not an individual physician acting unilaterally at the bedside (*see* Chapter 30). Asserting that such interventions are futile closes off this difficult but essential debate (11).

PRACTICAL PROBLEMS WITH THE CONCEPT OF FUTILITY

Several problems occur in practice when physicians make unilateral decisions to withhold "futile" interventions.

JUDGMENTS OF FUTILITY ARE OFTEN MISTAKEN OR PROBLEMATIC

Physicians often err when they claim that an intervention has a very low probability of success. One study analyzed cases in which residents had written DNAR orders on the basis of a probabilistic definition of futility (9). In 32% of such cases, residents estimated the probability of survival after CPR to be 5% or higher. In 20% of cases, the estimated probability of survival after CPR was 10% or greater. Thus, the term futility was applied inappropriately when the probability of success was considered much greater than the 1% threshold for futility proposed in the literature. Problems also occur when determinations of futility are based on quality of life. When residents judged that CPR would be futile because of unacceptable quality of life, they discussed quality of life with only 65% of competent patients (9). It is ethically problematic for physicians to judge a competent patient's quality of life without talking to the patient because doctors underestimate the extent to which patients believe their lives are worth living (12).

UNILATERAL PHYSICIANS DECISIONS POLARIZE DISAGREEMENTS

Attempts by physicians to resolve disputes by claiming the power to act unilaterally commonly antagonize patients and surrogates. Many surrogates do not agree with physicians' judgments of prognosis. In one small study, almost two thirds of surrogates of patients in critical care units doubted the accuracy of physician's predictions of futility, and almost a third would continue life support with less than a 1% estimate of survival (13). A larger study of relatives of patients who required mechanical ventilation and had a high probability of dying illuminated why relatives might reject physician's estimates of prognosis. Less than 2% of surrogates based that their beliefs about the patients' prognoses exclusively on prognostic information from physicians. Other additional factors included the patient's character and will to live, the patient's history of illness and survival, the surrogate's observations of the patient's appearance, and the surrogate's optimism, intuition, and faith (14). Furthermore, declaring one intervention futile might not settle other important issues in a case. For instance, a unilateral decision by physicians to withhold CPR in Case 9.2 might worsen disagreements about other interventions, such as mechanical ventilation, vasopressor support, and antibiotics for infection.

PHYSICIANS CONFUSE FUTILITY AND BEST INTERESTS

Physicians commonly confuse futility and best interests as a basis for their decisions (4). Even if an intervention cannot be termed futile in a strict sense, physicians may recommend against it because the burdens outweigh the benefits, according to the patient's values and goals, and try to persuade the patient or surrogate that the intervention is not in the patient's best interests. Chapter 4 discusses in detail the concept of best interests.

SAFEGUARDS IF INTERVENTIONS ARE DEEMED FUTILE

Procedural safeguards ensure that physicians' unilateral decisions to withhold "futile" interventions are appropriate. Open discussions help guard against errors and abuses. In the original meaning of "futile," there is no controversy that a leaky bucket will not hold water. Similarly, it should not be difficult for a physician to persuade colleagues, the patient or surrogate that an intervention is futile in a particular case.

OBTAIN A SECOND OPINION

The physician who is considering a unilateral decision to forego a "futile" treatment should obtain a second opinion from a colleague or from the institutional ethics committee, to guard against inappropriate interpretations of futility.

DISCUSS THE INTERVENTION WITH THE PATIENT OR SURROGATE

Some physicians believe that they need not discuss futile interventions with the patient or surrogate. To be sure, in Case 9.3 a vast array of interventions would be futile in a strict sense, such as cancer chemotherapy. It would be pointless to tell patients or surrogates of interventions that are irrelevant to the illness at hand. In some cases, however, physicians might not discuss pertinent interventions because they fear that the patient or surrogate will not agree they are futile. Physicians might use the idea of unilateral decisions about futility to avoid unpleasant discussions (15). The best approach, however, is more discussion, not less.

Discussing "futile" treatments with patients or surrogates shows respect for patients and surrogates and clarifies their expectations, goals, values, concerns, and needs. It also helps physicians understand the patient-specific considerations that surrogates consider when they assess prognosis (14). Sometimes after physicians better understand the values and goals of the patient, they are more willing to continue interventions. Alternatively, after such discussions patients and families usually agree with the physicians that the interventions are highly unlikely to achieve the patient's goals or that the burdens and risks are disproportionately heavy (16). Chapter 14 gives specific suggestions for such discussions.

ESTABLISH GUIDELINES AND PROCEDURES ON FUTILITY

Hospitals should develop written guidelines about futile interventions (15, 17). Written institutional guidelines demonstrate that unilateral decisions to forego futile interventions are based on carefully considered standards, not on *ad hoc* reasoning. Several states and cities have developed futility policies and procedures (15, 17).

Texas established a nonjudicial procedure for resolving disputes when a physician regards an intervention as "not medically indicated" and the patient or family disagrees (18, 19). This is a broader category than futile interventions and similarly ambiguous. A hospital medical or ethics committee must be convened, and the patient or family must be notified and invited to the meeting. If the committee agrees that the intervention is not medically indicated but the family disagrees, the hospital must try to work with the family to find another physician or institution willing to provide the intervention. After 10 days, if a transfer of the patient cannot be arranged, the physician and hospital is legally permitted to withhold or withdraw the intervention. The patient or family, however, may ask the courts to order that the intervention be continued beyond the 10-day period if it is likely that they will find a provider willing to accept the patient.

A study of the Texas law found that in 30% of cases, the committee determined that the intervention was medically appropriate and in another 3% of cases, the patient improved. Thus in one third of cases, the physician's initial judgment of medically inappropriate was not confirmed (20). In an additional 18% of cases, the intervention continued after the 10-day period. During the 10-day waiting period, 42% of patients died, and the family agreed to discontinue the intervention in 38% of cases (20). The Texas experience also raises concerns about unfairness because a disproportionately high percentage of cases involved ethnic minorities (21, 22). The Texas experience illustrates the need for policies and procedures to review cases when physicians seek to forego life-sustaining interventions over the objections of the patient or surrogate.

SUMMARY

1. The concepts of futility and "not medically indicated" are intuitively appealing but need to be used extremely carefully.
2. When futility is strictly defined, physicians may—and indeed should—make unilateral decisions to withhold interventions.

REFERENCES

1. Schneiderman LJ, Jecker NS, Jonsen AR. Medical futility: its meaning and ethical implications. *Ann Intern Med.* 1990;112:949–954.
2. Lo B. Unanswered questions about DNR orders. *JAMA.* 1991;265:1874–1875.
3. Helft PR, Siegler M, Lantos J. The rise and fall of the futility movement. *N Engl J Med.* 2000;343:293–296.
4. Kite S, Wilkinson S. Beyond futility: to what extent is the concept of futility useful in clinical decision-making about CPR? *Lancet Oncol.* 2002;3:638–642.
5. Lantos JD, Singer PA, Walker RM, et al. The illusion of futility in clinical practice. *Am J Med.* 1989;87:81–84.
6. Truog RD, Brett AS, Frader J. The problem with futility. *N Engl J Med.* 1992;326:1560–1564.
7. Schneiderman LJ, Jecker NS, Jonsen AR. Medical futility: response to critiques. *Ann Intern Med.* 1996;125:669–674.
8. Prendergast TJ, Luce JM. Increasing incidence of withholding and withdrawal of life support from the critically ill. *Am Rev Resp Dis Crit Care Med.* 1997;155:15–20.
9. Curtis JR, Park DR, Krone MR, et al. The use of the medical futility rationale in do not attempt resuscitation orders. *JAMA.* 1995;273:124–128.
10. Cruzan v. Harmon. 760 S.W.2d 408.

11. Alpers A, Lo B. Futility: not just a medical issue. *Law Med Health Care.* 1992;20:327–329.
12. Ubel PA, Loewenstein G, Schwarz N, et al. Misimagining the unimaginable: the disability paradox and health care decision making. *Health Psychol.* 2005;24:S57–S62.
13. Zier LS, Burack JH, Micco G, et al. Surrogate decision makers' responses to physicians' predictions of medical futility. *Chest.* 2009;136:110–117.
14. Boyd EA, Lo B, Evans LR, et al. "It is not just what the doctor tells me:" factors that influence surrogate decision-makers' perceptions of prognosis. *Crit Care Med.* 2010;38:1270–1275.
15. Council on Ethical and Judicial Affairs, AMA. Medical futility in end-of-life care. *JAMA.* 1999;281:937–941.
16. Smedira NG, Evans BH, Grais LS, et al. Withholding and withdrawing of life support from the critically ill. *N Engl J Med.* 1990;322:309–315.
17. Halevy A, Brody B. A multi-institutional collaborative policy on medical futility. *JAMA.* 1996;276:571–574.
18. Fine RL, Mayo TW. Resolution of futility by due process: early experience with the Texas Advance Directives Act. *Ann Intern Med.* 2003;138:743–746.
19. Fine RL. Point: the Texas advance directives act effectively and ethically resolves disputes about medical futility. *Chest.* 2009;136:963–967.
20. Smith ML, Gremillion G, Slomka J, et al. Texas hospitals' experience with the Texas Advance Directives Act. *Crit Care Med.* 2007;35:1271–1276.
21. Truog RD. Tackling medical futility in Texas. *N Engl J Med.* 2007;357:1–3.
22. Truog RD. Counterpoint: the Texas advance directives act is ethically flawed: medical futility disputes must be resolved by a fair process. *Chest.* 2009;136:968–971; discussion 971–973.

ANNOTATED BIBLIOGRAPHY

1. Kite S, Wilkinson S. Beyond futility: to what extent is the concept of futility useful in clinical decision-making about CPR? *Lancet Oncol.* 2002;3:638–642.
   Helft PR, Siegler M, Lantos J. The rise and fall of the futility movement. *N Engl J Med.* 2000;343:293–296.
   Two articles that argue that the concept of futility has limited usefulness in clinical practice.
2. Curtis JR, Park DR, Krone MR, et al. The use of the medical futility rationale in do not attempt resuscitation orders. *JAMA.* 1995;273:124–128.
   Empirical study documenting problems and mistakes that occur when physicians claim that CPR would be futile.
3. Boyd EA, Lo B, Evans LR, et al. "It is not just what the doctor tells me:" factors that influence surrogate decision-makers perceptions of prognosis. *Crit Care Med.* 2010;38:1270–1275.
   Empirical study showing how the vast majority of surrogates take into account factors other than prognostic information from the physician.
4. Smith ML, Gremillion G, Slomka J, et al. Texas hospitals' experience with the Texas Advance Directives Act. *Crit Care Med.* 2007;35:1271–1276.
   Empirical study of a statewide futility law that refers intractable disagreements over medically inappropriate interventions to the hospital ethics or medical committee. In over one half of cases, an intervention that the physician originally judged to be inappropriate was continued.

Decision-Making Capacity

P hysicians must respect the autonomous choices of patients; however, illness or medications can impair the capacity of patients to make decisions about their health care. Such patients might be unable to make decisions, or their decisions contradict their best interests and cause them serious harm. Decision-making ability falls along a continuum, with no natural threshold for adequate decision-making capacity. Nevertheless, for every patient a binary decision needs to be made: either a patient has adequate decision-making capacity and her choices should be respected, or she does not and someone else should decide (1). The following case illustrates how it might be difficult to decide whether decision-making power should be taken away from a patient.

CASE 10.1   **Refusal to explain a decision**

Mrs. C, a 74-year-old widow with mild dementia, is admitted for congestive heart failure and angina pectoris that has progressed despite maximal medical therapy. In the past 3 years, she has suffered two myocardial infarctions. Her physician recommends coronary angiography and, if possible, angioplasty.

Mrs. C recognizes her primary care physician, but seldom knows the date or the name of the clinic. She has forgotten to come to several clinic appointments. Her mental functioning gets worse when she is hospitalized. A nephew, her only relative, pays a woman to shop, cook, and clean house for her. He reports that Mrs. C enjoys watching television, attending the senior center, and sitting in the park.

When asked about her wishes for care, Mrs. C says that she wants to go home. After many discussions, the cardiology team convinces her to have the angiogram. On the morning of the procedure, however, she changes her mind, saying that she doesn't want anyone to put a tube into her heart and that she has been in the hospital long enough. Her nephew believes that angioplasty would be best for her, but is reluctant to contradict her wishes because she has always been independent and stubborn. Mrs. C is generally adverse to medical interventions. She refused mammography, even though she has a family history of breast cancer. She also refused treatment for a cholesterol level of 318 mg per dL.

The team asks a psychiatrist to see her. On a mental status examination, she does not know the date, the name of the hospital, or the city. She recalls only one of three objects and cannot perform serial subtraction. She refuses to talk further with the psychiatrist, saying that she is not crazy.

In this case, Mrs. C's mental functioning is obviously impaired. Is it so impaired that her nephew should assume the authority to make medical decisions for her? Her refusal did not seem so unreasonable to some physicians and nurses. Furthermore, some nurses asked why her consent to angiography was not questioned, but only her refusal (2).

This chapter analyzes how physicians should assess whether patients like Mrs. C have the capacity to make decisions about their care. This book uses the term *competent* to refer to patients who have the capacity to make informed decisions about medical interventions. Strictly speaking, all adults are considered competent to make such decisions unless a court has declared them *incompetent*. In everyday practice, however, physicians make *de facto* determinations that patients lack decision-making capacity and arrange for surrogates to make decisions, without involving the courts (3–6). This clinical approach has been defended because routine judicial intervention imposes unacceptable delays and generally involves only superficial hearings. This book uses the phrase *lacks decision-making capacity* if a physician, rather than a court, determines that the patient is unable to make informed decisions about health care (3).

ETHICAL IMPLICATIONS OF DECISION-MAKING CAPACITY

Caring for patients whose decision-making capacity is questionable involves two conflicting ethical guidelines. On the one hand, physicians must respect the authority of competent patients to make decisions that others might regard as foolish, unwise, or harmful (*see* Chapter 11). On the other hand, physicians should act in their patients' best interests (*see* Chapter 4). If patients who lack decision-making capacity make decisions that are contrary to their best interests, they need to be protected from serious harm (6). The patient's decision-making capacity is therefore crucial. If it is intact, then the patient's decisions will be respected. If it is seriously impaired, then decision-making power is taken from the patient and given to a surrogate.

Generally, a patient's decision-making capacity is not challenged if he or she agrees with the physician. On its face, this practice suggests that patients are only incapacitated when they disagree with physicians. It makes sense to raise more questions about decision-making capacity, however, when patients refuse a beneficial intervention than when they consent to it. When Mrs. C accepts angiography, her care would be the same whether or not she has decision-making capacity. If she has adequate decision-making capacity, her consent to angioplasty would be valid. If she lacks it, her physician and surrogate agree that angiography was in her best interests. Now consider Mrs. C's refusal of angiography (assuming that she had not previously given an informed refusal). If she has decision-making capacity, then her refusal would have to be respected. If she lacks it, then a surrogate would assume decision-making power. The physician and her nephew agree that angiography is in her best interests. Hence, if she refuses, then her management hinges on whether her decision-making capacity is considered impaired. Thus, it is appropriate that Mrs. C's refusal of recommended interventions triggers questions about her capacity to make medical decisions. Such a refusal, however, does not by itself prove that she lacks such capacity.

LEGAL STANDARDS FOR COMPETENCE

The courts have not articulated clear standards for competency to make medical decisions (4, 5). Many older legal cases viewed incompetence in general or global terms. Either the patient was competent in all aspects of life or the patient was not competent in any sphere. The courts inferred incompetence from a person's overall ability to function in life, medical diagnoses, general mental functioning, and personal appearance.

In reality, a person might be capable of performing some tasks adequately but not others (6); for example, a person might be capable of making informed medical decisions, but not informed financial decisions. A patient with Alzheimer disease who lacked capacity to consent to a clinical trial of a new drug may still have the capacity to appoint a surrogate to make decisions for them. Thus, it is more appropriate to consider a person competent or incompetent for specific tasks rather than in all aspects of life (5). The modern legal and ethical consensus is that a person should be considered competent to make medical decisions if he or she is capable of giving informed consent (5); that is, she appreciates the diagnosis and prognosis, the nature of the tests or treatments proposed, the alternatives, the risks and benefits of each, and the probable consequences. Chapter 3 discusses informed consent in detail.

CLINICAL STANDARDS FOR DECISION-MAKING CAPACITY

A patient's decision-making capacity should be subjected to scrutiny in several situations. As in Case 10.1, the patient might refuse a treatment that the physician strongly recommends or vacillate in making a decision. In other cases, patients might have conditions that commonly impair decision-making capacity, such as dementia, schizophrenia, or depression. Although these conditions justify closer scrutiny of the patient's decision-making capacity, they do not necessarily impair decision-making capacity. Physicians need to test directly the individual patient's ability to give informed consent for the proposed intervention (4–8). Decision-making capacity requires a cluster of abilities (Table 10-1).

THE PATIENT MAKES AND COMMUNICATES A CHOICE

A patient must appreciate that he or she—and not the physician or family members—has ultimate decision-making power. In addition, the patient must be willing to choose among the alternative courses of care. A patient who vacillates repeatedly between consent and refusal is incapable of making a decision, let alone an informed one. Such profound indecision must be distinguished from changing one's mind as the situation changes, as the patient receives more information or advice, or after the patient deliberates.

The patient must communicate his or her choice. A patient who is unable to speak because she is on a ventilator does not necessarily lack decision-making capacity. She might be able to communicate through writing messages, using an alphabet board, or blinking or nodding in response to questions.

THE PATIENT UNDERSTANDS PERTINENT INFORMATION AND APPRECIATES ITS RELEVANCE

A patient needs to understand the medical situation and prognosis, the nature of the proposed intervention, the alternatives, the risks and benefits, and the likely consequences of each alternative. In addition, the patient needs to appreciate that she has the disorder and what the consequences of the intervention (or no intervention) would be for her. The patient needs to appreciate that the information that the physician discussed is relevant to her own situation. In Case 10.1, the health

TABLE 10-1   Clinical Standards for Decision-Making Capacity
The patient makes and communicates a choice.

The patient understands the following information and appreciates its
    • relevance to the situation
    • the medical situation and prognosis
    • the nature of the recommended care
    • alternative courses of care
    • the risks, benefits, and consequences of each alternative

Decisions are consistent with the patient's values and goals.
Decisions do not result from delusions.
The patient uses reasoning to make a choice.

care team could not determine whether Mrs. C understood that angioplasty usually relieves chest pain, but has certain risks.

DECISIONS ARE CONSISTENT WITH THE PATIENT'S VALUES AND GOALS

Choices should be consistent with the patient's character and core values. If Mrs. C wants to be more active without pain, then refusing surgery or angioplasty would be inconsistent with her goals. Many patients, however, do not have well-articulated values and goals or might have multiple, conflicting goals. Mrs. C might want not only to return home but also to be more active and pain free. A choice might be consistent with some goals, but not with others. People do not necessarily have a fixed hierarchy of goals and values. Mrs. C might define her goals or set priorities only by deciding about angiography. Thus, physicians should not regard a patient as lacking decision-making capacity merely because that patient cannot articulate a set of general values or goals.

DECISIONS DO NOT RESULT FROM DELUSIONS

Some patients have delusions that preclude informed decision making. Delusions are defined as false beliefs or incorrect inferences in the face of incontrovertible or obvious evidence to the contrary. For instance, Mary Northern was an elderly woman who refused amputation of her gangrenous legs, denying that gangrene had caused her feet to be "dead, black, shriveled, rotting and stinking" (9). Instead, she believed that they were merely blackened by soot or dust. The court declared her incompetent because she was "incapable of recognizing facts which would be obvious to a person of normal perception" (9). The court said that if she had acknowledged that her legs were gangrenous but refused amputation because she preferred death to the loss of her feet, she would have been considered competent to refuse the surgery.

THE PATIENT USES REASONING TO MAKE A CHOICE

Processing information logically is another element of decision-making capacity. Patients should compare and weigh the various options for care (7). This requirement does not require the patient to choose what most people consider reasonable in the situation. Unconventional decisions do not necessarily imply lack of decision-making capacity. Expectations for reasoning must take into account that many people do not deliberate, but instead rely on emotional or intuitive factors in making important decisions.

ASSESSMENTS OF DECISION-MAKING CAPACITY SHOULD TAKE INTO ACCOUNT THE CLINICAL CONTEXT

Assessments must consider the patient's functional abilities, the demands of the specific clinical situation, and the harm that might result from her choice. Some writers have suggested that a patient who chooses an option that has great risk and little prospect of benefit should meet higher standards for decision-making capacity than a patient who chooses an option that has great prospect of benefit and little risk (6, 7, 10). The benefits and risks of alternatives should also be taken into account; a patient who chooses an option that has less benefit and greater risk than the alternatives should be held to a stricter standard of decision-making capacity. Also, the nature of the intervention might be important. A patient might be given more leeway to refuse disfiguring surgery, such as amputation, than treatments with less drastic side effects. Such a sliding scale offers more protection to patients when the potential harm resulting from their decisions is greater. According to this view, it seems plausible in Case 10.1 to apply a more rigorous standard of capacity when Mrs. C refuses treatment for symptomatic, life-threatening cardiac disease than when she refuses screening tests or preventive measures for cardiac risk factors. Although such a sliding scale is intuitively appealing, it might be problematic in practice. People are likely to disagree over what risks are serious and over what standard should be required for a particular decision. A sliding scale might allow physicians to exercise inappropriate control over patients with whom they disagree. To guard against such problems, physicians need to define explicitly the criteria they are using in assessing a patient's decision-making capacity.

ASSESSING THE CAPACITY TO MAKE DECISIONS

Table 10-2 offers practical suggestions for determining decision-making capacity (7, 8). The assessment requires that the patient has received adequate information about her condition and the interventions. Physicians should keep in mind that beliefs that others consider "unwise, foolish, or ridiculous" do not render a person incompetent (11). Indeed, informed consent would be meaningless if such individualistic refusals were not respected, even though they conflicted with medical recommendations or popular wisdom.

In addition, it is helpful to talk to family and friends, nurses, and other physicians caring for the patient, particularly when the physician does not know the patient well. These persons can clarify whether the patient's mental function or choices have changed over time.

THE ROLE OF MENTAL STATUS TESTING

Clinicians often use mental status tests when assessing a patient's capacity to make medical decisions. Such tests evaluate orientation of the subject to person, place, and time; attention span; immediate recall; short-term and long-term memory; ability to perform simple calculations; and language skills.

Mental status tests are less useful, however, than directly assessing whether the patient understands the nature of the intervention, the risks and benefits, the alternatives, and the consequences (12). For example, Mrs. C scored poorly on standard mental status tests, but if she appreciates that angioplasty would probably improve her chest pain and shortness of breath, she has the capacity to make an informed refusal. Mental status testing is helpful when scores are very low (below 19 on the Mini Mental Status Exam), indicating such severe cognitive impairments that patients cannot appreciate the benefits of treatment and lack the ability to reason (10).

In several court rulings, patients with abnormal mental status tests were found competent to make decisions about health care. For example, a 72-year-old man who withdrew his consent for amputation of his gangrenous legs was found competent even though one psychiatrist found that he was disoriented to the place and to the people around him and had visual hallucinations (13). The probate judge found that "his conversation did wander occasionally but to no greater extent than would be expected of a 72-year-old man in his circumstances." The patient hoped "for a miracle" but realized that "there is no great likelihood of its occurrence."

TABLE 10-2	Helpful Questions in Assessing Decision-Making Capacity

Does the Patient Understand the Disclosed Information?

- "Tell me what you believe is wrong with your health now."
- "What is angiography likely to do for you?"

Does the Patient Appreciate the Consequences of His or Her Choices?

- "What do you believe will happen if you do not have angiography?"
- "I've described the possible benefits and risks of angiography. If these benefits or risks occurred, then how would your everyday activities be affected?"

Does the Patient Use Reasoning to Make a Choice?

- "Tell me how you reached your decision...."
- "Help me understand how you decided to refuse the angiogram."
- "Tell me what makes angiography seem worse than the alternatives."

In another case, a 77-year-old woman was found competent to refuse amputation of her leg for gangrene (14). Testimony indicated that she was "lucid on some matters and confused on others," that her "train of thought sometimes wanders," and that "her conception of time is distorted." One psychiatrist claimed that her refusal to discuss the amputation with him indicated that "she was unable to face up to the problem." The court found that she understood that in "rejecting the amputation she is, in effect, choosing death over life."

CONSULTATION BY PSYCHIATRISTS

Psychiatrists can be helpful in evaluating patients whose decision-making capacity is questionable (15). Psychiatrists are skilled at interviewing patients with mental impairment and engaging them in discussions. In addition, psychiatrists specialize in diagnosing and treating mental illnesses that might impair a decision-making capacity.

Attending physicians can readily acquire the skills to assess patients' decision-making capacity, and routine psychiatric consultation is not necessary (12). Ultimately, attending physicians are responsible for judging whether the patient lacks decision-making capacity.

ENHANCING THE CAPACITY OF PATIENTS TO MAKE DECISIONS

Impairments in decision-making capacity might be reversible if underlying medical or psychiatric conditions are treated. In addition, physicians can enhance a patient's understanding of pertinent information by presenting information in simple language, in small chunks, slowly and repeatedly over time (16). Diagrams and videotapes might improve comprehension. Furthermore, family members or friends can help reduce anxiety, correct misunderstandings, and focus the discussion on the salient issues.

ENGAGING THE PATIENT IN DISCUSSIONS

Patients like Mrs. C who refuse to answer questions or explain their decisions might be angry at losing control or resent being badgered. Repeated attempts to assess decision-making capacity or to persuade them might be counterproductive and frustrate health care workers. Patients need to be told clearly and sympathetically that to get the physicians to do what they want, they need to answer some questions.

DECISION-MAKING CAPACITY IN SPECIFIC CLINICAL SITUATIONS

MENTAL ILLNESS IMPAIRING DECISION-MAKING CAPACITY

Many patients with mental illness are competent to make decisions about their medical care; however, lacking decision-making capacity is more common in certain psychiatric conditions. Patients with schizophrenia or depression commonly fail to appreciate the relevance of information to their situation. According to one study, among inpatients with schizophrenia, 35% did not acknowledge their symptoms and diagnosis (17). Furthermore, 13% to 14% of patients with schizophrenia or major depression denied the potential benefit of treatment.

Psychiatric illness might also impair decision-making capacity more subtly (18). Patients who are depressed might overemphasize the risks of treatment, underestimate the benefits, believe that treatment is less likely to be successful for them than for others, or feel unworthy of the intervention.

Psychiatric patients might be so gravely disabled or unable to care for themselves that they might be involuntarily committed (*see* Chapter 40); however, involuntary commitment does not empower physicians to give whatever medical treatment they consider advisable. If such a patient refuses treatment for medical problems, then an appropriate surrogate or a separate court order is needed to authorize treatment.

UNCONVENTIONAL DECISIONS BASED ON RELIGIOUS BELIEFS

Patients might refuse effective medical treatments because of their religious beliefs. In the United States, a person's religious beliefs are deeply respected. Religious beliefs often form the foundation of a person's value system and provide meaning in their lives (19). Physicians should not judge whether a patient's religious beliefs are true or false or try to change them. Because religion is based on faith, empirical evidence and rational arguments are unlikely to change people's beliefs. Doctors have no expertise in religious matters, and patients do not seek them for religious advice. Thus, refusals of treatment by competent adults on religious grounds are accepted. (Parental refusals of highly effective treatment for children, however, may be overridden, as discussed in Chapter 37.)

If, however, a patient refuses highly effective treatment for religiously based reasons, then the physician should not simply accept the refusal. Instead, the physician should respectfully explore whether the refusal is consistent with the patient's prior decisions and actions and is shared by other members of her faith tradition (20). Chapter 11 discusses how to carry out such discussions with Jehovah's Witnesses regarding refusal of blood transfusions. Furthermore, the physician should examine if other aspects of decision-making are problematic. Some patients have religious delusions or hallucinations. For example, a patient might believe that he is Christ and must die to redeem the world, that the devil is tempting him to take medicine, or that she should refuse surgery because it is God's will that she suffer. The physicians should arrange for the patient to talk with other members of the faith tradition and consider psychiatric evaluation and medication or counseling (20).

EMERGENCIES

A patient with questionable decision-making capacity might present with an emergency condition that requires immediate treatment. Rather than evaluating the patient's decision-making capacity, physicians should provide emergency care unless it is known that the patient or surrogate would refuse such care. This approach is justified by implied consent to emergency care (*see* Chapter 3).

CARING FOR PATIENTS WHO LACK DECISION-MAKING CAPACITY

After physicians determine that a patient lacks decision-making capacity, advance directives, or surrogate decision-making should guide further care (*see* Chapters 12 and 13).

Even if a patient lacks the capacity to make decisions, his or her stated preferences should be given substantial consideration. For instance, mentally incapacitated patients might balk at phlebotomy or x-rays, sometimes screaming their refusal. Even if the courts declared such a patient incompetent, it would be morally and emotionally repugnant to force interventions on an unwilling patient who cannot understand how the interventions are helping him (21). Health care workers might consider it inhumane to force a patient to undergo a highly invasive intervention when he or she cannot understand its purpose and benefits. Furthermore, future cooperation might be undermined. Physicians should try to obtain the patient's assent to interventions decided on by a surrogate or court, even if that patient cannot give informed consent. Persuasion, cajoling, and asking family members and friends to talk to the patient are acceptable ways to try to gain the patient's cooperation. Often, a patient will agree to treatment after caregivers have listened to his or her objections, modified the treatment plans, or changed the hospital routine.

SUMMARY

1. Physicians commonly determine that patients lack the capacity to make informed decisions about their care without resorting to the courts.
2. Physicians need to understand the clinical standards for decision-making capacity and be able to apply them in specific cases.

REFERENCES

1. Brock DW, ed. *Life and Death: Philosophical Essays in Biomedical Ethics*. New York, NY: Cambridge University Press; 1993.
2. Lo B. Assessing decision-making capacity. *Law Med Health Care*. 1990;18:193–201.
3. President's Commission for the Study of Ethical Problems in Medicine and Biomedical and Behavioral Research. *Making Health Care Decisions*. Washington, DC: U.S. Government Printing Office; 1982.
4. Berg JW, Lidz CW, Appelbaum PS. *Informed Consent: Legal Theory and Clinical Practice*. 2nd ed. New York, NY: Oxford University Press; 2001.
5. Meisel A. *The Right to Die*. 2nd ed. New York, NY: John Wiley & Sons; 1995.
6. Buchanan AE, Brock DW. *Deciding for Others*. Cambridge, UK: Cambridge University Press; 1989.
7. Grisso T, Appelbaum P. *Assessing Competence to Consent to Treatment: A Guide for Physicians and Other Health Professionals*. New York, NY: Oxford University Press; 1998.
8. Jeste DV, Saks E. Decisional capacity in mental illness and substance use disorders: empirical database and policy implications. *Behav Sci Law*. 2006;24:607–628.
9. *State Department of Human Resources v. Northern*, 563 S.W.2d 197 (Tenn. Ct. App. 1978).
10. Kim SY. When does decisional impairment become decisional incompetence? Ethical and methodological issues in capacity research in schizophrenia. *Schizophr Bull*. 2006;32:92–97.
11. *In re Brooks*, 32 Ill.2d 361, 205 N.E.2d 435 (1965).
12. Grisso T, Appelbaum P. *Assessing Competence to Consent to Treatment: A Guide for Physicians and Other Health Professionals*. New York, NY: Oxford University Press; 1998:90–91.
13. *In re Quackenbush*, 156 N.J. Super. 282, 383 A.2d 785 (1978).
14. *Lane v. Candura*, 6 Mass. App. 377,376 N.E.2d 1232 (1978).
15. Appelbaum PS, Grisso T. Assessing patient's capacities to consent to treatment. *N Engl J Med*. 1988;319:1635–1638.
16. Eyler LT, Jeste DV. Enhancing the informed consent process: a conceptual overview. *Behav Sci Law*. 2006;24:553–568.
17. Appelbaum PS, Grisso T. The macarthur treatment competence study, I: mental illness and competence to consent to treatment. *Law Hum Behav*. 1995;19:105–126.
18. Bursztajn HJ, Gutheil TG, Brodsky A. Affective disorders, competence, and decision making. In: Gutheil TG, Bursztajn HJ, Brodsky A, et al., eds. *Decision Making in Psychiatry and the Law*. Baltimore, MD: Williams & Wilkins; 1991:153–170.
19. Martin AM. Tales publicly allowed: competence, capacity, and religious belief. *Hastings Cent Rep*. 2007;37:33–40.
20. Cochrane TI. Religious delusions and the limits of spirituality in decision-making. *Am J Bioeth*. 2007;7:14–15.
21. The President's Council on Bioethics. *Taking Care: Ethical Caregiving in Our Aging Society*. Washington, DC: The President's Council on Bioethics; 2005.

ANNOTATED BIBLIOGRAPHY

1. Grisso T, Appelbaum P. Assessing Competence to Consent to Treatment: A Guide for Physicians and Other Health Professionals. New York, NY: Oxford University Press; 1998.
   Lucid, practical, and comprehensive discussion of how to assess decision-making capacity.
2. Buchanan AE, Brock DW. Deciding for Others. Cambridge, UK: Cambridge University Press; 1989.
   Comprehensive discussion of different definitions and standards for decision-making capacity.
3. Kim, SYH. *Evaluation of Capacity to Consent to Treatment and Research*. New York, NY: Oxford University Press; 2010.
   Detailed information on how to assess decision-making capacity.

Refusal of Treatment by Competent, Informed Patients

Competent and informed patients may refuse interventions that their physicians recommend. In some cases, physicians may hesitate to accept refusals that jeopardize the patient's life or health. Although concern for a patient's well-being is commendable, as discussed in Chapter 4, it is important for physicians to understand the compelling ethical and legal reasons for respecting refusals made by informed, competent patients. This chapter discusses the reasons for respecting such refusals, specific clinical examples of refusal of treatment, and restrictions on patient refusal.

REASONS FOR RESPECTING PATIENT REFUSALS

RESPECT FOR PATIENT AUTONOMY

Honoring refusal of treatment by competent, informed patients respects their autonomy to make decisions about their care and to be free of unwanted medical interventions (1–3). The option of declining treatment is fundamental to the concept of informed consent. If patients must consent to treatment, then logically they have the right to decline treatment. The US Supreme Court has suggested that the Constitution protects a competent patient's refusal of life-sustaining treatment (4). A large body of case law supports the right of competent, informed patients to refuse treatment (5).

IMPOSING MEDICAL INTERVENTIONS WOULD BE UNACCEPTABLE

On a practical level, it is difficult to impose unwanted interventions on a competent patient. Sedating or restraining patients to impose treatment over their objections seems intrusive and inhumane. Most people would reject such means, even if they disagree with the patient's refusal.

SCOPE OF REFUSAL

Competent patients are permitted to refuse virtually any treatment, even highly beneficial ones with few side effects. The range of interventions includes surgery, mechanical ventilation, renal dialysis, antibiotics, cardiopulmonary resuscitation, and tube feedings (5). Competent patients may refuse treatment even if such a refusal might shorten their lives or lead to their deaths. They are not required to have a terminal illness as a condition for refusing treatment.

Competent patients may refuse treatment even if their family, friends, or physicians disagree with them. As one court ruling declared, even decisions that are unwise or foolish might need to be respected (6). Indeed, informed consent would be meaningless unless patients could refuse interventions for highly personal reasons or make decisions that conflict with medical or popular wisdom.

JEHOVAH'S WITNESS CASES

Jehovah's Witnesses do not accept blood transfusions, basing their refusal on an interpretation of the Bible (7). They believe that although a blood transfusion might save their corporeal life, it will deprive them of everlasting salvation. Their refusals usually are clearly articulated, steadfast over time, and are supported by their family and friends. Jehovah's Witnesses generally consent to other interventions, such as surgery, if transfusions are not used.

Reactions of Health Care Providers

Refusals of blood transfusions by Jehovah's Witnesses might distress some physicians because the clinical benefits of transfusion are great and the medical risks very small (8). Many patients are young, previously healthy, and can be restored to perfect health. Physicians might feel that Jehovah's Witnesses, by refusing transfusions but agreeing to other care, unnecessarily compromise medical outcomes and require the physician to provide substandard care. Physicians might believe that they are being asked to accomplish the goal of saving the patient's life without using the best available means. Some surgeons complain that operating on a Jehovah's Witness without transfusions is like having to operate with one hand tied behind their back or being painted into a corner because they have less margin for error or complications (8). On a psychological level, some physicians resent the loss of control over the patient's care. Some health care workers might also blame the patient for making their jobs more complicated. Many surgeons and anesthesiologists prefer not to treat Jehovah's Witnesses. Often, however, transferring such patients to another institution or physician is impractical.

Frustrated health care workers sometimes develop ingenious plans for administering blood to Jehovah's Witnesses. Some physicians suggest waiting until such patients are unconscious and then asking if they object to a transfusion (8). Because patients are then no longer able to refuse, these physicians would administer blood. Other physicians advocate simply giving transfusions after patients are under anesthesia and not telling them about it. Such deceptive actions are unacceptable and undermine trust in physicians.

Health care workers need to appreciate that without transfusions, medical outcomes for Jehovah's Witness are often quite good. For example, outcomes after open heart surgery on Jehovah's Witnesses are good (9), using normovolemic hemodilution, intraoperative cell salvage, or other blood conservation techniques (10).

Legal Issues

The courts have consistently upheld refusals of blood transfusions by competent adult Jehovah's Witnesses (5, 11). Recent controversies have involved incompetent Jehovah's Witnesses. Many patients signed wallet cards declaring they would refuse transfusions. Some physicians, however, question whether patients have been coerced by peer pressure and whether they were informed about the risks and benefits of transfusions (12).

Practical Suggestions

Physicians caring for adult Jehovah's Witnesses should take several steps to ensure that the patient's refusal of transfusions is informed, voluntary, and steadfast. First, to minimize the possibility of undue influence, the physician should ask the patient about transfusions when no family members, friends, or religious advisors are present. When alone, some Jehovah's Witnesses will agree to transfusions (10). Second, the physician should ask patients whether they would accept transfusions if they are ordered by a court. Some Jehovah's Witnesses will accept a transfusion as long as they do not personally consent to it. Under these circumstances, many judges are willing to order that transfusions be given. Third, Jehovah's Witnesses vary in what types of transfusion they will refuse. Some refuse all blood products, but others accept various blood components. Most will accept epoietin and blood substitutes. Fourth, physicians should ask whether the patient has any other concerns about receiving blood, such as a risk of HIV infection or hepatitis. If the underlying reason for refusal is really a fear of infection, this concern should be addressed directly (10).

Having ensured that the refusal is free and informed, health care workers should respect the patient's decision. From the point of view of a Jehovah's Witness, the decision to refuse transfusions is simple. They would be pleased to survive the hospitalization, but as one patient put it, "What good is a few years of life compared to everlasting damnation?" (13). Even if health care workers do not agree with this belief, they need to respect it. Continuing to try to convince a Jehovah's Witness shows disrespect.

When an adult Jehovah's Witness, who requires a transfusion, lacks decision-making capacity, the situation is more complicated. Advance directives that reflect informed decisions should be respected, as Chapter 12 discusses.

If the patient is a minor and parents are refusing medically indicated transfusions, physicians should ask a court to order the transfusions (*see* Chapter 37). As one court declared, parents are "not free to make martyrs of their children" (14).

RENAL DIALYSIS

About 15% of deaths in patients on renal dialysis occur after a decision to withhold dialysis (15). The patient might have a very limited prognosis, unacceptable quality of life, or technical difficulties, such as poor venous access. When the possibility of withholding dialysis is considered, physicians need to ensure that the decision is informed and voluntary. Furthermore, physicians need to palliate for the symptoms of uremia (15).

PACEMAKERS AND IMPLANTED DEFIBRILLATORS

Some patients physicians are reluctant to deactivate these cardiac devices because they feel that turning off the device would be suicide or euthanasia (16). As Chapter 15 discusses, although such emotions are understandable, respecting informed and voluntary refusal by a patient is ethically and legally distinguishable from killing the patient. Physicians need to ensure that the patient's decision is informed and consistent with the patient's goals for care. For example, deactivating a pacemaker, particularly a sequential dual-chamber pacemaker, may lead to symptoms of shortness of breath, dizziness, and fatigue, rather than a peaceful death from arrhythmia.

RESTRICTIONS ON REFUSAL

The right of competent, informed patients to refuse medical treatment may be limited in certain situations.

COMMUNICABLE DISEASES

In certain circumstances, competent patients may be required to undergo treatment against their wishes to prevent harm to third parties. For example, tuberculosis can be transmitted by casual contact (17, 18). To reduce the risk of transmitting this infection to other persons, infected individuals may be required to be treated or be quarantined.

COMPELLED TREATMENT OF PREGNANT WOMEN

In several cases, the courts have ordered pregnant women to undergo cesarean deliveries or blood transfusions over their objections, allegedly to protect the health of the fetus. These rulings, however, have been sharply criticized for violating the woman's bodily integrity and right of self-determination. Recent court rulings have generally rejected interventions against the wishes of the pregnant woman (19–21). In other situations, compelled treatment in pregnancy is not feasible. In diabetes or drug addiction, interventions must be continued over an extended period, the cooperation of the pregnant woman is needed, and the infringement of her autonomy caused by ongoing forced treatment is substantial.

TREATING COMPETENT PATIENTS FOR THEIR OWN BENEFIT

Providing interventions over the objections of a competent patient to prevent harm to third parties needs to be clearly distinguished from providing treatment to prevent harm to the patient. The physician's duty to prevent harm to competent patients is weaker than the duty to prevent harm to unsuspecting third parties. Physicians should try to persuade patients and to negotiate a mutually acceptable plan of care (*see* Chapter 4). They may not, however, override the informed decisions of a competent patient because they believe it would be better for that patient.

In some situations, physicians might want to administer treatment to save the life of a patient who refuses treatment, for example to give antibiotics to patient with bacterial meningitis who shows no indication of impaired decision-making capacity other than his "enigmatic refusal" of treatment (22). Although it is troubling to allow a patient to die from an easily treatable infection, it is also troubling to override the a patient's refusal when the only evidence of impaired decision-making capacity is the refusal itself. It is appropriate to examine closely whether a patient refusing such life-saving treatment is competent and informed. It is ethically problematic to allow physicians to override patients who cannot provide satisfactory reasons for refusing treatment.

SUMMARY

1. There are cogent ethical and legal reasons to accept refusals of treatment by competent and informed patients.
2. Physicians can try to persuade patients to accept beneficial interventions while respecting their right to refuse.

REFERENCES

1. Lo B, Jonsen AR. Clinical decisions to limit treatment. *Ann Intern Med.* 1980;93:764–768.
2. President's Commission for the Study of Ethical Problems in Medicine and Biomedical and Behavioral Research. *Making Health Care Decisions.* Washington, DC: U.S. Government Printing Office; 1982.
3. President's Commission for the Study of Ethical Problems in Medicine and Biomedical and Behavioral Research. *Deciding to Forego Life-Sustaining Treatment.* Washington, DC: U.S. Government Printing Office; 1983.
4. Lo B, Steinbrook R. Beyond the Cruzan case: the U.S. Supreme Court and medical practice. *Ann Intern Med.* 1991;114:895–901.
5. Meisel A, Cerminara, K. *The Right to Die: The Law of End of Life Decision Making.* 3rd ed. New York, NY: Aspen Publishers; 2004.
6. *In re Brooks Estate,* 32 III.2d 361, 205 N.E.2d 435 (1965).
7. Sheldon M. Ethical issues in the forced transfusion of Jehovah's Witness children. *J Emer Med.* 1996;14:251–257.
8. Jones JW, McCullough LB, Richman BW. Painted into a corner: unexpected complications in treating a Jehovah's Witness. *J Vasc Surg.* 2006;44:425–428.
9. Stamou SC, White T, Barnett S, et al. Comparisons of cardiac surgery outcomes in Jehovah's versus Non-Jehovah's Witnesses. *Am J Cardiol.* 2006;98:1223–1225.
10. Rogers DM, Crookston KP. The approach to the patient who refuses blood transfusion. *Transfusion.* 2006;46:1471–1477.
11. Furrow BR, Johnson SH, Jost TS, et al. *Health Law: Cases, Materials and Problems.* St. Paul, MN: West Publishing Co.; 1991.
12. Migden DR, Braen GR. The Jehovah's Witness blood refusal card: ethical and medicolegal considerations for emergency physicians. *Acad Emerg Med.* 1998;5:815–824.
13. *In re Osborne,* 294 A.2d 372 (D.C. 1972).
14. *Prince v. Massachusetts,* 321 U.S. 158 (1944).
15. Cohen LM, Germain MJ, Poppel DM. Practical considerations in dialysis withdrawal: "to have that option is a blessing." *JAMA.* 2003;289:2113–2119.
16. Lampert R, Hayes DL, Annas GJ, et al. HRS expert consensus statement on the management of cardiovascular implantable electronic devices (CIEDs) in patients nearing end of life or requesting withdrawal of therapy. *Heart Rhythm.* 2010;7:1008–1026.
17. Oscherwitz T, Tulsky JP, Roger S, et al. Detention of persistently nonadherent patients with tuberculosis. *JAMA.* 1997;278:843–846.

18. Gasner MR, Maw KL, Feldman GE, et al. The use of legal action in New York city to ensure treatment of tuberculosis. *N Engl J Med.* 1999;340:359–366.

19. Curran WJ. Court-ordered cesarean sections receive judicial defeat. *N Engl J Med.* 1990;323:489–492.

20. Levy JK. Jehovah's Witnesses, pregnancy, and blood transfusions: a paradigm for the autonomy of all pregnant women. *J Law Med Ethics.* 1999;27:171–189.

21. Goldblatt AD. Commentary: no more jurisdiction over Jehovah. *J Law Med Ethics.* 1999;27:190–193.

22. Jonsen A, Siegler M, Winslade W. *Clinical Ethics.* 3rd ed. New York, NY: Macmillan Publishing Co.; 1991:61–63.

ANNOTATED BIBLIOGRAPHY

1. President's Commission for the Study of Ethical Problems in Medicine and Biomedical and Behavioral Research. *Deciding to Forego Life-Sustaining Treatment.* Washington, DC: U.S. Government Printing Office,1983.
   Lucid and thoughtful exposition of refusal of treatment by patients.

2. Meisel A, Cerminara, K. *The Right to Die: The Law of End of Life Decision Making.* 3rd ed. New York, NY: Aspen Publishers, 2004.
   Comprehensive legal treatise that describes court rulings permitting competent patients to refuse treatment.

3. Jones JW, McCullough LB, Richman BW. Painted into a corner: unexpected complications in treating a Jehovah's Witness. *J Vasc Surg.* 2006;44:425–428.
   Clear discussion of refusal of transfusions by Jehovah's Witnesses, from the perspective of a surgeon.

4. Lampert R, Hayes DL, Annas GJ, et al. HRS expert consensus statement on the management of cardiovascular implantable electronic devices (CIEDs) in patients nearing end of life or requesting withdrawal of therapy. *Heart Rhythm.* 2010;7:1008–1026.
   Consensus guidelines on the deactivation of implanted cardioverter defibrillators.

CHAPTER 12

Standards for Decisions When Patients Lack Decision-Making Capacity

When patients lack decision-making capacity, physicians must address two questions:

- What standards should be used when patients cannot give informed consent or refusal?
- Who should act as surrogate?

This chapter addresses the first question. Traditionally, these standards were viewed as a hierarchy: advance directives take priority over substituted judgments, which in turn supersede best interests. However, exceptions to this hierarchy can be justified. Chapter 13 addresses the choice of surrogates.

ADVANCE DIRECTIVES

Many patients fear that they will lose control over care if their decision-making capacity is lost. In advance directives, competent patients indicate *who* should act as surrogate or *what* interventions they would accept or refuse if they should lose their decision-making capacity. Advance directives respect patients by allowing their preferences and values to guide care even when they can no longer make informed decisions. In addition, advance directives relieve stress on family members who must make decisions.

HISTORY OF ADVANCE DIRECTIVES

Proof of principle and feasibility of advance directives were established early in the AIDS epidemic (1). Before antiretorivals were developed, persons with AIDS commonly died from opportunistic infections. Antibiotics were often not effective and at best only postponed a refractory opportunistic infection. Many persons with AIDS had watched friends die and had strong, informed preferences to forego mechanical ventilation for Pneumocystis carinii pneumonia or antibiotics for central nervous system opportunistic infections, preferring palliative care instead. Only by executing a durable power of attorney for health care could homosexual men with AIDS make such preferences legally binding and appoint their partner or a close friend as proxy, rather than relatives who did not know about their medical condition, were not familiar with AIDS, or were estranged from them. Lawyers volunteered to help patients complete these legal documents.

The ruling in the Nancy Cruzan case made an unwarranted conceptual jump: Although advance directives are useful in some cases, it does not follow that the only justification for limiting life-sustaining in patients who lack decision-making capacity is a written advance directive or an oral statement declining the intervention in the specific clinical situation (*see* Chapter 22). The Cruzan case spurred measures to encourage written advance directives, including new state laws authorizing them and the federal Patient Self-Determination Act to inform patients about them.

TYPES OF ADVANCE DIRECTIVES

The following case illustrates the usefulness and limitations of advance directives.

CASE 12.1   Advance directives

Mrs. A, a 76-year-old widow with Alzheimer disease, lives with her daughter. She cannot be left alone safely because she sometimes forgets to turn off the stove or wanders away. When she was still lucid, she told her children and her friends many times that she wanted "no heroics" if she became senile. After visiting a neighbor who was in a nursing home, poorly responsive after a severe stroke, she told her son, "That is not living. I would never live in a nursing home, unable to recognize my family and depending on others to take care of me. The smell is terrible. If I'm like that, just let me die in peace." She signed a POLST form, specifying that she did not want to be resuscitated or hospitalized (except if needed for comfort measures). She also wrote by hand, NO SURGERY, NO INTENSIVE CARE.

Mrs. A's children cannot afford to pay an attendant during the day while they are at work. Adult day health programs were cut back and are not available. Unable to care for Mrs. A safely at home, her children reluctantly consider placement.

Oral Statements to Family Members or Friends

Conversations with relatives or friends are the most common advance directives and, in clinical practice, frequently guide decisions for patients who have lost decision-making capacity.

Oral Statements to Physicians

Discussions with physicians are more common than written advance directives (2, 3). Unlike some oral statements to relatives or friends, directives to physicians are not casual comments. Moreover, physicians can check whether directives are informed, such as by eliciting a patient's reactions to clinical scenarios. For instance, Mrs. A's physician might point out that many patients with moderate dementia appear to enjoy activities and interactions with friends and family. In some states, oral statements to physicians appointing a proxy are legally binding for the duration of the illness or hospitalization.

Written Documents

All states have laws authorizing living wills or health care proxies (3, 4). Patients complete a formal legal document that must be witnessed or notarized. A lawyer is not needed to complete these documents. Many states honor forms from other states. Caregivers who follow written directives are given immunity from civil and criminal liability and professional disciplinary actions. Because statutes vary from state to state, caregivers and patients need to be familiar with their state's laws.

The courts consider written advance directives more reliable evidence of patient choices than oral statements because legal formalities make patients more likely to think seriously and appreciate the consequences. Only about 25% of patients, however, provide written advance directives (3).

Living wills. Patients direct their physicians to withhold or withdraw life-sustaining treatment if they develop a terminal condition or, in some states, enter a persistent vegetative state (PVS). Various states define "terminal condition" differently, usually only in general terms. In most states, living wills would not cover conditions such as Alzheimer disease. Patients typically may refuse only interventions that "merely prolong the process of dying." People might disagree on whether this includes common scenarios such as antibiotics for pneumonia or sepsis. Some states do not allow patients to decline artificial nutrition and hydration through living wills. Living wills are less flexible and comprehensive than the health care proxy.

Health care proxy. Competent patients may appoint a health care proxy or agent, typically a relative or close friend, to make medical decisions if they lose decision-making capacity. In some states, this process is called executing a durable power of attorney for health care. As long as patients remain competent, they continue to make their own health care decisions. Because of conflicts of interest, certain people may not serve as surrogates, such as the treating physician or employees of the treating physician or institution unless they are relatives of the patient. The health care proxy applies to all situations in which the patient is incapable of making decisions, not just to terminal illness. Proxy decisions must be consistent with the patient's previously expressed choices or best interests. No additional evidence of the patient's wishes, however, is required. Appointing a health care proxy, supplemented with statements of what life-sustaining treatment the patient would want or refuse in various scenarios, is the best way to provide advance directives.

Physician orders for life-sustaining treatment (POLST). This standardized one-page order form directs first responders regarding such interventions as CPR and transport to hospital in urgent situations where there is no time to contact the responsible physician or proxy. The POLST form can be used in many settings, including a patient's home or nursing homes and can accompany a patient from one setting to another. It is signed by the patient or surrogate. Most states have authorized POLST forms (4).

POLST is more flexible than "do not attempt resuscitation" or "do not hospitalize" orders. There are three options regarding transfer to the hospital:

1. Comfort measures only; transfer to hospital only if comfort needs cannot be met in the current setting;
2. Limited additional measures, including antibiotics and other medical treatment as indicated, but no intubation and generally avoiding intensive care; an additional checkbox may be checked to transfer to hospital only if comfort needs cannot be met in the current setting; or
3. Full treatment as indicated, including intensive care.

Thus, POLST recognizes that the goal of patient comfort may require hospitalization or limited noninvasive care.

Written advance directives are particularly useful if patients have strong preferences about specific medical interventions or anticipate disagreements over who should serve as surrogate.

LIMITATIONS OF ADVANCE DIRECTIVES

Statements Might Not Be Intended to Guide Care

People might comment about the care of other people without intending to direct their own future care or might state views without thinking deeply about them.

Advance Directives Might Not Be Informed

Even after discussions with physicians, patients commonly have serious misconceptions about life-sustaining interventions (5). Only 33% of patients know that patients on a ventilator cannot talk, and about one half believe that ventilators are oxygen tanks. More than one fourth cannot identify any basic characteristics of cardiopulmonary resuscitation (CPR), such as chest compressions or assisted breathing. Only one third know that if CPR succeeds in restarting the heart, a breathing machine is usually needed. Thus, patients may express "strong preferences about treatments that they did not understand" (5).

Patients commonly overestimate their prognosis. In a cohort of patients with metastatic lung or colon cancer, who had a 6-month survival of 45%, most patients were decidedly overoptimistic: 59% believed that their chance of surviving 6 months was greater than 90% (6).

People generally cannot predict how they will respond to future medical conditions, underestimating the extent to which people cope and adapt to new situations (7). Thus, their choices when healthy may differ from what they would decide later if they actually are in the situation.

Many people do not have preexisting preferences regarding life-prolonging interventions in various clinical situations, developing them only when faced with an actual decision (8).

Patients Might Change Their Minds

Patient willingness to accept potentially life-sustaining therapy that is highly burdensome or would result in a severely disabled condition is only moderately stable over time (9). Although some of this change may be related to declines in health, there is considerable unexplained variation.

Interpretations of Advance Directives Might Be Problematical

Vague terms. Advance directives often contain vague terms such as *heroic* or *extraordinary* care. Physicians are commonly directed to refuse interventions when "the burdens outweigh the benefits of care." These terms must be interpreted. When does "senility" commence: When Mrs. A can no longer pursue her favorite activities, such as reading? When she sometimes or usually does not recognize family members? Or only when she no longer responds at all? Patients' choices in specific scenarios cannot be accurately predicted from their general preferences and goals (10, 11).

Application to similar situations. In Case 12.1, Mrs. A gave advance directives about one situation (stroke), but developed a different condition (dementia). Patients differ in how much leeway surrogates should have. In one study, 39% of patients wanted their directives to be followed literally, but 31% of patients wanted their surrogates to override their advance directives if their surrogates believed it was best for them (12).

Unrealistic expectations. Advance directives enable patients to have some control over health care decisions if they lose decision-making capacity. It is unrealistic, however, for patients to expect to control all future care through advance directives. No one can anticipate what specific clinical decisions will need to be made in the future, or whether her overall health or life situation will change significantly.

Advance Directives Might Conflict With the Patient's Best Interests

Following a patient's advance directives might not be in her current best interests. For example, surrogates and physicians might wish to override prior refusal of care if a new, short-term intervention with few side effects is virtually certain to restore the patient to previous health (13, 14). Alternatively, wishes to receive an intervention may become impractical if the patient no longer takes oral medicines regularly or cannot cooperate with a postoperative regimen. In addition, when giving advance directives, patients make implicit assumptions about their prognosis or situation that later may no longer hold true.

More fundamentally, the incompetent person might have changed so much since giving advance directives that she is essentially a different person, and her previous statements may no longer be relevant (15).

Despite many limitations, advance directives are valuable to begin important discussions about end-of-life care among patients, family members, and physicians. They promote respect for patients as unique individuals. Furthermore, they offer a means for patients to express strongly held, informed choices that they want surrogates to follow closely.

TRUSTWORTHINESS OF ADVANCE DIRECTIVES

In light of the limitations of advance directives, physicians and surrogates need to assess how much weight to give them when patients no longer have decision-making capacity. Advance directives are more trustworthy and should be given more weight if

- the directive indicates what *specific treatments* the patient would want or not want *in particular clinical situations*;
- the directive is *informed*, for example, because the patient has experienced the intervention or discussed it with a physician;

- the directive is *repeated* over time, in different situations, to various individuals; or
- the directive does not clearly contradict the patient's current best interests.

RATIONALE FOR DISCUSSING ADVANCE DIRECTIVES

Most patients—between 59% and 85% of outpatients and 42% and 81% of hospitalized patients—want to talk with their physicians about life-sustaining interventions before a clinical crisis occurs (1, 2, 16–18), yet few have done so. When thinking or talking about life-sustaining interventions, most patients feel in control, relieved, or cared for (16). Even patients who feel sad or anxious when thinking about life-sustaining treatment still want to have such conversations (1, 16). Most patients want physicians to take the initiative in discussing advance directives (16, 19). Physician can help patients understand the limitations of advance directives.

PROBLEMS WITH DISCUSSIONS ABOUT ADVANCE DIRECTIVES

Currently, discussions between patients and physicians about advance directives are problematic. In one study, only 11% of patients who had executed advance directives had discussed them with their physician (20). Almost all discussions concerned general attitudes and feelings rather than specific interventions (20).

Even when discussions occur, they rarely give patients enough information to make informed decisions (21). When discussing hypothetical scenarios with patients, physicians usually pose dire scenarios in which patients would not survive outside an intensive care unit or reversible scenarios in which patients are expected to recover their previous health. Physicians seldom pose more difficult—and more common—situations, such as when recovery is uncertain or serious disability might persist.

Physicians also use vague language, asking patients what they would want if they were "very, very sick" or "had something that was very serious." Doctors rarely define such terms or ascertain how patients interpret them. Physicians commonly discuss specific interventions, usually CPR or mechanical ventilation, without learning what patients know about them. In discussing outcomes, physicians seldom give numerical probabilities of success or mention outcomes other than death and complete recovery.

Physicians rarely elicit patients' values, goals for care, and reasons for choices. Most commonly, physicians simply ask whether patients want interventions in scenarios without exploring their reasoning. Even when reasons are discussed, physicians rarely ask patients to clarify what they mean by a poor quality of life or being a burden to their family, which are frequent reasons for refusing interventions.

ADVANCE CARE PLANNING

Because advance directives overemphasize legal formalities and specific interventions, an alternative approach called advance care planning focuses instead on (22)

- discussions among patients, physicians and surrogates, rather than legal documents;
- the patient's values, goals, hopes, and fears, rather than a specific clinical scenario such as cardiopulmonary resuscitation. Starting with these topics generally makes it easier to reach agreement on specific decisions and may not take much more time;
- the patient's preferences and hopes for a "good death," such as how the patient would like to be remembered, what they would like to say to their family, and what they would like the family to say to them. This shifts attention from withholding of medical interventions to reaching closure at the end of life. These discussions also help address the emotional needs of the patient and family (23); and
- the need for surrogates to exercise judgment and interpret the patient's previous statements, not simply implement literally the patient's directives. Surrogates should anticipate the need to make difficult decisions.

IMPROVING ADVANCE CARE PLANNING DISCUSSIONS

Physicians can resolve many problems with advance care planning by explicitly addressing the following issues (Table 12-1):

When Should Discussions Be Initiated?

Physicians should discuss advance care planning if it would not be surprising if the patient were to lose decision-making capacity or to die (24). Hence, physicians should target not only patients who are "terminal" or in a downhill course but also those with serious chronic illness, such as congestive heart failure, whose course is not so predictable. Patients usually want discussions to occur earlier in their illness and earlier in the patient–physician relationship (19).

In some cultures discussions might be problematic. Many traditional Chinese patients believe that giving directives implies that they do not trust their family to make decisions for them (25). Moreover, patients might believe that designating one person to make decisions violates the expectation of family decision-making. Furthermore, some patients believe that talking about future illness will anger ghosts or spirits, who will then bring about the illness or cause bad luck. Such reluctance to discuss advance care planning needs to be respected.

Who Should Serve as Proxy?

Most patients find it easier to discuss the choice of proxy than to discuss preferences regarding care. Straightforward questions can broach the topic: "I ask all my elderly patients how they want decisions to be made. Who would you want to make decisions for you in case you are too sick to talk with me directly?" Patients who do not wish to discuss this topics can easily demur. Patients need to select someone whose judgment they trust. It is unrealistic to think that the proxy can simply follow the patient's previous statements.

What Are the Patient's Goals and Values?

Although many physicians focus on specific medical decisions, such as Do Not Attempt Resuscitation (DNAR) orders, discussing the patient's values and goals first generally helps make these specific decisions (23). Open-ended questions help elicit the patient's perspective (23, 26):

- "When you think of serious illness, what concerns you the most?" Alternatively, "When you think of serious illness, what is most important to you?"
- "Sometimes your family might need to make decisions about your medical care. What things would you want them to take into account?" These questions elicit how the patient defines his or her best interests or an acceptable quality of life.
- "Are there situations in which you would not want life-prolonging interventions?"

What Are the Patient's Preferences in Specific Clinical Situations?

It is unrealistic to try to discuss all future medical situations. The goal of discussions is not to be exhaustive, but to elicit informed choices about highly likely scenarios and to understand what considerations are important to the patient.

TABLE 12-1 Topics to Discuss in Advance Care Planning
Who should serve as proxy?
What are the patient's goals and values?
What are the patient's preferences in specific clinical situations?
How should advance directives be interpreted?
How do patients want to be treated near the end of life?

Discuss scenarios that are likely to occur. Rather than discussing dire or completely reversible situations, physicians should discuss common scenarios in which the outcome is uncertain, return to previous health is unlikely, and interventions are burdensome (5). What types of intervention would the patient be willing to accept, for how long, and for what likelihood, magnitude, and duration of improvement?

Physicians need to describe interventions and their likely outcomes. For mechanical ventilation, patients need to understand that they will have a tube in their throat, will not be able to speak, and will need sedation. Discussions should be tailored to the patient's condition. With elderly patients, physicians should discuss severe dementia and stroke. Would the patient want infections treated with antibiotics or intensive care? Would the patient want a feeding tube if he or she could not swallow food? How would the patient characterize severe dementia or stroke?

Correct unrealistic expectations. For example, a woman with lung cancer metastatic to liver and bone might say that she wants everything done. In such cases, physicians should elicit expectations, concerns, and emotions, using open-ended questions. The physician could say, "What do you think happens to patients whose cancer spreads like that?" or "I wish that were the case. Unfortunately when cancer has spread that much, even breathing machines don't help patients live much longer" (23, 27).

Physicians also need to point out that patients often adapt to situations that seem devastating to healthy persons. For instance, many patients with dementia or stroke find enjoyment and value in their lives, even though they would not have chosen that situation (15).

How Should Directives Be Interpreted?

Because advance care planning cannot cover all contingencies, it is important to understand how the patient would want the surrogate and physician to interpret her preferences. Physicians need to clarify ambiguous statements: "Can you tell me what you mean by 'no heroic treatment'?"

Physicians should also ask patients how much leeway they would allow surrogates to interpret their statements, extrapolate directives to unforeseen situations, take into account unforeseen changes in their situation, or override their directives if it seemed in their best interests (12). The patient might want their directives simply to be preferences or suggestions to be taken into account, but not binding. Alternatively, the patient may want directives followed unless there are compelling reasons to do the opposite. Finally, there may be some specific directives that the patient wants to be followed literally, even if the proxy believes they are contrary to what is best for the patient. Doctors should clarify, however, that it might not be possible to carry out directives, as discussed later.

How Do Patients Want to Be Treated Near the End of Life?

In some advance care planning forms, patients may indicate that they want their families to know that "I love them," "I wish to be forgiven for the times I might have hurt them," and "I forgive them for what they have done to me" (28). In addition, patients can fill out what they would like their family to say if anyone asks how they want to be remembered. These issues shift the focus from making clinical decisions to reaching closure at the end of life.

CONTINUE DISCUSSIONS OVER TIME

Physicians should not expect to advance care planning to be completed in a single conversation. In addition, patients' choices and values might change as their illness or life situation changes. If patients change their mind, then they should tell both the surrogate and the physician, destroy all copies of written advance directives, and complete a new advance directive.

Recommend Written Directives

Physicians should tell patients about the advantages of written advance directives and encourage patients to complete them.

TABLE 12-2	Resolving Conflicts Between Advance Directives and Best Interests of Patients Who Lack Decision-Making Capacity

When the patient gave advance directives, did she consider that

- her preferences might change?
- her proxy might believe that following her directives conflicted with her best interests?

Did the patient grant her surrogate leeway in making decisions?

Does the patient's current behavior suggest that her values and preferences have changed?

Does the patient's current situation present burdens or constraints that she did not foresee when giving advance directives?

For example, directives to provide interventions become problematic if the patient refuses to have blood drawn, pulls out intravenous lines, or cannot comply with postoperative rehabilitation.

Document Discussions in the Medical Record

The physician's note should describe the patient's decision-making capacity as well as the issues in Table 12-2. It is not necessary for the patient to sign the record.

CASE 12.1	*Continued*

Mrs. A's physician needs to discuss with her family whether she repeated these preferences over time. Furthermore, he needs to clarify what she objected to—Was it the nursing home itself or her friend's loss of awareness? The doctor should also explain that advance directives cannot be binding if they are not feasible.

Even though placement is not a medical decision, advance care planning helped her family think through the issues regarding placement. After discussing Mrs. A's statements in other contexts, it became clear that she strongly wanted to live in her own home and feared a loss of independence. To try to honor her directives, her family searched for alternatives to a nursing home. They explored switching off gas to the stove when they were away from home and setting up a GPS device connected to an alarm if she went beyond her yard. Ultimately, they found a residential care facility where Mrs. A seemed to like the caregivers.

In retrospect, when Mrs. A signed her POLST, it would have been desirable to have additional discussions. Did she realize that some nursing home residents appear contented even though they had strongly preferred not to live there? Did she realize that for some patients with severe dementia, living at home can endanger themselves and others? Although it is reasonable for her family to promise that will do their best to keep her out of a nursing home, they cannot promise to never to place her.

SUBSTITUTED JUDGMENT

Often patients have given only general directives or no indication of their preferences, so that someone else needs to make the decision.

In the absence of clear and specific advance directives, surrogates can try to construct the decision that the patient would make under the circumstances, taking into account all they know about the patient. The surrogate might imagine that the patient miraculously regains decision-making capacity. What care would the patient choose under the circumstances? Reconstructing patients' choices is ethically justified because it respects their individuality to the extent that this is possible (29). It respects the integrity, authenticity, and coherence of the patient's life as a unique individual

CASE 12.2　Disagreements over substituted judgment

Mr. S, a 76-year-old widower, suffers a massive stroke and aphasia. One week later, he still has paralysis of his right arm and leg. He does not respond consistently to simple requests or questions, but sometimes smiles when his hand is held. He develops pneumonia.

Throughout his life, he had been reluctant to see physicians and did not regularly take prescribed medications to lower his cholesterol. He loved to take walks and work in his garden. When his wife died of a sudden heart attack, he said, "Death isn't the enemy. She wanted to be active and healthy to the end, and the good Lord granted her wish." He was a proud and independent man who was reluctant to accept help from others. He has given no oral or written advance directives. His son and daughter believe Mr. S would refuse antibiotics for his pneumonia, even though he might still improve from his stroke. "He disliked being dependent on others and would hate being in a nursing home. In this condition, he can't do any of the things he loved in life."

(30). The metaphor of narrative has been suggested—the more coherent the narrative, the better. However, there might be a number of endings that are consistent with the patient's life story, and the choice of one ending among alternatives requires a subjective judgment and interpretation. Finally, surrogates should not dismiss the possibility of substantial change or growth near the end of life.

PROBLEMS WITH SUBSTITUTED JUDGMENT

Inconsistency

Reasonable people acting in good faith may disagree over what the patient would want. For example, Mr. S's sister might believe that he would want antibiotics. "He's been a fighter all his life and never gave up." She recalled that as a young man, Mr. S had overcome tremendous odds to come to America and get a college education.

Inaccuracy

Neither family members nor physicians can accurately state a competent patient's choices regarding future life-sustaining treatment (31). About one third of surrogates incorrectly state the patient's preferences (31). This level of agreement between proxies and patients would be expected by chance alone. Proxies' statements about patients' preferences are closer to what *they* would want in the situation than to what the patient actually wants (32). Even an intensive intervention to facilitate discussions between the patient and proxy about the patient's wishes for end-of-life care failed to increase the level of agreement (33).

Questionable Considerations

A competent patient might not want to be a burden or might want to spare the family the expenses and stress of terminal care. A patient also might prefer to provide a college fund for a granddaughter than to spend down savings to cover nursing home costs. It seems reasonable for surrogates to consider these factors when the patient himself has already done so, but it might be self-serving for surrogates to consider them when patients have not indicated their importance (34). Family members might confound what they would want with what the patient would want.

Unavoidable Speculation

Substituted judgments are inherently less certain than advance directives (35–37). Mr. S's comments about his wife do not necessarily express his own desires for medical care. In Case 12.2, the children's reasoning is unconvincing when applied to the converse situation. If a patient had seen physicians regularly, had taken medications faithfully, and was content with a sedentary life, it would not be logical to infer that he wanted all life-sustaining interventions in his current situation.

Conflicts With the Patient's Best Interests

In some cases, substituted judgments might lead to decisions that contradict the patient's current best interest. Suppose Mr. S's stroke were less severe and he had definitely improved; the family's reasoning that he would not want medical treatment for pneumonia and to be dependent on others would seem contrary to his best interests. It might be appropriate to withhold treatment in this situation on the basis of a clear and specific advance directive from a patient to reject antibiotics even though he might regain a high level of functioning. It would be problematic, however, to decline antibiotics in this situation solely on the basis of substituted judgment.

Despite the limitations of substituted judgments, they are still desirable because they respect the patient's individuality as a person with unique values and preferences and focus surrogates on what the patient would want, not what they might want for themselves (29).

CASE 12.2   *Continued*

First, Mr. S's physicians need to clarify the probability of his recovering to be able to be independent and do the things he enjoyed in life. Second, the doctors need to clarify his values and preferences. Mr. S's comments about his wife do not necessarily express his own choices for medical care. Even if he could no longer take walks and read, he might adapt to his illness and find life worthwhile. Many people learn to accept disabilities and assistance from others. His children's reasoning is unconvincing when applied to the converse situation. If a patient had seen physicians regularly, had taken medications faithfully, and had no active hobbies, it would not be logical to infer that he wanted all life-sustaining interventions in this situation.

The physician might pose the dilemma as how much burden Mr. S would accept for what probability and degree of recovery, and for how long. It might be reasonable to allow more time for him to recover, but to forego life-sustaining interventions in the future if the likelihood of an acceptable recovery of function is small.

BEST INTERESTS

A best interests standard may be appropriate in several situations. For some patients who have not given advance directives, a substituted judgment may be so speculative that it would be more honest for the surrogate and physician to acknowledge that they are basing decisions on what they believe is best for the patient (15). The ethical guideline of beneficence requires physicians to act weigh the benefits and burdens of interventions for the patient and for the patient's best interests. Best interests must be determined for the particular patient in a specific situation in light of the available options under the circumstances, which are often less than ideal (38). The best interests standard does not require physicians or surrogates to extend a patient's life as long as medically possible (15).

ASSESSING BEST INTERESTS

Problems may arise when surrogates make judgments about what is best for the patient based on their own values and preferences, rather than the patient's. For example, other people tend to underestimate how patients perceive their quality of life (*see* Chapter 4 for more details). Other questionable considerations arise when surrogates consider the interests of third parties, as discussed in the section on substituted judgment.

May the surrogate's own interests and needs be taken into account? Family members cannot be expected to ignore their own needs and interests. Best interests must be based on what is feasible, not on some theoretical ideal. Surrogates cannot be expected to put all their effort and resources to keeping a patient with dementia out of a nursing home, even though it would be best for the patient to reside with family.

Other dilemmas occur if surrogates request painful interventions that will only prolong the patient's life for a few days because they believe that suffering serves a spiritual purpose or that biologic life should be prolonged even if the interventions required are very burdensome. Decisions based on such beliefs need to be scrutinized carefully (39). Did the patient hold such views, as opposed to the surrogate? Did the patient say explicitly that he would accept painful interventions in this situation and decline palliative relief? Many patients who believe their illness serves a spiritual purpose still decline burdensome interventions. Health care workers might believe that they are acting inhumanely and causing the patient to suffer if they do not provide standard, effective palliative care when a patient is in great distress (39, 40). The ethical guideline of nonmaleficence allows health care workers to refrain from interventions that cause significant suffering and prolong the patient's life for only a few hours or days (*see* Chapter 14).

Incompetent patients who have not given advance directives and have no surrogates often pose difficult cases (41). Some doctors believe all life-sustaining interventions that are technically feasible should be provided to such patients unless they are futile. Insisting on life-sustaining interventions, however, simply because it is not certain that the patient would decline them would impose burdensome interventions on many patients and make them "prisoners of technology" (42). In this situation, it is appropriate for physicians to make decisions on the basis of what they believe is in the patient's best interests. Obtaining a second opinion from another physician or from the hospital ethics committee helps assure that the decision is not an idiosyncratic reflection of the physician's own personal views.

CONFLICTS BEWTEEN ADVANCE DIRECTIVES BEST INTERESTS

In some cases, an incapacitated patient's advance directives may conflict with his current best interests.

CASE 12.1   *Continued*

Several years later, Mrs. A's dementia has progressed. Because she required assistance with dressing, bathing, eating, and toileting, she had to be moved to a nursing home. She seems content there much of the time, socializing with other residents, watching television, and participating in group activities. However, she often complains about the food and staff, sometimes refusing to eat, and curses at aides who are helping her dress and bathe. She usually smiles when her children and grandchildren visit, although she frequently does not recognize them.

Mrs. A falls, has left hip pain, and cannot bear weight. Most likely she has a hip fracture. The on-call physician does not know Mrs. A and her family and cannot contact her primary physician or daughter. Her POLST specifies no intubation, no intensive care, no surgery, and hospitalization only for comfort measures. The on-call physician believes that it is in Mrs. A's best interests to have her hip stabilized surgically. Without surgery, she will have pain whenever she moves her leg, decreased mobility, and worse functioning and quality of life.

A person's values and preferences may change after he develops an incapacitating illness. People generally cannot anticipate how they will react to a radically different situation (7). Healthy persons tend to underestimate how persons with disabilities adapt and find meaning when living with disabilities (43). More radically, some scholars believe that preferences expressed by a young, healthy person should not carry much weight many years later after she develops severe dementia. In this view, she has changed so much that she should be considered a different person from the healthy person who provided the advance directives (15).

The mere possibility that a person's values and preferences may have changed after developing a disabling illness does not justify ignoring her advance directives. Table 12-2 presents a framework for resolving conflicts between advance directives and best interests. An advance directive should be followed unless there is a good reason to override it. Advance directives, however, should carry less weight the less relevant they are to the current situation and the more leeway the patient gave surrogates in making decisions.

CASE 12.1 | *Continued*

Table 12-2 suggests how to think through whether to override Mrs. A's advance directives to repair her hip fracture and how to discuss these issues with her family. First, when Mrs. A completed her POLST, did she realize that her preferences might change or that her directives might conflict with her best interests? If she did not, as is usually the case, her directives should carry less weight. Because they failed to take into account key features of her current situation, they are now less pertinent. Second, did Mrs. A grant her surrogate leeway in making decisions? If so, this is also a reason for her directive to carry less weight. Third, does Mrs. A's current behavior suggest that her values and preferences have changed? Sometimes, Mrs. A seems content in the nursing home, which must be balanced against her complaints and noncooperation. To the extent that her family believes that she finds value in her life at the nursing home, her values seem to have changed, and her previous directives would be less pertinent. Fourth, Mrs. A's current situation presents burdens and constraints that she did not foresee when giving advance directives. Surgery would prevent pain and loss of function, assuming that no serious complications occur. Again, her directives would be less pertinent to this unforeseen situation.

Most likely, when she completed the POLST, there was no discussion of how surgery for a hip fracture might be considered palliative care. Because outcomes are better if hip fracture is repaired promptly, the physician transfers Mrs. A to the hospital while continuing to try to contact her daughter to give permission for surgery.

SUMMARY

1. Advance directives encourage patients to think about what values and goals are important to them to discuss them with their physicians and family members. Furthermore, advance directives allow patients to identify whom they trust to make decisions for them.
2. Surrogates often must take responsibility for making difficult decisions regarding what the patient would have wanted or what is best for the patient in her current situation.
3. Physicians and surrogates need to guard against two types of errors: withholding treatments that would likely provide a net benefit or continuing treatments that the patient would not want or whose burdens outweigh the benefits.

REFERENCES

1. Steinbrook R, Lo B, Moulton J, et al. Preferences of homosexual men with AIDS for life-sustaining treatment. *N Engl J Med.* 1986;314:457–460.
2. Emanuel LL, Barry MJ, Stoeckle JD, et al. Advance directives for medical care—a case for greater use. *N Engl J Med.* 1991;324:889–895.
3. Lo B, Steinbrook RL. Resuscitating advance directives. *Arch Intern Med.* 2004;164:1501–1506.
4. Sabatino CP. The evolution of health care advance planning law and policy. *Milbank Q.* 2010;88:211–239.
5. Fischer GS, Tulsky JA, Rose MR, et al. Patient knowledge and physician predications of treatment preferences after discussions of advance directives. *J Gen Intern Med.* 1998;13:447–454.
6. Weeks JC, Cook EF, O'Day SJ, et al. Relationship between cancer patients' predictions of prognosis and their treatment preferences. *JAMA.* 1998;279:1709–1714.
7. Halpern J, Arnold RM. Affective forecasting: an unrecognized challenge in making serious health decisions. *J Gen Intern Med.* 2008;23:1708–1712.

8. Perkins HS. Controlling death: the false promise of advance directives. *Ann Intern Med.* 2007;147:51–57.

9. Fried TR, Van Ness PH, Byers AL, et al. Changes in preferences for life-sustaining treatment among older persons with advanced illness. *J Gen Intern Med.* 2007;22:495–501.

10. Schneiderman LJ, Kronick R, Kaplan RM, et al. Effects of offering advance directives on medical treatments and costs. *Ann Intern Med.* 1992;117:599–606.

11. Fischer GS, Alpert HR, Stoeckle JD, et al. Can goals of care be used to predict intervention preferences in an advance directive? *Arch Intern Med.* 1997;157:810–807.

12. Sehgal A, Galbraith A, Chesney M, et al. How strictly do dialysis patients want their advance directives followed. *JAMA.* 1992;267:59–63.

13. Brock DW, Wartman, S.A. When competent patients make irrational choices. *N Engl J Med.* 1990;322:1595–1599.

14. Swanson JW, McCrary SV, Swartz MS, et al. Superseding psychiatric advance directives: ethical and legal considerations. *J Am Acad Psychiatry Law.* 2006;34:385–394.

15. The President's Council on Bioethics. *Taking Care: Ethical Caregiving in Our Aging Society.* Washington, DC: The President's Council on Bioethics; 2005.

16. Lo B, Mc Leod G, Saika G. Patient attitudes towards discussing life-sustaining treatment. *Arch Intern Med.* 1986;146:1613–1615.

17. Reilly BM, Magnussen CR, Ross J, et al. Can we talk? Inpatient discussions about advance directives in a community hospital. Attending physicians' attitudes, their inpatients' wishes, and reported experience. *Arch Intern Med.* 1994;154:2299–2308.

18. Hoffman JC, Wenger NS, Davis RH, et al. Patient preferences for communication with physicians about end-of-life decisions. *Ann Intern Med.* 1997;127:1–12.

19. Johnston SC, Pfeifer MP, McNutt R. The discussion about advance directives. Patient and physician opinions regarding when and how it should be conducted. End of Life Study Group. *Arch Intern Med.* 1995;155:1025–1030.

20. Virmani J, Schneiderman LJ, Kaplan RM. Relationship of advance directives to physician–patient communication. *Arch Intern Med.* 1994;154:909–913.

21. Tulsky JA, Fischer GS, Rose MR, et al. Opening the black box: how do physicians communicate about advance directives. *Ann Intern Med.* 1998;129:441–449.

22. Sudore RL, Fried TR. Redefining the "planning" in advance care planning: preparing for end-of-life decision making. *Ann Intern Med.* 2010;153:256–261.

23. Tulsky JA. Beyond advance directives: importance of communication skills at the end of life. *JAMA.* 2005;294:359–365.

24. Lynn J, Schuster JL. *Improving Care for the End of Life: A Sourcebook for Health Care Managers and Clinicians.* New York, NY: Oxford University Press; 1999.

25. Bowman KW, Singer PA. Chinese seniors' perspective on end-of-life decisions. *Soc Sci Med.* 2001;53:455–464.

26. Lo B, Snyder L, Sox H. Care at the end of life: guiding practice where there are no easy answers. *Ann Intern Med.* 1999;130:772–774.

27. Back AL, Arnold RM, Quill TE. Hope for the best, and prepare for the worst. *Ann Intern Med.* 2003;138:439–443.

28. Aging with Dignity. *Five Wishes.* http://www.agingwithdignity.org/. Accessed October 12, 2007.

29. Blustein J. Choosing for others as continuing a life story: the problem of personal identity revisited. *J Law Med Ethics.* 1999;27:13–19.

30. Brudney D. Choosing for another: beyond autonomy and best interests. *Hastings Cent Rep.* 2009;39:31–37.

31. Shalowitz DI, Garrett-Mayer E, Wendler D. The accuracy of surrogate decision makers: a systematic review. *Arch Intern Med.* 2006;166:493–497.

32. Fagerlin A, Ditto PH, Danks JH, et al. Projection in surrogate decisions about life-sustaining medical treatments. *Health Psychol.* 2001;20:166–175.

33. Ditto PH, Danks JH, Smucker WD, et al. Advance directives as acts of communication: a randomized controlled trial. *Arch Intern Med.* 2001;161:421–430.

34. Lo B. Caring for the incompetent patient: is there a doctor in the house? *Law Med Health Care.* 1990;17:214–220.

35. Buchanan AE, Brock DW. *Deciding for Others.* Cambridge, UK: Cambridge University Press; 1989.

36. Annas GJ. Quality of life in the courts: earle spring in fantasyland. *Hastings Cent Rep.* 1980;10:9–10.

37. Annas GJ. The case of Mary Hier: when substituted judgment becomes sleight of hand. *Hastings Cent Rep.* 1984;14:23–25.

38. Kopelman LM. The best interests standard for incompetent or incapacitated persons of all ages. *J Law Med Ethics.* 2007;35:187–196.

39. Alpers A, Lo B. Avoiding family feuds: responding to surrogates' demands for life-sustaining treatment. *J Law Med Ethics.* 1999;27:74–80.

40. Braithwaite S, Thomasma DC. New guidelines on foregoing life-sustaining treatment in incompetent patients: an anti-cruelty policy. *Ann Intern Med.* 1986;104:711–715.

41. White DB, Curtis JR, Wolf LE, et al. Life support for patients without a surrogate decision maker: who decides? *Ann Intern Med.* 2007;147:34–40.

42. Angell M. Prisoners of technology: the case of Nancy Cruzan. *N Engl J Med.* 1990;322:1226–1228.

43. Ubel PA, Loewenstein G, Schwarz N, et al. Misimagining the unimaginable: the disability paradox and health care decision making. *Health Psychol.* 2005;24:S57–S62.

ANNOTATED BIBLIOGRAPHY

1. Lo B, Steinbrook RL. Resuscitating advance directives. *Arch Intern Med.* 2004;164:1501–1506.

Castillo LS, Williams BA, Hooper SM, et al. Lost in translation: the unintended consequences of advance directive law on clinical care. *Ann Intern Med.* 2011;154:121–128.

Analyzes limitations of advance directives and argues that emphasis should be on appointing a proxy whom the patient trusts to make decisions.

2. Brudney D. Choosing for another: beyond autonomy and best interests. *Hastings Cent Rep.* 2009;39:31–37.

Analyzes standards for decisions regarding incompetent patients. Argues that authenticity rather than autonomy should make decisions for patients who lack decision-making capacity.

3. Tulsky JA. Beyond advance directives: importance of communication skills at the end of life. *JAMA.* 2005;294:359–365.

Sudore RL, Fried TR. Redefining the "planning" in advance care planning: preparing for end-of-life decision making. *Ann Intern Med.* 2010;153:256–261.

Advance planning should focus more on goals of care than on specific treatments and address the patient's and family's emotional needs.

4. The President's Council on Bioethics. *Taking Care: Ethical Caregiving in Our Aging Society.* Washington, DC: The President's Council on Bioethics; 2005.

Discusses the difficulties in determining what is best in a specific situation for a patient who lacks decision-making capacity. Argues for a case-by-case determination at the bedside by the family and physician.

13

Surrogate Decision Making

When patients lack decision-making capacity, physicians turn to surrogates to make decisions on their behalf. Traditionally, family members serve as surrogate decision makers for such patients. This book uses the term *surrogate* for anyone who makes decisions for a patient who lacks decision-making capacity and reserves the term *proxy* for a surrogate appointed by the patient. This distinction is most helpful when there is disagreement over who should make decisions for the patient. This chapter deals with who should serve as surrogate and how physicians should discuss decisions with surrogates. Chapter 12 discusses the related issue of what standards should be used in making decisions for patients who lack decision-making capacity.

CASE 13.1	Disagreement between family members

Mrs. R is a 72-year-old widow with severe Alzheimer disease. She does not recognize her family, but often smiles when someone holds her hand or gives her a hug. She lives with her sister, who provides help with all activities of daily living together with an attendant. Mrs. R develops pneumonia. She had never signed an advance directive indicating what she would want in such a situation or whom she would want to make decisions for her. Her sister believes that Mrs. R would not want her life prolonged in this condition because she prized her independence and asks the physician to withhold antibiotics. Mrs. R's only child is a son who visits once or twice a year. He is outraged at this request. He asserts, "Life is sacred; it's God's gift. We can't just snuff it out."

Because Mrs. R had not indicated what she would care she would accept or refuse, a surrogate needs to make decisions on care. Both the sister and the son desire to act as her surrogate. The sister asserts priority because she cared for Mrs. R and has been close to her sister most of her life, yet the son has closer ties of kinship. What considerations justify selecting one surrogate over the other?

WHO SHOULD SERVE AS SURROGATE?

Among potential surrogates, there is a hierarchy that physicians should keep in mind. These decisions, however, are often best made by consensus rather than by giving one potential surrogate unilateral power.

COURT-APPOINTED GUARDIANS

Court-appointed guardians have legal priority over other potential surrogates. The courts have legal authority to declare a patient incompetent and to appoint a guardian to make medical decisions for the patient. The legal system offers procedural safeguards, such as notice to all parties, the right to call and cross-examine witnesses, impartial judges, explicit justification for decisions, and an appeals process. Involving the courts routinely in decisions, however, has serious drawbacks (1, 2). First, the courts intrude on highly personal and private issues. The adversarial judicial system might polarize families and physicians rather than foster a mutually acceptable decision. Second, guardianship hearings are usually superficial, and courts do not monitor guardians' decisions (3). Finally, intolerable delays would occur if the courts were frequently involved in decisions on life-sustaining treatment. As one court decision declared, "Courts are not the proper place to resolve the agonizing personal problems that underlie these cases. Our legal system cannot replace the more intimate struggle that must be borne by the patient, those caring for the patient, and those who care about the patient" (4). Physicians and hospitals should seek court intervention only as a last resort, when disputes cannot be resolved in a clinical setting.

SURROGATES SELECTED BY PATIENTS

As Chapter 12 discusses, all states allow competent patients to appoint a health care proxy with legal authority to make decisions if they lose decision-making capacity (5, 6). Generally, the patient must complete a form and have it witnessed or notarized. In California and several other states, a patient may appoint a proxy through an oral statement to a physician. Many patients find it easier to select who should act as proxy rather than anticipate what their preference is in future scenarios. Appointing a proxy commonly prevents future disputes among potential surrogates.

FAMILY MEMBERS

Decisions by families of patients who lack decision-making capacity are standard medical practice (7). There are compelling ethical justifications for family decision making (8).

Most People Want Family Members to Serve as Surrogates

In one survey, 30% of respondents wanted their families to make medical decisions for them if they became incapacitated, and an additional 53% wanted their family to make decisions together with their physician (9). Only 3% of respondents wanted the courts to decide. Patients trust family members to do their best under circumstances that could not be foreseen (10).

Family Members Often Know What the Patient Would Want

Because family members generally have close relationships with patients, they are more likely than other people to have discussed life-sustaining interventions with patients.

Family Members Are Presumed to Act in the Patient's Best Interests

Ties of kinship and affection generally lead relatives to care about the patient, deliberate carefully, and do what is best for the patient (8). Social, cultural, and religious norms encourage family members to subordinate their own interests for the sake of relatives in need. The term *family* should be interpreted in light of the large number of unmarried couples living together. Ethically, the crucial issue is not the relationship's legal status, but whether it is reasonable to presume that the partner will act in the patient's best interests.

Decision Making by the Family as a Group

For many families, singling out one person as a surrogate would be inappropriate. Family connections have both ethical and practical significance. Proponents of an ethics of care (*see* Chapter 1) argue that more attention should be paid to how decisions affect various relationships and that families should have a stronger voice in decisions (11, 12). In this view, surviving relatives have continuing relationships that deserve respect, and physicians should try to maintain family harmony. From a pragmatic viewpoint, many proxies who are appointed by the patient are reluctant to contradict the views of close relatives. They might feel torn between what they think is best for the patient and what other family members want to do (13, 14).

NO FAMILY MEMBERS AVAILABLE

Decisions are most difficult when patients with impaired decision-making capacity have no advance directives and no family members. In some cases, a friend would be an appropriate surrogate. If the friend has an emotional bond with the patient, then it is plausible to presume that the friend will act in the patient's best interests.

If no one is available as surrogate, then physicians do not need to administer burdensome interventions that offer little prospect of benefit just because there is no surrogate to decline them on behalf of the patient. In this situation, physicians may forego interventions that they do not consider to be in the patient's best interests. When there is no surrogate, it is advisable for physicians to consult with the hospital ethics committee or another physician (15). Simply explaining one's reasoning to another person can clarify thinking, identify unwarranted assumptions and unconvincing arguments, and suggest new options for care.

LEGAL ISSUES

Most states have laws that specify which relatives have priority to act as surrogates for incapacitated patients who have not provided advance directives (5, 6). Generally, the patient's spouse takes priority over adult children, followed by adult siblings. Some states give domestic partners the same authority as spouses or allow close friends as surrogates if there are no relatives. Such laws, however, might lead to ethically troubling results, such as favoring the distant son in Case 13.1 over the sister who has a closer day-to-day relationship with the patient. These laws might also be problematic when a spouse is estranged but not legally divorced or when the patient has a domestic partner who is not recognized by the surrogate statute.

In some cases, the patient indicates the selection of a surrogate to the physician but does not complete a legal document appointing the person. If this person and the surrogate under state law disagree over plans for care, ethically speaking, the person whom the patient wanted to serve as surrogate should have priority. The physician should try to persuade the surrogate named in the state law to respect the patient's choice of proxy.

PROBLEMS WITH SURROGATE DECISION MAKING

EMOTIONAL BARRIERS TO DECISIONS

At least one third of surrogates experience adverse emotional consequences, most commonly stress, guilt over the decision that was made, or doubt whether they made the right decision (16).

DECISIONS INCONSISTENT WITH PATIENT'S VALUES

In Case 13.1, if Mrs. R held such views on prolonging life, then they would be followed out of respect for her autonomy (*see* Chapter 4). If, however, she disagreed with her son's beliefs about the sanctity of life, it would be inappropriate for a surrogate to impose his own values on the patient rather than respect the patient's choices and values. Thus, the physician needs to inquire whether the patient herself held such religious views.

CONFLICTS OF INTEREST

In some cases, relatives might promote their own interests, not the patient's (17). Unscrupulous family members might try to gain control of an inheritance or a pension. When it comes to the basis for their decisions, surrogates are given less leeway than competent patients. For example, patients may choose to forego interventions to spare family members emotional distress or to preserve an inheritance. Such refusals are heeded to respect patient autonomy. As Chapter 12 discusses, however, claims by surrogates that the patient would refuse beneficial interventions for these reasons might be self-serving and need to be based on statements by the patient.

Family members cannot be expected to ignore their own needs and interests. Caring for a relative with serious chronic illness can cause emotional distress, fatigue, financial burdens, or conflicts with other responsibilities (18, 19). Most family members subordinate their interests to those of the patient and make considerable sacrifices. Physicians should not be overly suspicious about surrogates. Respecting close family relationships is an important social value, and physicians should support families who are trying to deal with difficult situations as best as they can. Simply making sacrifices to care for a relative or being mentioned in a will is not a conflict of interest.

DISAGREEMENTS AMONG POTENTIAL SURROGATES

Case 13.1 illustrates how family members might disagree over decisions. Some physicians withhold interventions only when all family members agree. Giving every relative a veto, however, might impose interventions that are not in the patient's best interests. Furthermore, it is problematic to give distant or estranged relatives a voice equal to that of those with the closest relationship to the patient. Realistically, physicians often make decisions with family consensus rather than unanimity (20). Relatives are often willing to accept a decision made by the rest of the family, even though they would have decided differently themselves.

IMPROVING SURROGATE DECISION MAKING

Table 13.1 provides several suggestions for improving surrogate decision making.

DISCUSS THE DECISION-MAKING PROCESS

A family meeting can help relatives understand and accept the medical situation (21, 22). Physicians should acknowledge that decisions are difficult and that people with good intentions might disagree. Doctors can help families express their preferred role in decision making, articulate their emotions, and cope with their grief (21). In an ICU, the vast majority of surrogates of intubated patients want to play an active role in decision making (23). Physicians should remind everybody that decisions should be based on the patient's preferences and interests, not on what surrogates or doctors would choose for themselves.

GIVE A RECOMMENDATION

Physicians should not merely list options and leave it to surrogates to decide. Doctors can help surrogates deliberate by summarizing and reframing surrogates' statements about the patient's values and links values to decisions at hand (24). Going further, doctors should offer to make a recommendation on the basis of what is known about the patient's preferences and values. About 40% of surrogates, however, prefer not to receive a recommendation (25). It may be helpful for physicians to give the family permission to let the patient die if that is consistent with the patient's values. In some cases, when surrogates are unwilling to limit life-sustaining interventions because they do not want to take responsibility for the patient's death, the physician might ask surrogates to assent to foregoing life-sustaining interventions: The physician will take responsibility for writing such an order unless the surrogates object (26).

TABLE 13-1   Suggestions for Improving Surrogate Decision Making
Discuss the decision-making process.
Give a recommendation.
Get help from other health care workers.

GET HELP FROM OTHER HEALTH CARE WORKERS

A nurse, social worker, or chaplain can often help the family address their spiritual needs, accept the medical situation and work through past antagonisms with the patient or among themselves, as well as provide support.

CASE 13.1   *Continued*

First Mrs. R's physician asked the family what they believed Mrs. R's medical situation was and what concerns they had about her condition. The doctor then framed task as making decisions consistent with her values and best interests, which might not be what the family would want for themselves. He asked what she would regard as important to consider in this situation. He asked specifically about prior statements she had made and her religious views. He also said that this illness is usually hard on family members and asked how they were feeling caring for or watching Mr. R. He planned to have repeated discussions with them and suggested they might talk to others who might have insight about her views, for example, her religious or spiritual advisor.

SUMMARY

1. Surrogates should be willing to respect the patient's preferences and act in the patient's best interests.
2. In most cases, the standard clinical practice of family decision making is ethically appropriate.
3. When family members disagree, physicians should try to achieve consensus.

REFERENCES

1. Lo B, Rouse F, Dornbrand L. Family decision-making on trial: who decides for incompetent patients? *N Engl J Med* 1990;322:1228–1231.
2. Bandy RJ, Helft PR, Bandy RW, et al. Medical decision-making during the guardianship process for incapacitated, hospitalized adults: a descriptive cohort study. *J Gen Intern Med* 2010;25:1003–1008.
3. Bulcroft K, Kielkopf MR, Tripp K. Elderly wards and their legal guardians: analysis of county probate records in Ohio and Washington. *Gerontologist* 1991;31:156–164.
4. In re Jobes. 529 A. 2d 434 (N.J. 1987).
5. Commission on Law and Aging. Default Surrogate Consent Statutes as of November 2009. Available at: http:// new.abanet.org/aging/Pages/HealthDecisions.aspx. Accessed October 29, 2011.
6. Lo B, Steinbrook RL. Resuscitating advance directives. *Arch Intern Med* 2004;164:1501–1506.
7. Meisel A. *The Right to Die*. 3rd ed. New York NY: Aspen Publishers; 2004.
8. Arnold RM, Kellum J. Moral justifications for surrogate decision making in the intensive care unit: implications and limitations. *Crit Care Med* 2003;31:S347–353.
9. Blendon RJ, Szalay US, Knox RA. Should physicians aid their patients in dying? The public perspective. *JAMA* 1992;267:2658–2662.
10. Singer PA, Martin DK, Lavery JV, et al. Reconceptualizing advance care planning from the patient's perspective. *Arch Intern Med* 1998;158:879–884.
11. Jecker N. The role of intimate others in medical decision making. *Gerontologist* 1990;30:65–71.
12. Hardwig J. What about the family? *Hastings Center Report* 1990;20:5–10.
13. Alpers A, Lo B. Avoiding family feuds: responding to surrogates' demands for life–sustaining treatment. *Journal of Law, Medicine & Ethics* 1999;27:74–80.
14. Vig EK, Starks H, Taylor JS, et al. Surviving surrogate decision–making: what helps and hampers the experience of making medical decisions for others. *J Gen Intern Med* 2007;22:1274–1279.
15. White DB, Curtis JR, Wolf LE, et al. Life support for patients without a surrogate decision maker: who decides? *Ann Intern Med* 2007;147:34–40.
16. Wendler D, Rid A. Systematic review: the effect on surrogates of making treatment decisions for others. *Ann Intern Med* 2011;154:336–346.
17. Lo B. Caring for the incompetent patient: is there a doctor in the house? *Law, Medcine, & Health Care* 1989;17:214–220.

18. Covinsky KE, Goldman L, Cook FS, et al. The impact of serious illness on patients' families. *JAMA* 1994;272:1839–1844.

19. Covinsky KE, Landefeld CS, Teno J, et al. Is economic hardship on the families of the seriously ill associated with patient and surrogate care preferences? *Arch Intern Med* 1996;156:1737–1741.

20. Torke AM, Alexander GC, Lantos J, et al. The physician-surrogate relationship. *Arch Intern Med* 2007;167:1117–1121.

21. Curtis JR, White DB. Practical guidance for evidence-based ICU family conferences. *Chest* 2008;134:835–843.

22. Lilly CM, Daly BJ. The healing power of listening in the ICU. *N Engl J Med* 2007;356:513–515.

23. Johnson SK, Bautista CA, Hong SY, et al. An empirical study of surrogates' preferred level of control over value-laden life support decisions in intensive care units. *Am J Respir Crit Care Med* 2011;183:915–921.

24. White DB, Malvar G, Karr J, et al. Expanding the paradigm of the physician's role in surrogate decision-making: an empirically derived framework. *Crit Care Med* 2010;38:743–750.

25. White DB, Evans LR, Bautista CA, et al. Are physicians' recommendations to limit life support beneficial or burdensome? Bringing empirical data to the debate. *Am J Respir Crit Care Med* 2009;180:320–325.

26. Curtis JR, Burt RA. Point: the ethics of unilateral "do not resuscitate" orders: the role of "informed assent". *Chest* 2007;132:748–751.

ANNOTATED BIBLIOGRAPHY

1. Lo B, Rouse F, Dornbrand L. Family decision making on trial: who decides for incompetent patients? *N Engl J Med*. 1990;322:1228–1231.
Argues that families should be presumed to be appropriate decision makers for patients who lack decision-making capacity.

2. Buchanan AE, Brock DW. *Deciding for Others: The Ethics of Surrogate Decision Making*. Cambridge, UK: Cambridge University Press; 1989.
Detailed ethical analysis of surrogate decision making.

3. Commission on Law and Aging Default Surrogate Consent Statutes as of November 2009. http://new.abanet.org/aging/Pages/HealthDecisions.aspx. Accessed October 29, 2011.
Recent analysis of state laws regarding surrogate decision making.

4. Arnold RM, Kellum J. Moral justifications for surrogate decision making in the intensive care unit: implications and limitations. *Crit Care Med*. 2003;31:S347–S353.
Clear and thoughtful review of surrogate decision making.

5. Torke AM, Alexander GC, Lantos J, et al. The physician–surrogate relationship. *Arch Intern Med*. 2007;167:1117–1121.
Analysis of the relationship between the physician and surrogate of a patient who lacks decision-making capacity, with suggestions on how to strengthen it.

Persistent Disagreements Over Care

Disagreements over life-sustaining interventions are common, occurring in as many as one-half of ICU cases (1). Although disagreements are resolved in almost all cases (2, 3), in a few cases sharp disagreements persist. This chapter discusses cases in which either physicians or patients or their surrogates insist on interventions that the other party considers inappropriate.

Other chapters discuss related issues. Chapter 4 analyzes patient refusals that are not in their best interests. Chapter 9 discusses demands by patients or surrogates for "futile" interventions.

PATIENT OR SURROGATE INSISTENCE ON LIFE-SUSTAINING INTERVENTIONS

CLINICAL CONSIDERATIONS

Physicians are exhorted to improve palliative care near the end of life and help patients achieve a peaceful death (4–6). In some cases, however, patients or surrogates insist on life-sustaining interventions that physicians believe cause suffering (5, 6).

CASE 14.1	Desire for cardiopulmonary resuscitation (CPR) and mechanical ventilation in end-stage lung disease

Mr. H was a 29-year-old man with end-stage cystic fibrosis who was admitted to the hospital for antibiotics and respiratory therapy. He was emaciated, required home oxygen, and was dyspneic walking around his home. During conversations, he often paused to catch his breath or to cough up thick secretions. Lung transplantation was not an option for him because of recurrent aspiration pneumonia. He understood that his shortness of breath would get worse. He appreciated that physicians believed that CPR or mechanical ventilation had very little chance of success. He further realized that the physicians believed that if he required intubation and mechanical ventilation, he could not be weaned off the ventilator. He responded, "My entire life has been a struggle. No one thought I would live this long. I've always beaten the odds. I've always been a fighter. I'll keep fighting until the man upstairs tells me it's time to stop."

Mr. H rejected a palliative approach and was willing to accept a very small hope of success. His core values included overcoming situations that others believed were hopeless. Other patients also want life-sustaining interventions that offer a very small hope of success.

The SUPPORT study documented shortcomings in palliative care at the end of life. This study enrolled more than 9,000 hospitalized patients with an advanced stage of one of nine illnesses (4). These patients had a hospital mortality of more than 25% and a 6-month mortality of almost 50%. For many patients who died, their last days included "undesirable states": 38% spent at least 10 days in an intensive care unit, 46% received mechanical ventilation within 3 days before death, and 45% were unconscious during their last 3 days of life (4, 7). Relatives reported that 50% of conscious dying patients experienced moderate or severe pain during their last 3 days of life. These findings were widely interpreted inappropriately as aggressive use of technology and failure to relieve suffering near the end of life (4–6).

The SUPPORT study also showed that many seriously ill patients desire interventions that have a low likelihood of success, perhaps because of overly optimistic estimates of prognosis. One study analyzed patients with metastatic cancer whose physicians predicted a 6-month survival of 10%. Thirty-six percent of such patients preferred life-extending therapy rather than relief of pain and discomfort as the primary goal of care (8). Among those patients who believed that they had a 90% chance of surviving for 6 months, 61% wanted life-extending therapy, compared with only 15% of patients who estimated their chance for surviving 6 months to be less than 90%.

ETHICAL CONSIDERATIONS

The ethical guideline of beneficence requires physicians to refrain from interventions that would not improve outcomes, particularly if they would cause serious suffering. In this section, we analyze three difficult situations: requests that "everything" be done, requests based on religious beliefs, and requests for interventions that cause suffering with little prospect of medical benefit.

CASE 14.2   **Family insistence that everything be done**

Bishop P is a 60-year-old African American man with diabetes, quadriplegia, and persistent infections. One year ago, he developed Staphylococcus aureus meningitis, epidural abscess, and pneumonia. During his hospitalization, he developed quadriplegia, respiratory failure, renal failure, and persistent fevers.

Ten months later, Bishop P was rehospitalized with urosepsis from Enterobacter cloacae. Hypotension, respiratory failure, renal failure, stroke, and seizures complicated his course. He required mechanical ventilation and dialysis. Despite multiple courses of antibiotics, his blood cultures remained positive for E. cloacae, resistant to all antibiotics. A drug reaction caused a total body rash, and his skin sheared away around his bandages and electrocardiographic leads. The physicians and nurses believed that further interventions would be inhumane and disfiguring, that he would not survive the hospitalization or attempts at CPR.

Bishop P's Pentecostalist church emphasizes faith healing. Bishop P was obtunded and could not state his preferences for care. His family insisted that everything be done because he believed that all life was sacred.

Bishop P's family wanted to act in accordance with his lifelong values, appropriately making a substituted judgment (*see* Chapter 12) (9).

Requests That "Everything" Be Done

When a patient or family requests that "everything" be done, physicians should first clarify what patients or surrogates mean by "everything." Many do not want literally everything done, acknowledging that some interventions might cause more suffering or harm than benefit. It is also useful to elicit the values and concerns that animate such requests. Some patients or surrogates might be concerned that if they do not insist on interventions, beneficial treatments will be withheld. Such concerns can be addressed directly.

Insistence on Interventions Based on Religion or Culture

As in Case 14.2, many patients base decisions about life-sustaining interventions on their religious, spiritual, or cultural beliefs (10, 11). Religiously based reasons deserve special respect because they reflect a person's core values and identity (9). Some patients or surrogates might want any intervention that prolongs life, even for a very short time. They may believe that life is a good in itself, regardless of its quality, and that human beings must preserve and prolong life until God determines its end (12). Other patients or surrogates might believe that a miraculous recovery will occur if their faith is strong enough. Insisting on interventions might be a way of demonstrating their faith.

To many African Americans, spiritual beliefs are an important source of comfort and a means of coping with illness (13). Many believe prayer has the power to promote healing and that miracles might occur. See Chapter 44 for a more extensive discussion of how cultural factors lead many African Americans to insist on life-sustaining interventions that physicians regard as medically inappropriate. African Americans might mistrust physicians and hospitals because of a history of discrimination and limited access to medical care (14).

Physicians need sufficient information about the patient's religious beliefs to understand their impact on specific clinical decisions. Individual beliefs might differ from official doctrines. People who hold a general belief, such as the sacredness of life, may differ in their preferences regarding specific interventions (15). To inquire how religion shapes a patient's decisions, a physician might say, "I understand that religion plays an important part in your father's life. Please tell me more about his beliefs." Physicians might need to understand the patient's specific beliefs regarding miracles, prayer, and divine intervention (16).

Request for Interventions That Cause the Patient Suffering

In Case 14.2, the family's request for CPR troubled caregivers, who believed that further medical interventions were causing pain and mutilation without improving his prognosis. The ethical guideline of nonmaleficence, as well as professional integrity, allows health care workers not to provide interventions that cause significant suffering but prolong the patient's life only briefly (9, 17). This rationale justifies overriding surrogate preferences and withholding interventions in exceptional cases.

Some surrogates state that the patient believes suffering serves a spiritual purpose. Caregivers should examine carefully surrogates' claims about the redemptive nature of suffering. The family's views might differ from the patient's. Many patients who believe their illness serves a spiritual purpose will still accept medications for pain and decline highly burdensome interventions (9).

RECOMMENDATIONS

Physicians can respond to requests by patients or families for life-sustaining interventions in several constructive ways (Table 14-1). The suggestions in Chapter 5 on informed consent might also be helpful.

Understand the Patient's or Surrogate's Perspective

When patients or surrogates continue to request life-sustaining interventions that the physician considers inadvisable, the doctor should first try to understand their perspective, including their understanding of the illness, concerns, goals, and expectations for care (18, 19). This approach is generally more effective than immediately trying to persuade them about specific clinical decisions

TABLE 14-1   Recommendations for Responding to Requests for Life-Sustaining Interventions
Understand the patient's or surrogate's perpective.
Respond to the patient's or surrogate's needs and emotions.
Be sensitive to cultural and religious issues.
Use time constructively.
Find common ground for ongoing care.

such as a Do Not Attempt Resuscitation order (20). Open-ended questions are helpful to elicit the patient's concerns and emotions (20):

- "What concerns you most about your illness?"
- "How is treatment going for you (your family)?"
- "As you think about your illness, what is the best and the worst that might happen?"
- "What has been most difficult about this illness for you?"
- "What are your hopes (your expectations, your fears) for the future?"
- "As you think about the future, what is most important to you (what matters the most to you)?"

Respond to the Patient's or Surrogate's Needs and Emotions

Empathic comments, which reflect the speaker's emotions, encourage patients or surrogates to explore emotions and to discuss difficult topics (20–22). In Case 14.1, when Mr. H has difficulty completing sentences, the physician might say, "It can be frightening to not get enough air." Some physicians might fear that exploring emotions might arouse in the patient and family feelings of anger, hopelessness, or sadness that doctors are powerless to alleviate. Patients and families, however, will have these emotions whether or not physicians choose to probe them. After these emotions are discussed openly, the patient and family no longer must face them alone. Talking about emotional reactions to serious illness is frequently therapeutic and helps patients and families accept a grave prognosis. Furthermore, anxiety and depression can be treated once they are identified. It is valuable for physicians to listen to patients and families. In turn, patients who feel they are understood might then be more willing to listen to the physician's perspective.

Physicians can respond to unrealistic expectations without destroying hope. One approach is to "Hope for the best, and prepare for the worst" (23). Also, physicians can use "I wish statements" to align with hopes of the patient or family, while suggesting that the desired outcome is unlikely (23, 24). In Case 14.1, the physician might say, "I wish I could make the odds be in your favor."

Be Sensitive to Cultural and Religious Issues

Bishop P and his family were African Americans. African Americans might mistrust physicians and hospitals because of a history of discrimination and limited access to medical care (14).

In Case 14.2, rather than leave concerns about discrimination and undertreatment unspoken, physicians might ask explicitly about the underlying issue of trust. "Many African Americans worry that they will not receive the care they need. Have you ever experienced that?" Physicians should not immediately try to reassure the family that all appropriate care will be provided (25). Reassurance is premature and generally ineffective until patients have discussed their concerns and emotions in detail (26).

Other cultural and religious traditions also have beliefs about the nature of suffering, the definition of death, the refusal of life-sustaining interventions, or the acceptance of pain (27–29). Physicians cannot be expected to have in-depth knowledge of every culture or religion; however, doctors can ask open-ended questions to understand the cultural and religious values that impact on a patient's or family's decisions (10, 11). "How does religion or spirituality play a role in your life?" Or, "In your religion or culture, is there anything that should be done now? Is there any ceremony that should be carried out?"

Use Time Constructively

Patients or surrogates frequently have little time to adjust to a new situation before making decisions about life-sustaining interventions. Rather than trying to make a definitive decision immediately, physicians might consider how to use time to help persuade them to forego life-sustaining interventions that are more burdensome than beneficial. Physicians might suggest a time-limited trial of interventions, setting parameters for improvement or worsening and a time frame to reassess outcomes (30). Also physicians can direct attention to palliative care. Doctors might say, "Your father is so seriously ill that it's possible that he might die in the hospital. Are there things that would be left undone if he were to die suddenly?" Social workers, chaplains, or the hospital ethics committee can also help the family reach closure.

Find Common Ground for Ongoing Care

The process of negotiation requires that both sides are willing to compromise (19, 30b). When patients or surrogates insist on life-sustaining interventions, a common compromise is to not add or increase interventions but also to not withdraw them (31). Although law and ethics do not distinguish between withholding life support and withdrawing it, the emotional difference might be significant to families.

In almost all cases, physicians eventually can reach an agreement with patients or surrogates on an acceptable plan of care (2, 3). In rare instances, physicians might conclude, after repeated discussions and an ethics committee consultation, that they cannot agree with the patient's or surrogate's request. If the physician is considered unilateral decisions to forego life-sustaining interventions, the procedures suggested in Chapter 9 should be followed. The patient or surrogate should be notified, invited to the ethics committee meeting, and informed of their right to seek another provider.

CASE 14.2   *Continued*

It is helpful to schedule regular family meetings, have one physician serve as spokesperson, and have different teams give consistent messages (32). Physicians should try to spend more time listening than talking. To ascertain the perspective of Bishop P's family and their needs, the physician might ask, "What are your feelings when you see your father so sick?" The doctor can also ask what they understand his skin condition is and whether they think it is painful. The physician should ask about their preferred role in making decisions. Because many surrogates find it stressful to make decisions, physicians might say, "Tell me what is most difficult about making decisions for your husband." If emotions like anxiety, fear, or guilt are identified, they should be explored further (33).

The physician should also ask if the family is hoping for a miracle. If so, the doctor should acknowledge that many families hope for that but also ask the family to clarify what they mean by a miracle (34). Rather than flatly disagreeing with the family's hopes, the physician might say, "I wish that we had more effective medicines for his infection."

While continuing life support, doctors might also "preparing for the possibility that the treatment doesn't work out as we all hope" (23). They might also say, "Your father is so seriously ill that no one would be surprised if he died in the hospital. What would be left undone if he were to die suddenly?" Consultation with palliative care or ethics committee generally is helpful.

PHYSICIAN INSISTENCE ON LIFE-SUSTAINING INTERVENTIONS

Physicians and hospitals might seek to administer life-sustaining interventions to an unwilling patient. This section focuses on insistence on interventions based on the physician's conscience or religious beliefs. Chapter 24 discusses conscience-based refusals to provide medical interventions.

CASE 14.3   Withdrawal of mechanical ventilation

William Bartling was a 70-year-old man with chronic obstructive lung disease. A needle aspirate of a new pulmonary nodule revealed adenocarcinoma. After the procedure, he suffered a pneumothorax and required a chest tube and mechanical ventilation. During the next 2 months, he could not be weaned from the respirator. Mr. Bartling requested that the respirator be disconnected and signed a living will, a durable power of attorney for health care, and a declaration of his wishes. His family also signed documents releasing the physicians and hospital from liability.

The hospital and physicians refused Mr. Bartling's request, arguing that they had an ethical duty to preserve life and that withholding life-sustaining treatment was incompatible with their own born-again Christian prolife beliefs. Attempts to transfer the patient to another hospital that would comply with his wishes were unsuccessful. The Bartling case posed the question of whether the caregivers may insist on providing life-sustaining interventions over a patient's refusal (35).

ARGUMENTS FOR INSISTENCE BY CAREGIVERS ON INTERVENTIONS

Respect the Autonomy of Caregivers

Health care professionals are moral agents with values, rights, and consciences. In this view, just as patients have the right to refuse interventions, physicians should also have the right to refuse to violate their professional ethics or personal morality. Because the United States respects freedom of religion, it would be particularly repugnant to require health care workers to carry out actions that violate their religious beliefs. Also, it would be counterproductive to require physicians to act against their moral views. A grudging or antagonistic doctor–patient relationship would not be therapeutic.

Respect the Mission of Health Care Institutions

Health care institutions might have a mission statement that expresses their goals and values. Hospices have an explicit philosophy of palliative care. Catholic hospitals have policies that forbid abortions. Many people believe that a pluralistic society should encourage such statements of mission so that patients can seek care at institutions whose moral and spiritual views match their own (36, 37).

OBJECTIONS TO INSISTENCE BY CAREGIVERS ON INTERVENTIONS

Insistence by caregivers on providing interventions over the informed objections of patients is ethically troubling for several reasons (Table 14-2).

Undermining the Right of Refusal

If caregivers could insist on treatment, the right of patients to refuse medical interventions would in effect be nullified. In Case 14.3, the court ruled that the patient's refusal of treatment must be respected: "If the right of the patient to self-determination as to his own medical treatment is to have any meaning at all, it must be paramount to the interests of the patient's hospital and doctors" (38).

Confusion Between Negative and Positive Rights

Philosophers make a distinction between negative and positive rights. *Negative rights* are claims to be left alone, to be free from unwanted interference or intrusions. An example is the constitutional right to be free of unreasonable searches and seizures. Negative rights might require other people to refrain from intervening, exerting control, or thwarting the person holding the rights. Patients claim the negative right to be free of unwanted medical interventions. To be exercised, this negative right requires physicians to refrain from providing the treatment.

Positive or *affirmative rights*, on the other hand, are claims to receive something or act in a certain way. Positive rights might require others to take action or provide means or resources, not simply to refrain from interfering (39). In Case 14.3, the physicians claimed the positive right to continue medical interventions, even though Mr. Bartling did not want it.

TABLE 14-2   Objections to Caregivers' Insistence on Life-Sustaining Interventions
Undermining the right of refusal
Confusion between negative and positive rights
Lack of timely and clear notification of patients

Negative rights are generally considered to carry more moral weight than positive rights (40). Usually, negative liberty is limited only by promises or special role-specific obligations; for example, parents cannot claim a negative right to be freed from providing their children's basic needs. In contrast, positive rights are more difficult to justify and enforce because they generally require other people to do something or interfere with the negative rights of others.

RECOMMENDATIONS WHEN PHYSICIANS INSIST ON INTERVENTIONS
Timely and Clear Notification of Patients

Physicians who work in a situation in which this conflict is likely to arise should make their position known before starting a doctor–patient relationship. Such notification would enable patients to make informed plans for their care and to seek another provider. Similarly, institutions that have policies insisting on certain interventions should describe in their publicity and notify patients on admission. Patients may have no option to seek another provider if they are brought by ambulance or are restricted by insurance.

Transferring Care of the Patient

Health care workers should be permitted to withdraw from a case in which they have deep moral objections to the plan of care, but they also have professional obligations not to abandon patients (*see* Chapter 24). Thus, they should facilitate transfer of the patient to a health care worker or an institution that is willing to forego withdrawal of the intervention in question.

Some physicians might not want to inform the surrogate of the option of transfer of care because they believe this would constitute cooperation with an immoral act. Physicians have an obligation, however, to inform patients (or surrogates) of alternatives to the proposed treatment. Generally, even if a physician personally would not carry out a medical intervention, the physician still needs to mention it if a respected minority of physicians would do so. The obligation would be even stronger if the intervention were generally considered an acceptable option. If the physician did not want to provide the information personally, then he or she could ask another physician or the ethics committee to do so.

Even when transfer of care can be arranged, it might be very burdensome for patients or their families. Patients might face a tragic choice if they must either accept unwanted interventions or else leave caregivers with whom they have developed a long-term relationship. In the Requena case, a 57-year-old woman with amyotrophic lateral sclerosis wanted tube feedings withheld if she could no longer swallow. The hospital asserted that her decision conflicted with its prolife values and sought to transfer her to another local hospital that would respect her decision. When she refused to accept the transfer, the hospital went to court to force her to leave. According to the court, because she had lived in the hospital for 17 months transfer would be upsetting and burdensome for her. The trial court judge suggested that "by rethinking their own attitudes," the hospital staff "might find it possible to be more fully accepting and supportive of Ms. Requena's decision." The court continued, "It is fairer to ask the health care workers to bend than to ask Ms. Requena to bend" (41).

SUMMARY

1. Health care workers almost always can find common ground with patients or surrogates.
2. In disagreements, physicians need to understand the patient's or surrogate's perspective.
3. As a last resort, physicians may withdraw from the case and transfer care to another provider.

REFERENCES

1. Breen CM, Abernethy AP, Abbott KH, et al. Conflict associated with decisions to limit life-sustaining treatment in intensive care units. *J Gen Intern Med.* 2001;16:283–289.
2. Smedira NG, Evans BH, Grais LS, et al. Withholding and withdrawing of life support from the critically ill. *N Engl J Med.* 1990;322:309–315.

3. Prendergast TJ, Luce JM. Increasing incidence of withholding and withdrawal of life support from the critically ill. *Am Rev Resp Dis Crit Care Med.* 1997;155:15–20.

4. The SUPPORT Principal Investigators. A controlled trial to improve care for seriously ill hospitalized patients. The study to understand prognoses and preferences for outcomes and risks of treatments (SUPPORT). *JAMA.* 1995;274:1591–1598.

5. Lo B. End-of-life care after termination of SUPPORT. *Hastings Cent Rep.* 1995;25:S6–S8.

6. Lo B. Improving care near the end of life: why is it so hard? *JAMA.* 1995;274:1634–1636.

7. Lynn J, Teno JM, Phillips RS, et al. Perceptions by family members of the dying experience of older and seriously ill patients. *Ann Intern Med.* 1997;126:97–106.

8. Weeks JC, Cook EF, O'Day SJ, et al. Relationship between cancer patients' predictions of prognosis and their treatment preferences. *JAMA.* 1998;279:1709–1714.

9. Alpers A, Lo B. Avoiding family feuds: responding to surrogates' demands for life-sustaining treatment. *J Law Med Ethics.* 1999;27:74–80.

10. Lo B, Ruston D, Kates LW, et al. Discussing religious and spiritual issues at the end of life: a practical guide for physicians. *JAMA.* 2002;287:749–754.

11. Lo B, Kates LW, Ruston D, et al. Responding to requests regarding prayer and religious ceremonies by patients near the end of life and their families. *J Palliat Med.* 2003;6:409–415.

12. Boozang KM. An intimate passing: restoring the role of family and religion in dying. *Univ Pittsbg Law Rev.* 1997;58:549–617.

13. Johnson KS, Elbert-Avila KI, Tulsky JA. The influence of spiritual beliefs and practices on the treatment preferences of African Americans: a review of the literature. *J Am Geriatr Soc.* 2005;53:711–719.

14. Crawley LM, Marshall PA, Lo B, et al. Strategies for culturally effective end-of-life care. *Ann Intern Med.* 2002;136:673–679.

15. Dworkin R. *Life's Dominion: An Argument about Abortion, Euthanasia and Individual Freedom.* New York, NY: Alfred A. Knopf; 1993.

16. Orr RD, Genesen LB. Requests for "inappropriate" treatment based on religious beliefs. *J Med Ethics.* 1997;23:142–147.

17. Braithwaite S, Thomasma DC. New guidelines on foregoing life-sustaining treatment in incompetent patients: an anti-cruelty policy. *Ann Intern Med.* 1986;104:711–715.

18. Kleinman A, Eisenberg L, Good B. Culture, illness and care: clinical lessons from anthropologic and cross cultural research. *Ann Intern Med.* 1978;89:251–258.

19. Quill TE. Partnerships in patient care: a contractual approach. *Ann Intern Med.* 1983;98:228–234.

20. Lo B, Snyder L, Sox H. Care at the end of life: guiding practice where there are no easy answers. *Ann Intern Med.* 1999;130:772–774.

21. Buckman R. *How to Break Bad News: a guide for health care professionals.* Baltimore, MD: Johns Hopkins University Press; 1992.

22. Suchman AL, Markakis K, Beckman HB, et al. A model of empathic communication in the medical interview. *JAMA.* 1997;277:678–682.

23. Back AL, Arnold RM, Quill TE. Hope for the best, and prepare for the worst. *Ann Intern Med.* 2003;138:439–443.

24. Quill TE, Arnold RM, Platt FW. "I wish things were different": expressing wishes in response to loss, futility, and unrealistic hopes. *Ann Intern Med.* 2001;135:51–55.

25. Lo B, Quill T, Tulsky J. Discussing palliative care with patients. *Ann Intern Med.* 1999;130:744–749.

26. Maguire P, Faulkner A, Booth K, et al. Helping cancer patients disclose their concerns. *European J Cancer.* 1996;32A:78–81.

27. Firth S. End-of-life: a Hindu view. *Lancet.* 2005;366:682–686.

28. Keown D. End-of-life: the Buddhist view. *Lancet.* 2005;366:952–955.

29. Sachedina A. End-of-life: the Islamic view. *Lancet.* 2005;366:774–779.

30. Quill TE, Holloway R. Time-limited trials near the end of life. *JAMA* 2011;306:1483–1484.

30b. Fisher R, Ury W, Patton, B. *Getting to Yes: Negotiating agreement without giving in.* 2nd ed. New York, NY: Penguin Books; 1991.

31. Christakis NA, Asch DA. Biases in how physicians choose to withdraw life support. *Lancet.* 1993;342:642–646.

32. Curtis JR, Vincent JL. Ethics and end-of-life care for adults in the intensive care unit. *Lancet* 2010;376:1347–1353

33. Quill TE, Arnold R, Back AL. Discussing treatment preferences with patients who want "everything". *Ann Intern Med* 2009;151:345–349.

34. Widera EW, Rosenfeld KE, Fromme EK, et al. Approaching patients and family members who hope for a miracle. *J Pain Symptom Manage* 2011;42:119–125.

35. Lo B. The Bartling case: protecting patients from harm while respecting their wishes. *J Am Geriatr Soc.* 1986;34:44–48.

36. Miles SH, Singer PA, Siegler M. Conflicts between patients' wishes to forgo treatment and the policies of health care facilities. *N Engl J Med.* 1989;321:48–50.

37. Engelhardt HT. *The Foundations of Bioethics.* New York, NY: Oxford University Press; 1986.

38. *Bartling v. Superior Court,* 209 Cal. Rptr. 220 163 Cal. App. 3d 186 (1984).

39. Collopy BJ. Autonomy in long term care: some crucial distinctions. *Gerontologist.* 1988;28(supp.):10–17.
40. Beauchamp TL, Childress JF. *Principles of Biomedical Ethics.* 5th ed. New York, NY: Oxford University Press; 2001.
41. *In re Requena,* 517 A.2d 869 (N.J. Sup. Ct. App. Div. 1986).

ANNOTATED BIBLIOGRAPHY

1. Lo B, Quill T, Tulsky J. Discussing palliative care with patients. *Ann Intern Med.* 1999;130:744–749.
   Back AL, Arnold RM, Baile WF, et al. Approaching difficult communication tasks in oncology. *CA Cancer J Clin.* 2005;55:164–177.
   Quill TE, Arnold R, Back AL. Discussing treatment preferences with patients who want "everything." *Ann Intern Med.* 2009;151:345–349.
   Suggestions for communicating with patients and familes, emphasizing how the physician can use empathic comments and open-ended questions to understand their perceptions of illness, concerns, and emotions.
2. Lo B, Ruston D, Kates LW, et al. Discussing religious and spiritual issues at the end of life: a practical guide for physicians. *JAMA.* 2002;287:749–754.
   Lo B, Kates LW, Ruston D, et al. Responding to requests regarding prayer and religious ceremonies by patients near the end of life and their families. *J Palliat Med.* 2003;6:417–424.
   Two articles that discuss how physicians might respond in disagreements in which the patient's religious concerns or beliefs are salient.
3. Curtis JR, Vincent JL. Ethics and end-of-life care for adults in the intensive care unit. *Lancet.* 2010;376:1347–1353.
   Suggestions for improving family meetings about end-of-life decisions.
4. Sachedina A. End-of-life: the Islamic view. *Lancet.* 2005;366:774–779.
   Keown D. End-of-life: the Buddhist view. *Lancet.* 2005;366:952–955.
   Firth S. End-of-life: a Hindu view. *Lancet.* 2005;366:682–686.
   Articles on how three non-Western faith traditions approach end-of-life decisions.

Decisions About Life-Sustaining Interventions

SECTION II

Decisions About
Life-Sustaining
Interventions

CHAPTER 15

Confusing Ethical Distinctions

In discussions about life-sustaining interventions, physicians often draw distinctions that seem intuitively plausible, but prove problematic on closer analysis. Examples are distinctions between withdrawing and withholding interventions and between extraordinary (or heroic) and ordinary care. However, some distinctions, although less intuitive, are nonetheless ethically valid. For instance, there is an important distinction between providing very high doses of opioids to relieve symptoms in a patient with terminal illness and intentionally administering opioids to kill the patient (1). Failure to appreciate which distinctions are ethically meaningful and which are not leads to confusion and poor care.

CASE 15.1 **Withdrawal of mechanical ventilation**

Mr. C, a 68-year-old man with severe chronic obstructive lung disease, developed respiratory failure. He had told his outpatient physician repeatedly that he was willing to be on a ventilator in the intensive care unit, but only for a brief period. If he did not recover, then he wanted the physicians to let him die in peace. After 2 weeks on antibiotics, bronchodilators, and mechanical ventilation, Mr. C showed little improvement and was still in respiratory failure. He asked his physicians to discontinue the ventilator and to keep him comfortable while he died. His family and primary physician believed that his decision was informed.

Some health care workers objected that although a patient may refuse life-sustaining interventions, removing them would be tantamount to murder. Other health care workers believed that it would be appropriate to discontinue heroic treatments, such as the mechanical ventilation, but that ordinary treatments, such as antibiotics and intravenous fluids, needed to be continued. Still others objected to the use of sedating doses of opioids for the relief of dyspnea after the ventilator was withdrawn because they would hasten death.

WITHDRAWING AND WITHHOLDING INTERVENTIONS

Many physicians and nurses are more willing to withhold interventions than to withdraw them once they have been started (2). In a recent study, only 78% of physicians and 57% of pediatric intensive care unit (PICU) nurses agreed that withholding and withdrawing are ethically the same (3). This distinction seems plausible because discontinuing the ventilator is frequently characterized as a positive action, but not starting the ventilator might seem more passive and, therefore, less reprehensible. In everyday life, people generally are held more responsible for their actions than for their omissions. This distinction between acting and refraining from action, however, is not tenable in clinical medicine. Philosophers have devised ingenious examples to illustrate how the distinction between acting and refraining from acting cannot, by itself, be decisive (4). Suppose that the ventilator is accidentally disconnected from the patient. It is problematic to argue that it was permissible to refrain from reconnecting the ventilator, but not to take action to disconnect it. In either situation, the physician has an ethical obligation to respect the patient's preferences and to act in the patient's best interests. If the patient wishes the ventilator continued and the physician does not reconnect it, then it is morally wrong, even though the physician might be said to withhold the ventilator or refrain from acting. Conversely, if a patient wishes to discontinue mechanical ventilation, as in Case 15.1, then respecting the patient's wishes requires the physician to withdraw it. What is decisive is the patient's informed preferences, not the distinction between withdrawing and withholding. The considerations that justify not initiating a treatment—in Case 15.1 informed refusal by a competent patient—also justify discontinuing it.

In many cases, justifications for withdrawing treatment are actually stronger than reasons to not initiate it. Additional information might become available after treatment has started—for example, the patient did not want treatment or has end-stage disease. Furthermore, a hoped-for benefit might not materialize, as shown in Case 15.1 (5). Typically, decisions on life-sustaining treatment must be made when the patient's prognosis is still uncertain. A time-limited trial of intensive therapy might be appropriate in this situation. If a treatment proves ineffective, then there is no point in continuing it. However, if people were unable to discontinue a treatment once it was started, then they might not even try interventions that might prove beneficial (6). The courts have consistently ruled that there is no distinction between discontinuing medical interventions and not initiating them (7, 8). In this book, we use the term *forego* to include both withholding and withdrawing interventions.

Discontinuing implantable cardiac defibrillators (ICDs) and pacemakers raise similar concerns, even though there is a longer time between the decision to withhold the intervention and the patient's death. ICDs effectively deliver electroshocks if ventricular arrhythmias occur and can prolong survival. If deactivation of the ICD or a Do Not Attempt Resuscitation (DNAR) order is considered, the physician needs to clarify the goals for care. Discontinuing pacemakers, especially dual chamber pacemakers, may cause symptoms of light-headedness and shortness of breath. Some health care workers, patients, or family members may be reluctant to discontinue cardiac devices because they believe it would be suicide or euthanasia; however, recent consensus guidelines carefully explain why this is not the case (9).

EXTRAORDINARY OR HEROIC CARE

People might intuitively distinguish between extraordinary and ordinary care. Interventions that are highly technologic, invasive, complicated, expensive, or unusual are sometimes regarded as "heroic" or "extraordinary." Examples are mechanical ventilation and renal dialysis. In contrast, antibiotics, intravenous fluids, and tube feedings are typically considered "ordinary" care. Some ordinary measures are commonly considered basic care or a standard nursing measure, such as a warm, dry bed. Often, it is argued that extraordinary treatments may be withheld or withdrawn, but not ordinary ones. In an older survey, 74% of doctors and nurses found this distinction helpful in making decisions (10).

This distinction, however, is neither logical nor a reliable guide to decisions (11). In some settings, such as during general anesthesia, mechanical ventilation is highly effective, desired by patients, and universally used. It is indeed appropriate to withdraw mechanical ventilation from Mr. C in Case 15.1. The reason, however, is not that the ventilator can be characterized as extraordinary or heroic, but rather that the burdens outweigh the benefits and the patient does not want it. Instead of trying to determine whether the technology should be considered extraordinary or ordinary, physicians should examine the benefits and burdens of the intervention in the particular case, as well as the patient's preferences. The courts have rejected distinctions between ordinary and extraordinary interventions (7, 8). Numerous rulings have declared that interventions ranging from ventilators to tube feedings may be withheld or withdrawn in appropriate circumstances. Chapter 20 discusses tube feedings in more detail.

RELIEVING SYMPTOMS WITH HIGH DOSES OF OPIOIDS AND SEDATIVES

Relief of pain and other symptoms in terminal illness, such as shortness of breath, is often inadequate. In the SUPPORT study of seriously ill patients, 50% of patients who died experienced moderate to severe pain in their last 3 days of life (12). Doctors might be reluctant to prescribe opioids in sufficient doses to relieve symptoms, or nurses might be reluctant to administer them (13). Some health care workers withhold high doses of opioids because they fear patients will become addicted. However, addiction rarely develops in terminal illness and should not be a primary consideration under these circumstances. Another concern is that a high dose of opioids required to relieve symptoms might hasten the patient's death by suppressing respiration or causing hypotension and, therefore, cross the line to active euthanasia or murder.

In 1996, the US Supreme Court declared, "A patient who is suffering from a terminal illness and who is experiencing great pain has no legal barriers to obtaining medication from qualified physicians, even to the point of causing unconsciousness and hastening death." Physicians, therefore, need to understand the distinctions between high-dose opioids and sedatives to relieve symptoms in patients with terminal illness and active euthanasia. One survey found that almost 90% of physicians and nurses agreed that it is appropriate to administer medication to relieve pain even if the medication hastens a patient's death (10). The doctrine of double effect, long-standing in Catholic moral philosophy, addresses this issue.

THE DOCTRINE OF DOUBLE EFFECT

Like all interventions, opioids and sedatives have both intended effects and unintended adverse effects. The doctrine of double effect distinguishes effects that are intended from those that are foreseen but unintended (14–17). In this view, intentionally causing death is wrong; however, physicians may provide high doses of opioids and sedatives to relieve suffering, provided that they do not intend the patient's death. Such high doses are permitted even if the risk of hastening death is foreseen, but not intended. The intended benefit must be proportionate to the risk of the foreseen side effect. There must be no less harmful means to accomplish the intended effect. Furthermore, the bad effect (the patient's death) may not be the means to accomplish the intended effect (relief of suffering). In addition, the unintended but foreseen bad effect must be proportional to the intended good effect. For a patient who is experiencing refractory and distressing symptoms, the doctrine of double effect justifies high doses of opioids and sedatives if alternative means to relieve symptoms are ineffective or not tolerated and if the physician's intention is to relieve symptoms, not shorten the patient's life. If the patient is close to death because of the underlying illness, it is very unlikely that these medications significantly shorten the patient's survival.

PROBLEMS WITH THE DOUBLE EFFECT DOCTRINE

The doctrine of double effect, although widely accepted, presents several problems (14–17). First, people commonly have multiple intentions (18). In one study, physicians who ordered sedatives and analgesics while withholding life-sustaining interventions said they intended both to decrease pain and to hasten death in about a third of cases (19). Second, the doctrine of double effect seems to focus on what physicians say rather than on what they do. It apparently implies that physicians may administer large doses of opioids if they can put out of mind the possibility that death might be hastened. Third, people generally are held accountable for consequences they foresee or should have foreseen, not merely for those consequences they intended (20).

The issue of intention is further clouded because refusal of medical interventions by a competent patient might involve the intention to hasten death in some cases. Many competent patients who forego life-sustaining interventions but hope nevertheless that they can live without them. However, some patients who refuse life support want to bring about their death. There is broad agreement that physicians should respect patient refusals of interventions, even when the patient's intention is to die. Thus, although intention is central to the doctrine of double effect, it should not be the only criterion for judging an action right or wrong.

Despite problems with the doctrine of double effect, it is useful because it provides a well-accepted rationale that allows persons who strongly oppose active euthanasia to support palliative sedation. Because of controversies surrounding the doctrine of double effect, it might be helpful to give an alternative justification for high doses of opioids and sedatives to relieve refractory symptoms. When terminally ill patients experience refractory symptoms, the physician is caught between two duties: to relieve suffering and not to cause the patient's death. In balancing these conflicting duties, proportionality is important. The risk of hastening death is warranted if lower doses have failed to relieve severe symptoms (20). In this situation, compassion impels the physician to give higher priority to relieving refractory symptoms than to prolonging a painful existence for a few hours or days, or, in our opinion, a few months.

PRACTICAL ASPECTS OF RELIEVING REFRACTORY SYMPTOMS

Intention is judged by a person's actions, as well as by her statements. Physicians cannot simply say that they intended to relieve pain; their actions must also be consistent with their statements (1). What approach to the use of opioids and sedatives is consistent with an intent to relieve pain but not to hasten death? If physicians intend to palliate symptoms, their actions must allow the possibility of relieving symptoms without hastening death. Thus, the starting dose for opioids and sedatives may not be lethal, and the criteria for increasing the dose must be reasonable.

If the physician intends only to palliate suffering, there is no warrant for increasing the dose of opioids or sedatives when the patient is comfortable. In conscious patients, the dose can be increased if the patient reports unacceptably severe symptoms. If patients are unconscious, physicians and nurses must assess whether patients are comfortable. Reasonable criteria for increasing the dose include restlessness, grimacing, withdrawal from pain, furrowed brow, hypertension, and tachycardia. These are criteria that nurses and physicians commonly use to adjust the level of anesthesia in the operating room or sedation in a patient on mechanical ventilation.

RESPONSES TO REFRACTORY SUFFERING

Some terminally ill patients might experience suffering that even excellent palliative care and high-dose opioids do not relieve. Examples are uncontrollable pain, dyspnea, bleeding, and inability to swallow oral secretions. How should physicians respond in such dire situations?

PALLIATIVE SEDATION

In terminal illness, symptom relief generally is achieved with the patient remaining conscious (21). In palliative sedation, sedatives and analgesics are administered, with doses increased as needed to control refractory symptoms, even if unconsciousness may result. The most commonly reported refractory symptoms leading to palliative sedation are agitation or restlessness, pain, confusion, respiratory distress, and myoclonus. In addition, all life-sustaining interventions are withheld. The patient dies of dehydration, starvation, or another intervening complication. Death occurs a few hours to days later, depending on clinical circumstances. The term *proportionate palliative sedation* is often used to emphasize that increasing the dose to that of unconsciousness is a last resort used only if expert palliative care has not relieved symptoms (22). The American Medical Association, American Academy of Hospice and Palliative Medicine, National Hospice and Palliative Care Organization, and Hospice and Palliative Care Nurses Organization all have supported proportionate palliative care sedation (22).

Broader uses of palliative sedation, however, are ethically controversial (17). Some persons object when it is combined with withdrawing other life-sustaining interventions, particularly artificial nutrition and hydration (23, 24). Critics note that the doctrine of double effect justifies only sedation: other reasons are needed to forego artificial hydration and nutrition.

Palliative sedation is also controversial when the refractory symptom is existential or spiritual suffering rather than physical symptoms (17, 24, 25). It is difficult to establish that existential suffering is refractory, and there is a perception that death is hastened (26, 27). Physicians are often unskilled at responding to such suffering (24) and fail to consider referral to a chaplain or the patient's spiritual or religious advisor (28, 29).

Palliative sedation sometimes is carried out without the express agreement of patients or surrogates or without explicit acknowledgement that other interventions will be withheld (17, 30, 31). This violates the principle of respect for patient autonomy. Patients have different preferences regarding sedation in their last hours or days. Some will want relief from intolerable distress even if totally sedated, whereas others will prefer to have some awareness. Thus, the patient (or the surrogate of a patient who lacks decision-making capacity) should give informed consent to palliative sedation as a means of relieving refractory symptoms, knowing that she is expected to die and will not regain consciousness.

Palliative sedation also has limitations as a response to refractory suffering (17). First, patients who wish to die in their own homes might not be able to arrange palliative sedation at home. Second, palliative sedation cannot relieve some symptoms, such as uncontrollable bleeding or inability to swallow secretions. Although patients are not conscious of these conditions once they are sedated, their death cannot be considered dignified or peaceful.

VOLUNTARY STOPPING OF EATING AND DRINKING

In response to refractory suffering, a patient with terminal illness may voluntarily stop eating and drinking and "allowed to die," primarily of dehydration or some intervening complication (31). Ethically and legally, the right of competent, informed patients to refuse life-prolonging interventions is firmly established. Forcibly feeding a competent patient who refuses food and fluids would violate the patient's autonomy. Stopping eating and drinking requires considerable patient resolve and is clearly voluntary. Stopping eating and drinking might seem natural because severe anorexia commonly occurs in the final stage of many illnesses.

Voluntary stopping of eating and drinking requires considerable resolve, might last for up to 2 weeks, and, therefore, might seem inhumane. Initially, the patient might experience thirst and hunger, which can be relived by ice chips, mouth care, and pain medication. Patients should be regularly offered the opportunity to eat and drink in case they change their minds, yet such offers might be viewed as undermining the patient's resolve. Patients typically lose mental clarity toward the end of this process, which might raise questions about voluntariness or seem unacceptable to some patients or families.

EMOTIONAL REACTIONS TO THESE DISTINCTIONS

Physicians need to appreciate that these topics in this chapter raise emotional, as well as philosophical issues. To many people, stopping a treatment is much more difficult emotionally than not starting it. Health care workers, particularly nurses, might feel that they are causing the patient's death by turning down ventilator settings, discontinuing vasopressors, turning off a implanted cardiac device, or administering large doses of opioids or sedatives. The shorter the time between the withdrawal of the intervention and the patient's death, the more responsible the health care worker might feel for the patient's death.

Doctors should routinely elicit the concerns, feelings, and objections of other health care workers, as well as patients or surrogates about these issues. Moreover, doctors need to acknowledge the depth and sincerity of such feelings. Team meetings and family meetings are often helpful for this purpose.

Strong emotional reactions might be a clue that further deliberation and discussion are needed. However, the fact that something is emotionally difficult does not necessarily mean that it is unethical. Health care workers should try to articulate the reasons for their reactions.

The concerns of nurses and house staff should be accommodated if reasonably possible. Nurses who have strong personal objections to the plan of care should not be required to carry it out if other arrangements can be made to care for the patient. Generally, other nurses will volunteer to care for the patient. The attending physician should closely monitor the administration of opioids and sedatives, rather than leave it completely to the nurses and house staff. Nurses and house officers appreciate the attending physician's presence at the bedside when mechanical ventilation is withdrawn.

UNPRECEDENTED CASES

A highly publicized episode during the Hurricane Katrina disaster in 2005 illustrates the importance of distinguishing clearly between euthanasia and palliative sedation (32–33).

CASE 15.2   Alleged active euthanasia during Hurricane Katrina

In August 2005, Hurricane Katrina caused widespread flooding in New Orleans. At Memorial Hospital, electricity was lost, the basement flooded, toilets overflowed, and the temperature reached over 100°. On the second day after the hurricane struck, all backup power was lost, and ventilators and other medical equipment, telephone lines, and computers failed. Although some patients were evacuated through private boats, there was no coordinated rescue plan. Usually the hospital had one death a day. The second night, 8 patients had a cardiopulmonary arrest, and the following night, 10 patients. The third morning after the hurricane, the hospital crisis manager allegedly announced that they expected no evacuation that day and that patients on a long-term care floor were not expected to survive and would not be evacuated.

The daughter of a 78-year-old patient receiving antibiotics on that floor for an infection following colon cancer surgery reported overhearing nurses saying that patients with DNR orders would not be evacuated. She reacted, "DNR means do not resuscitate. It does not mean do not rescue, do not take care of. I tried to rescind her DNR order, but no one paid attention."

The pharmacy director on the long-term floor alleged being told that no living patients would be left behind and seeing Dr. Anna Pou with syringes of morphine entering patients' room and closing the door. Several other doctors later said that they administered medications to patients to hasten their deaths.

Later on that third day, Coast Guard and private helicopters, as well as some private boats, arrived to transport patients.

In July 2006, the Attorney General of Louisiana recommended charges of second-degree murder be brought against Dr. Pou and two nurses for administering a "lethal cocktail" of morphine and midazolam to kill four patients. Dr. Pou responded in an interview, "I did not murder those patients....I do not believe in euthanasia. I don't think it's anyone's decision to make when a patient dies. However, what I do believe in is comfort care, and that means that we ensure that they do not suffer pain." Many New Orleans residents, as well as several medical organizations, strongly defended Dr. Pou. An ICU physician who spent a lot of time in Memorial Hospital visiting his grandmother on the extended-care floor said he gave morphine and midazolam to two or three patients who were taken off ventilators to relieve their gasping for breath. All survived. He called it "irresponsible" to assert that this combination of drugs was lethal. The coroner reported that because autopsies could not be carried out for over 2 weeks, he was unable to determine whether the patients died of natural causes or homicide. Charges against the two nurses were dropped in exchange for their testimony against Dr. Pou. In August 2007, the grand jury refused to indict Dr. Pou. After extensive press coverage, the coroner reviewed the cases in 2010 and called them "unclassified." Several civil suits are still pending.

KEEPING ETHICAL DISTINCTIONS CLEAR

The facts of this case are uncertain, because conflicting accounts have been reported (32,33) and there has been no testimony in court under oath and cross-examination. It is important, however, to distinguish active euthanasia from palliative sedation. Palliative sedation to relieve intractable symptoms is always appropriate. The Katrina case illustrates that special challenges arise if it is not feasible to monitor the patient closely, increase dosage as needed, and document the plan for care. As Chapter 19 discusses, active euthanasia, intentionally causing or hastening a patient's death, is illegal. For the sake of discussion, let us assume that Dr. Pou intended to carry out palliative sedation, not active euthanasia. How might such care have been improved?

SUGGESTIONS FOR DECISIONS DURING A CRISIS

The Katrina case is an extreme example of how cases involving refractory suffering and palliative sedation commonly involve great stress, time pressures, and strong emotions. The following suggestions will help ensure that decisions are sound.

Obtain the Agreement of Other Staff

Although clear communication is important in any clinical situation, it is particularly important during a disaster. The attending physician should anticipate objections and misunderstandings about palliative sedation. Some people will believe that it is the same as active euthanasia. There may seem to be no time for discussions in a crisis; however, other health care workers are more likely to work effectively toward the common goal and keep up their morale if they can voice their concerns and objections and understand the plan of care. Furthermore, other members of the health care team may suggest how to improve care. During an unprecedented crisis, crucial considerations may be overlooked. As in ordinary clinical care, health care workers may opt not to administer the medications for palliative sedation personally. Conversely, if most members of the team remain in strong disagreement, the attending physician should reconsider the plan.

Obtain the Agreement of the Patient or Surrogate

During a crisis, staff may feel that they lack time to spend with patients. Furthermore, it may be impossible to contact surrogates of patients who lack decision-making capacity. Health care workers may wish to protect patients from grim news; however, patients who are still sentient undoubtedly already realize that their situation is dire. Competent patients should be offered a choice regarding palliative sedation, as in usual clinical care. Some patients will welcome analgesia and sedation in such a crisis, whereas others may wish to remain as lucid as possible or hope that they will survive against unfavorable odds. The Katrina case illustrates how predictions during a disaster are uncertain. Although the consequences of the hurricane were far worse than expected, the appearance of rescue teams on the afternoon of the third day was much better than what was expected early that morning, when plans for the day were made.

Consider Other Actions to Relieve Distress

Palliative sedation is a means toward the goal of relieving intractable suffering, not a goal in itself. Caregivers also should consider other ways to relieve suffering. If patients will die because evacuation is not possible, then it may be critical for them to have the opportunity to reach closure, to say a prayer, or to voice their good-byes even if family cannot be present. Even if health care workers can spend only a few minutes, such actions may provide relief to the patient.

Plan for Disasters

Hurricane Katrina revealed a lack of disaster planning and training; hospitals and states need to better prepare for disasters that are inevitable in the future, for example, after an earthquake or epidemic (34-36). Without planning and staff training, health care workers will be unprepared to make life-and-death decisions.

CASE 15.2 *Continued*

Hurricane Katrina presented unprecedented circumstances, with severe staff shortages, lack of basic resources like electricity and telephones, and great uncertainty. Although usual standards of care were impossible, fundamental ethical principles need to be observed to the extent circumstances permitted (36). The distinction between palliative sedation and active euthanasia is still important. Furthermore, the preferences of the patient are still crucial, as some patients who were not expected to be evacuated or to survive might prefer to be lucid rather than sedated. Finally, during a crisis, communication among caregivers remains crucial. Although most MDs will never encounter such a crisis, clear thinking about general rules is essential before considering exceptions necessitated by an extraordinary situation.

SUMMARY

1. Several commonly held distinctions regarding life-sustaining interventions are not logically tenable.
2. Physicians should appreciate that it might be appropriate to withdraw interventions that have been started or that some persons consider ordinary care. In addition, administering high doses of opioids and sedatives is appropriate to relieve symptoms in patients who have a terminal illness or who have refused mechanical ventilation.

REFERENCES

1. Alpers A, Lo B. The Supreme Court addresses physician-assisted suicide. Can its decisions improve palliative care? *Arch Fam Pract.* 1999;8:200–205.
2. Farber NJ, Simpson P, Salam T, et al. Physicians' decisions to withhold and withdraw life-sustaining treatment. *Arch Intern Med.* 2006;166:560–564.
3. Burns JP, Mitchell C, Griffith JL, et al. End-of-life care in the pediatric intensive care unit: attitudes and practices of pediatric critical care physicians and nurses. *Crit Care Med.* 2001;29:658–564.
4. Brock D. Forgoing life-sustaining food and water: is it killing? In: Lynn J, ed. *By No Extraordinary Means.* Expanded ed. Bloomington, IN: Indiana University Press; 1989:117–131.
5. President's Commission for the Study of Ethical Problems in Medicine and Biomedical and Behavioral Research. *Deciding to Forego Life-Sustaining Treatment.* Washington, DC: U.S. Government Printing Office; 1983:73–77.
6. Lo B, Rouse F, Dornbrand L. Family decision-making on trial. Who decides for incompetent patients? *N Engl J Med.* 1990;322:1228–1231.
7. Meisel A. Legal myths about terminating life support. *Arch Intern Med.* 1991;151:1497–1502.
8. Meisel A. *The Right to Die.* 2nd ed. New York, NY: John Wiley & Sons; 1995.
9. Lampert R, Hayes DL, Annas GJ, et al. HRS expert consensus statement on the management of cardiovascular implantable electronic devices (CIEDs) in patients nearing end of life or requesting withdrawal of therapy. *Heart Rhythm.* 2010;7:1008–1026.
10. Solomon MZ, O'Donnell LO, Jennings B, et al. Decisions near the end of life: professional views on life-sustaining treatments. *Am J Public Health.* 1993;83:14–23.
11. President's Commission for the Study of Ethical Problems in Medicine and Biomedical and Behavioral Research. *Deciding to Forego Life-Sustaining Treatment.* Washington, DC: U.S. Government Printing Office; 1983:82–89.
12. The SUPPORT Investigators. A controlled trial to improve care for seriously ill hospitalized patients. *JAMA.* 1995;274:1591–1598.
13. Edwards MJ, Tolle SW. Disconnecting the ventilator at the request of a patient who knows he will then die: the doctor's anguish. *Ann Int Med.* 1992;117:254–256.
14. Quill TE, Dresser R, Brock DW. The rule of double effect—A critique of its role in end-of-life decision making. *N Engl J Med.* 1997;3337:1768–1771.
15. McIntyre A. The double life of double effect. *Theor Med Bioeth.* 2004;25:61–74.
16. Beauchamp TL, Childress JF. *Principles of Biomedical Ethics.* 5th ed. New York, NY: Oxford University Press; 2001:128–132.
17. Lo B, Rubenfeld G. Palliative sedation in dying patients: "we turn to it when everything else hasn't worked." *JAMA.* 2005;294:1810–1816.
18. Quill TE. Doctor, I want to die. Will you help me? *JAMA.* 1993;270:870–873.

19. Wilson WC, Smedira NG, Fink C, et al. Ordering and administration of sedatives and analgesics during the withholding and withdrawal of life support from critically ill patients. *JAMA.* 1992;267:949–953.
20. President's Commission for the Study of Ethical Problems in Medicine and Biomedical and Behavioral Research. *Deciding to Forego Life-Sustaining Treatment.* Washington, DC: U.S. Government Printing Office; 1983:73–89.
21. Sykes N, Thorns A. The use of opioids and sedatives at the end of life. *Lancet Oncol.* 2003;4:312–318.
22. Quill TE, Lo B, Brock DW, et al. Last-resort options for palliative sedation. *Ann Intern Med.* 2009;151:421–424.
23. Orentlicher D. The Supreme Court and physician-assisted suicide: rejecting physician-assisted suicide but embracing euthanasia. *N Engl J Med.* 1997;337:1236–1239.
24. Jansen LA, Sulmasy DP. Sedation, alimentation, hydration, and equivocation: careful conversation about care at the end of life. *Ann Intern Med.* 2002;136:845–849.
25. Braun TC, Hagen NA, Clark T. Development of a clinical practice guideline for palliative sedation. *J Palliat Med.* 2003;6:345–350.
26. Taylor BR, McCann RM. Controlled sedation for physical and existential suffering? *J Palliat Med.* 2005;8:144–147.
27. Rousseau P. Palliative sedation in the control of refractory symptoms. *J Palliat Med.* 2005;8:10–12.
28. Lo B, Ruston D, Kates LW, et al. Discussing religious and spiritual issues at the end of life: a practical guide for physicians. *JAMA.* 2002;287:749–754.
29. Lo B, Kates LW, Ruston D, et al. Responding to requests regarding prayer and religious ceremonies by patients near the end of life and their families. *J Palliat Med.* 2003;6:409–415.
30. Billings JA. Slow euthanasia. *J Palliat Care.* 1996;12:21–30.
31. Quill TE, Lo B, Brock DW. Palliative options of last resort: a comparison of voluntarily stopping eating and drinking, terminal sedation, physician-assisted suicide, and voluntary active euthanasia. *JAMA.* 1997;278:2099–2104.
32. Katrina One Year Later: For Dear Life. A five-part series from The Times-Picayune. http://www.nola.com/katrina/mercy/. Accessed July 25, 2008.
33. Fink S. The deadly choices at Memorial. http://www.propublica.org/article/the-deadly-choices-at-memorial-826. Accessed August 28, 2012.
34. Curiel TJ. Murder or mercy? Hurricane Katrina and the need for disaster training. *N Engl J Med.* 2006;355:2067–2069.
35. Okie S. Dr. Pou and the hurricane—Implications for patient care during disasters. *N Engl J Med.* 2008;358:1–5.
36. Altvogel B, Stroud C, Hanson SL, Hanfling D, Gostin LO. Guidance for Establishing Crisis Standards of Care for Use in Disaster Situations. 2009. http://www.nap.edu/catalog.php?record_id=12749&m=0003000740. Accessed December 9. 2011.

ANNOTATED BIBLIOGRAPHY

1. Lampert R, Hayes DL, Annas GJ, et al. HRS expert consensus statement on the management of cardiovascular implantable electronic devices (CIEDs) in patients nearing end of life or requesting withdrawal of therapy. *Heart Rhythm.* 2010;7:1008–1026.
   Comprehensive analysis of withdrawal of life-sustaining interventions.
2. Quill TE, Dresser R, Brock DW. The rule of double effect—A critique of its role in end-of-life decision making. *N Engl J Med.* 1997;3337:1768–1771.
   Analysis of the doctrine of double effect and its application to decisions on life-sustaining interventions.
3. Quill TE, Lo B, Brock DW. Palliative options of last resort: a comparison of voluntarily stopping eating and drinking, terminal sedation, physician-assisted suicide, and voluntary active euthanasia. *JAMA.* 1997;278:2099–2104.
   Analysis of different approaches to responding to refractory suffering at the end of life.
4. Lo B, Rubenfeld G. Palliative sedation in dying patients: "we turn to it when everything else hasn't worked." *JAMA.* 2005;294:1810–1816.
   Analysis of palliative sedation and the doctrine of double effect, which justifies it even for persons who believe that intentionally hastening death is unethical.
5. Okie S. Dr. Pou and the hurricane—Implications for patient care during disasters. *N Engl J Med.* 2008;358:1–5.
   Analysis of palliative sedation versus active euthanasia in the context of Hurricane Katrina.

CHAPTER 16

Ethics Consultations and Ethics Committees

E thical dilemmas in clinical practice can lead to deep disagreements and strong emotions. The Joint Commission requires health care institutions to have a mechanism to address ethical issues in patient care, such as an ethics committee or an ethics consultation service. Ethics case consultations might be carried out by the full ethics committee, by a smaller team, or by an individual consultant; we thus use the term "ethics consultant" to refer to all these options. Compared with court proceedings, such consultations are more timely and less adversarial. This chapter reviews the goals, problems, and effective procedures of ethics consultations. Although ethics committees usually have several tasks, such as educational activities and development of institutional policies, this chapter focuses only on their work as consultants.

GOALS OF ETHICS CONSULTATIONS

The goal of ethics consultations is to analyze and help resolve ethical problems in clinical care (1). Ethics consultations in intensive care unit (ICU) cases involving value conflicts reduce the length of hospitalization for patients who die during the hospitalization and are viewed as helpful by family members (2, 3).

CASE 16.1   **Disagreement between family and health care team**

A 76-year-old widower with severe Alzheimer disease is cared for by his two daughters and their families. He does not engage in conversations, but usually responds appropriately to simple questions. He often smiles when playing with his grandchildren and when watching television. For the third time in 6 months, he is hospitalized for pneumonia despite aspiration precautions.

The physicians believe that antibiotics are "futile" in this case and strongly recommend a palliative approach. The patient has not appointed a health care proxy, but had indicated to his primary physician that his daughters should make decisions for him. His daughters acknowledge that their father has limited life expectancy, but believe that he still has acceptable quality of life. "His family was always the most important thing to him. He always said that nothing made him happier than seeing his grandchildren grow up."

At the attending physician's request, two members of the ethics committee review the patient's medical record. They agree that antibiotics are futile in this situation. Family members are outraged. "Who are these people? They've never even spoken to us."

CLARIFY THE FACTS OF THE CASE

The first step in ethics consultations is to gather information about the medical situation and the ethical issues in the case. Ethics consultants should not uncritically accept secondhand data, which might omit important information or views (4). Moreover, conclusions and inferences might be presented rather than primary data. For instance, physicians or nurses might describe interventions as "futile" without explaining in what sense they are using this term. In Case 16.1, the ethics consultants need to gather information about previous statements by the patient about his values and wishes for care.

IDENTIFY AND ANALYZE UNCERTAINTY AND CONFLICT OVER ETHICAL ISSUES

Physicians, patients, and families commonly use ethical concepts and terms without analyzing them carefully. In Case 16.1, concepts needing clarification are futility (*see* Chapter 9), quality of life (*see* Chapter 4), and surrogate decision making (*see* Chapter 13).

BUILD CONSENSUS AMONG STAKEHOLDERS

Ethics case consultants should help the stakeholders arrive at decisions that are acceptable to them, within the bounds of acceptable ethical practice (5). Ethics consultants should not impose their own personal views about the course of action, but rather allow the stakeholders to reach a decision that is consistent with ethical guidelines, their own values, and the patient's values. This process usually requires discussion and negotiation (Table 16-1).

Help Stakeholders Express Their Views and Concerns

Patients and family members often feel that physicians are not listening to them. Conversely, physicians often complain that patients and family members do not hear their recommendations. Ethics consultants need to elicit the concerns and views of the various stakeholders. When patients and relatives feel their voices have been heard, they usually are more willing to listen to the physicians' assessment of the patient's prognosis and to recommendations. Moreover, physicians who hear the patient and family generally appreciate that their positions are based on deeply felt concerns and values.

Improve Communication

Many ethical dilemmas are exacerbated by breakdowns in communication. The ethics consultant can help improve communication through empathic listening and by summarizing each stakeholder's perspective. Furthermore, a frequent recommendation to health care providers is to spend more time understanding the patient's and family's concerns and needs; for example, by using open-ended questions, rather than trying to convince them to accept the physician's perspective.

Provide Emotional Support

In situations such as the one discussed in Case 16.1, emotions often are intense. In response to the patient's serious clinical situation, the children might have a variety of feelings, including grief, anxiety, and anger. The attending physician, house officers, and nurses in Case 16.1 felt frustrated at

TABLE 16-1	Goals of Ethics Case Consultations
Clarify the facts of the case.	
Identify and analyze uncertainty and conflict over ethical issues.	
Build consensus among stakeholders.	
Help stakeholders express their views and concerns	
Improve communication among clinical caregivers, patient, and family	
Provide emotional support	
Negotiate an acceptable resolution	

the repeated hospitalizations. Unless such feelings are acknowledged, discussion of substantive issues may not be fruitful.

Negotiate an Acceptable Resolution

Ethics consultants need to know how to lead a discussion, to assure that all views are presented, and to help parties appreciate other points of view (6). Bioethics training programs sometimes fail to teach these interpersonal skills. After such a discussion, parties who had been in conflict may be willing to go along with the plan for care, even if it is not the approach they would take personally.

POTENTIAL PROBLEMS WITH ETHICS CASE CONSULTATIONS

Although ethics consultations might help resolve disputes, they might also be problematic (Table 16-2) (4, 7), as the following continuation of Case 16.1 illustrates.

LACK OF PARTICIPATION OF PATIENTS OR SURROGATES

Patients or relatives usually feel outraged if ethical issues are resolved "behind closed doors" without their knowledge or participation and by people whom they have never met (4). They might feel that their decision-making responsibility has been usurped.

BIAS OR PERCEIVED BIAS

Patients or surrogates who disagree with physicians might regard an ethics consultation as serving the interests of the physician or institution. Ethics consultants are generally employees of the hospital and might be colleagues of the health care workers in the case. Hence, families might perceive them as biased in favor of the doctors, nurses, and hospital.

UNSOUND RECOMMENDATIONS

Agreement among ethics committee members or consultants does not guarantee that their recommendations are sound. In Case 16.1, the ethics committee members adopted a view of "futility" that is highly problematic (*see* Chapter 9). Antibiotics are effective in treating the episode of aspiration pneumonia, even though they have no impact on the course of dementia or the risk of further episodes of aspiration.

PROBLEMS BEYOND THE SCOPE OF AN ETHICS CONSULTATION

In some cases, the problems concern legal liability, staff grievances, or discharge planning, rather than strictly ethical issues. It is unwise for ethics committees and consultants to take on the duties of risk managers, hospital administrators, psychiatrists, or social workers.

PROCEDURES FOR ETHICS CASE CONSULTATIONS

For ethics case consultations to be widely accepted, they must be regarded as accessible and fair (4, 7).

TABLE 16-2   Potential Problems With Ethics Consultations

Lack of participation of patients or surrogates

Bias or perceived bias

Unsound recommendations

Problems beyond the scope of an ethics consultation

WHO CAN REQUEST ETHICS CASE CONSULTATIONS?

In addition to attending physicians, patients or their surrogates, nurses, and house officers should also be able to request case consultations. Disagreements over the need for a consultation generally indicate serious conflicts over patient care or ethical issues.

WHO PARTICIPATES IN CASE CONSULTATIONS?

All health care workers providing direct patient care should be invited to attend an ethics case consultation, including the attending physicians, consultant, trainees, nurses, and social workers. The patient and family also should attend. Broad attendance ensures that all pertinent information is presented and all viewpoints are represented. As a practical matter, people are more likely to accept recommendations if they are allowed to express their views and to hear the reasoning behind a decision. In some cases, health care workers need to think through the ethical concerns before meeting with the patient or family.

DOCUMENT RECOMMENDATIONS

Most consultants offer specific recommendations for resolving ethical dilemmas. For instance, in Case 16.1, the ethics consultation can recommend that more information about the patient's previous statements should be gathered. Recommendations should be written in the medical record, together with their rationale. Unwritten recommendations invite misunderstandings and reduce accountability. As with any consultation, the attending physician retains the power to follow or not to follow the recommendations. Ethically and legally, the attending should act as a reasonable physician would after receiving the recommendations.

SUMMARY

1. No single approach to ethics consultations is appropriate for all hospitals and situations.
2. Persons who conduct ethics case consultations need to be aware of the potential pitfalls and the steps that can be taken to avoid them.

REFERENCES

1. Dubler NN, Webber MP, Swiderski DM. Charting the future. Credentialing, privileging, quality, and evaluation in clinical ethics consultation. *Hastings Cent Rep.* 2009;39:23–33.
2. Schneiderman LJ, Gilmer T, Teetzel HD, et al. Effect of ethics consultations on non-beneficial life-sustaining treatments in the intensive care setting: a multi-center, prospective, randomized, controlled trial. *JAMA.* 2003;290:1166–1172.
3. Lo B. Answers and questions about ethics consultations. *JAMA.* 2003;290:298–299.
4. Lo B. Behind closed doors: promises and pitfalls of ethics committees. *N Engl J Med.* 1987;317:46–49.
5. Aulisio MP, Arnold RM, Youngner S, eds. *Ethics Consultation: From Theory to Practice.* Baltimore, MD: Johns Hopkins University Press; 2003.
6. Arnold RM, Silver MHW. Techniques for training ethics consultants: why traditional classroom methods are not enough. In: Aulisio MP, Arnold RM, Youngner SJ, eds. *Ethics Consultation: From Theory to Practice.* Baltimore, MD: John Hopkins University Press; 2003:70–87.
7. Fletcher JC, Moseley KL. The structure and process of ethics consultation services. In: Aulisio MP, Arnold RM, Youngner SJ, eds. *Ethics Consultation: From Theory to Practice.* Baltimore, MD: John Hopkins University Press; 2003:96–120.

ANNOTATED BIBLIOGRAPHY

1. Lo B. Behind closed doors: promises and pitfalls of ethics committees. *N Engl J Med.* 1987;317:46–49.
   Discusses potential problems with ethics committees, such as exclusion of patients and nurses, reliance on second-hand data, and groupthink.
2. Aulisio MP, Arnold RM, Youngner SJ. Health care ethics consultation: nature, goals and competencies. *Ann Intern Med.* 2000;133:59–69.

Report of an interdisciplinary task force to set standards for ethics consultations by ethics committees and individual consultants.

3. Schneiderman LJ, Gilmer T, Teetzel HD, et al. Effect of ethics consultations on non-beneficial life-sustaining treatments in the intensive care setting: a multi-center, prospective, randomized, controlled trial. *JAMA.* 2003; 290:1166–1172.

Lo B. Answers and questions about ethics consultations. *JAMA.* 2003;290:298–299.

Randomized clinical trial of ethics consultations in cases of value disagreements and accompanying editorial.

4. Dubler NN, Webber MP, Swiderski DM. Charting the future. Credentialing, privileging, quality, and evaluation in clinical ethics consultation. *Hastings Cent Rep.* 2009;39:23–33.

Argues that training, credentialing, and certification will improve the quality of clinical ethics consultations.

17

Do Not Attempt Resuscitation Orders

Everyone who dies suffers a cardiopulmonary arrest. Although cardiopulmonary resuscitation (CPR) might revive some patients after unexpected cardiopulmonary arrests, in severe illness CPR is much more likely to prolong dying than to reverse death. This chapter discusses the effectiveness of CPR, appropriate reasons for Do Not Attempt Resuscitation (DNAR) orders, the interpretation of such orders, and discussions with patients or surrogates about CPR.

CPR differs from other medical interventions in several ways. When a cardiopulmonary arrest occurs, physicians or nurses who might not know the patient must decide immediately whether to initiate CPR. Otherwise, the patient will certainly die. To avoid delays, CPR is attempted in every hospitalized patient who suffers a cardiopulmonary arrest unless a prior decision has been made not to do so. Unlike other medical interventions, CPR is initiated without a physician's order. Instead, a physician's order is required to withhold CPR—the DNAR order or the No CPR order.

THE EFFECTIVENESS OF CPR

To make informed decisions about CPR, patients (or their surrogates) need to understand that CPR has limited effectiveness in many clinical situations. When CPR is attempted in an acute-care hospital, spontaneous pulse is restored in 44% of cases (1). Of those initially resuscitated, over one third survive to discharge from the hospital. Thus, 17% of patients on whom CPR is attempted are discharged alive from the hospital (1, 2). In other words, even when CPR is attempted, about 83% of patients die. CPR is more effective when patients suffer cardiopulmonary arrests in the operating room or the cardiac catheterization laboratory (ICUs).

In certain patient groups, CPR is even less beneficial. Physicians have tried to identify subgroups for which the probability of successful CPR is close to zero. However, later studies have not confirmed early reports of very low survival in patient subgroups. In recent publications, 9.3% of patients on pressors when cardiopulmonary arrest occurred and 1.9% of patients with metastatic cancer survived to discharge (1, 2). Survival to discharge is 1.3% in patients above 75 years of age and 5.5% in sepsis (2).

Complications can occur in patients who are revived by CPR. A dreaded outcome of CPR is severe neurologic impairment due to anoxic brain damage. However, 86% of those who had highest category cognitive performance before CPR remained in that category. Functional status may also be impaired (1). In patients who received CPR, 84% lived at home preadmission and 51% returned home postdischarge (1). Although only 6% of CPR recipients were admitted from a nursing home or rehabilitation, 31% were discharged to one of these sites (1). Neurologic outcomes may be better after therapeutic hypothermia (3). Other medical complications may also occur during CPR, including fractured ribs or sternum or flail chest.

JUSTIFICATIONS FOR DNAR ORDERS

As with other medical interventions, there are several acceptable justifications for withholding CPR.

PATIENT REFUSES CPR

Competent, informed patients may not want CPR. Many patients wish to die peacefully rather than have physicians and nurses attempt to revive them. Such informed refusals should be respected (4).

SURROGATE REFUSES CPR

Surrogates may decline CPR for patients who lack decision-making capacity (4), based on the patient's preferences or best interests.

CPR IS FUTILE IN A STRICT SENSE

As Chapter 10 discusses, physicians may decide unilaterally to withhold interventions that are futile in a strict sense: CPR has no pathophysiologic rationale, it has already failed in the patient, or hypotension progresses despite maximal treatment. In these strictly defined situations, physicians appropriately make the decision to stop or withhold resuscitation and CPR should not be offered to patients or surrogates (5). Instead, physicians should inform them of the DNAR order or the termination of CPR and explain the reasons.

Problematic Appeals to Futility

Physicians often use futility in a looser sense to justify unilateral decisions by physicians to withhold CPR. Some physicians assert that they may withhold CPR unilaterally as "futile" when patients are highly likely to die even if CPR is attempted.

CASE 17.1	Family wants CPR even though survival would be highly unlikely

Mr. R is a 54-year-old man, bedridden with squamous cell carcinoma of the lung metastatic to liver and bone, is hospitalized for pneumonia and confusion. He has never indicated his preferences about CPR. The family insists on "full code," saying that even if he does not regain consciousness or survive the hospitalization, it is worth prolonging his life for even a few hours or days. The physicians, however, consider CPR futile because the medical literature reports that very few such patients are discharged alive after cardiopulmonary arrest. Furthermore, the doctors consider his quality of life extremely poor. In their view, prolonging the patient's life for a few hours or days is not an appropriate goal for care (6).

Unilateral DNAR orders based on low likelihood of success or quality of life, however, are problematic (*see* Chapter 9) (7). Physicians are inaccurate in predicting outcomes of CPR. One study found that physicians were no more accurate at identifying patients who would survive resuscitation than would be expected by chance alone (8). Moreover, physicians often define futility far more broadly than recommended in the literature. In a study of DNAR cases in which physicians believed CPR was futile, residents estimated the probability of the patient's survival after CPR as 5% or higher in 32% of higher (9). This threshold is far looser than the criteria for futility proposed in the literature—namely, 0 successes in the previous 100 cases (10, 11).

DISCUSSING DNAR ORDERS WITH PATIENTS

Patients or surrogates need to discuss CPR with physicians if they are to make informed decisions about it. Physicians cannot accurately determine patients' preferences about CPR without asking them directly. In a large multicenter study, physicians misunderstood patients' preferences about CPR in about 50% of cases (12).

BARRIERS TO DISCUSSIONS

Some physicians believe that patients do not want to discuss DNAR decisions. In fact, most ambulatory patients—between 67% and 85%—want to discuss life-sustaining treatment with physicians (13, 14). Among hospitalized patients, between 42% and 81% want to discuss end-of-life decisions with their physicians (15, 16).

Physicians sometimes hesitate to discuss DNAR orders with patients, fearing that they will lose hope, become depressed, refuse highly beneficial treatments, or even attempt suicide. Such adverse outcomes, however, rarely occur.

TARGETING DISCUSSIONS

Physicians typically discuss CPR only with patients whom they believe are at high risk for cardiopulmonary arrest. The prospect of cardiopulmonary arrest becomes more salient as a patient's condition worsens. If discussions are deferred, however, patients might become so sick that they are no longer capable of making medical decisions (17). In addition, targeting sicker patients for discussions about CPR reinforces the belief that DNAR discussions signify a bleak prognosis. For these reasons, physicians should routinely discuss CPR with all adult inpatients with serious illness. Ideally, such discussions would be initiated in the ambulatory setting. When patients lack decision-making capacity, physicians should conduct discussions about CPR with appropriate surrogates.

PATIENT MISUNDERSTANDINGS ABOUT CPR

Many patients misunderstand basic information about the nature of CPR. Few patients understand that mechanical ventilation is usually required after CPR and that patients on a ventilator are usually conscious but cannot talk (18). Patients substantially overestimate favorable outcomes after CPR (18), perhaps because of unrealistic portrayals on television (19). Many patients who initially want CPR change their minds after they are informed about the nature and outcomes of CPR (20, 21).

IMPROVING DISCUSSIONS ABOUT DNAR ORDERS

Better discussions with physicians will help patients make informed decisions, as Table 17-1 summarizes.

Place Discussions in Context

It is generally better to start with a discussion of the patient's understanding of the situation and his concerns and goals for care rather than the specific decision about CPR (22).

Routinely Invite Patients to Discuss CPR

Physicians can raise the issue of CPR in a straightforward manner. "I try to discuss with all patients what to do if they become too sick to talk with me directly. How would you feel about discussing this?" If the patient agrees, the physician can continue, "One important issue is CPR. Let me explain what CPR is…"

TABLE 17-1	Improving Discussions With Patients or Surrogates About DNAR Orders

Routinely invite patients to discuss CPR.

Provide information so that patients can make informed decisions.

Make explicit recommendations about CPR.

Reassure patients about ongoing care.

Allow time for decisions.

Provide Information so That Patients Can Make Informed Decisions

Often, doctors shroud DNAR discussions in euphemisms or technical jargon (23). Physicians sometimes ask patients, "If your heart or lungs stop, would you like us to start them up again?" Such phrasing mistakenly implies that CPR is as simple and effective as jump-starting an automobile battery or changing a light bulb. The question is whether patients want doctors to *try* to revive them, even though the likelihood of death is 83% or more. Physicians can be explicit without being blunt or offensive. To avoid bias due to framing effects, physicians should explain that if CPR is attempted, overall 17% of patients will survive the hospitalization and 83% will die. Doctors can describe CPR (including chest compressions, electroshock, and intubation) and the possible outcomes (including survival, persistent unconsciousness, and death). Some physicians try to dissuade patients from CPR by describing it in graphic detail, such as "pounding on your chest." Such biased information, however, undermines the goal of informed patient decision making. Even after discussions with physicians, patients often have serious misunderstandings about CPR.

Make Explicit Recommendations About CPR

Physicians can offer recommendations while still allowing patients ultimate decision-making power. In rare cases, if CPR would be futile in a strict sense, then physicians should not simply offer patients or surrogates a choice but instead inform them of the DNAR order, its rationale, and the procedures families can take if they disagree.

Reassure Patients About Ongoing Care

Some patients fear that after a DNAR order, physicians will give up on them. Physicians need to emphasize plans for treating other problems, seeing the patient regularly, and providing palliative care.

Allow Time for Decisions

Patients or surrogates often need time to think about issues and deal with their emotions. Even in the emergency department, physicians usually can give them some private time to reflect and return later to resume the discussion.

Physicians can improve their skills at DNAR discussions. Doctors seldom observe more experienced physicians carry out such discussions or have colleagues watch them (24). Asking the advice of colleagues about a particular situation, role playing, and reviewing videotapes of simulated discussions might be helpful.

CASE 17.1   *Continued*

If Mr. R were to suffer a cardiopulmonary arrest, his likelihood of survival would be even lower than the 2% figure for persons with metastatic cancer. However, the physicians need to try to work with the family on a plan that is mutually acceptable. The physicians should shift the focus of discussions from CPR to the goal of care. What were Mr. R's hopes and fears? What would remain unfinished if he were to die soon? Using an approach of "hope for the best but plan for the worst"(25 Note new reference (moved)), physicians might ask if there are relatives who should visit and say what they have not yet said to the patient. Doctors can also ask the family for suggestions on how to make the patient more comfortable. The physicians can also ask whether religion and spirituality were important to Mr. R, to ascertain his goals for care.

Such patient-centered discussions show respect for patients and families and may make them more receptive to the physicians' recommendations about what is best for the patient.

If such discussions do not lead to a mutually acceptable plan for care, the physician may request an ethics consultation or initiate the hospital procedures for foregoing life-sustaining interventions without the concurrence of surrogates.

IMPLEMENTING DNAR ORDERS

WRITING A DNAR ORDER

DNAR orders are common in critically and terminally ill patients. CPR is not attempted for 89% of seriously ill patients who die in acute care hospitals (26). To prevent misunderstandings, physicians should write DNAR orders in the medical record. In addition, the physician should explain in a progress note the rationale for the DNAR order, document the agreement of the patient or surrogate, and describe plans for further care. DNAR orders should be reviewed periodically, particularly if the patient's condition changes.

Oral DNAR orders might lead to mistakes, misunderstandings, and confusion. They create ethical quandaries and legal jeopardy for nurses and first responders to cardiopulmonary arrests. Generally considering an oral DNAR order indicates serious disagreements and a need for further discussions. A DNAR order over the telephone may be acceptable in an urgent situation, provided that the physician signs the order promptly.

INTERPRETATION OF DNAR ORDERS

Implications for Other Treatments

Strictly speaking, a DNAR order means only to withhold CPR. Other treatments, such as antibiotics, transfusions, and even intensive care, might still be appropriate. However, the same reasons that make CPR inappropriate might also render other interventions unsuitable. Many hospitals now require more detailed orders than simply "no CPR," for example, specifying on a checklist whether to provide mechanical ventilation, vasopressors, or antiarrhythmic drugs (27, 28). Such detailed orders clarify whether nurses should treat abnormalities, such as hypotension or ventricular arrhythmia, or allow them to progress, perhaps to cardiopulmonary arrest.

Noninvasive Ventilation (NIV) (29). As medical technology advances, physicians need to be even more specific about what they mean by a DNAR order. For example, NIV, also known as noninvasive positive pressure ventilation or BiPAP, which uses a tightly fitting mask rather than intubation, may allow time for treatments directed at the cause of respiratory failure or to delay death for a specific goal. Some patients find the mask unbearable, but deep sedation is not feasible. If a patient with chronic obstructive lung disease or congestive heart failure requests "no intubation," then physicians should clarify whether the patient would accept or decline NIV (29). Many patients are willing to try NPPV, with the understanding that it may be discontinued if it is unsuccessful or not tolerated.

"Limited" or "Partial" DNAR Orders

Some patients or surrogates may wish to withhold aspects of advanced life support, such as defibrillation or intubation. For instance, patients with chronic obstructive lung disease may decline mechanical ventilation but agree to other resuscitative measures. Such restrictions limit chances for survival. Even if basic CPR is ineffective, advanced life support might restore circulation, breathing, and consciousness. "Limited" DNAR orders are appropriate if an informed patient (or surrogate) consents to them or requests them.

Preventing Misunderstandings

Some physicians are reluctant to write DNAR orders because they fear that other health care workers—consultants, house staff, nurses, or respiratory therapists—might cease to provide needed care to the patient. Conversely, some nurses believe that after a DNAR order, physicians will stop rounding on patients or talking to them. Concerns that DNAR orders might lead to suboptimal care need to be addressed openly. Everyone needs to appreciate that DNAR orders do not mean "do not provide care."

Slow or Show Codes

"Slow codes" or "show codes" appear to provide CPR but actually do not—or do so in a way that is known to be ineffective (30, 31). For example, the code team is not paged immediately, only a few chest compressions are performed, or drugs are injected into the bed rather than into the patient. Such orders are usually given orally and not written down. Slow or show codes are commonly considered when the patient has a grim prognosis but an attending physician insists that CPR be attempted or the patient or surrogate insists that "everything" be done, as in Case 17.1. Show codes are unacceptable because they deceive patients or families, undermine public trust, compromise the ethical integrity of health care professionals, and cause confusion and cynicism among health care workers (32).

SPECIAL SETTINGS

Anesthesia for Surgery and Invasive Procedures

Patients with DNAR orders might undergo surgery for palliation or for conditions unrelated to their primary diagnosis. Many physicians want to "suspend" DNAR orders in the operating room, when the patient's vital functions are deliberately depressed by anesthesia and maintained using techniques similar to those of advanced cardiac life support (33–35). If resuscitation were not permitted, medications might be titrated to ensure greater hemodynamic stability but at the risk of lighter anesthesia, less analgesia, and less amnesia. CPR is much more successful in the operating room than elsewhere in the hospital. In one study, 65% of patients who had a cardiopulmonary arrest in the operating room and 92% of those whose arrest was caused by anesthesia survived to discharge (36). Another reason for suspending DNAR orders during surgery is the physician's sense of responsibility for intraoperative deaths (*see* Chapter 38).

If patients with DNAR orders undergo surgery or invasive procedures, then physicians should discuss how the DNAR orders will be interpreted perioperatively and document plans in the medical record. Similar considerations apply to DNAR orders in radiology during conscious sedation for procedures (37–39).

Emergency Medical Services

When emergency medical personnel are called to the home of a patient with serious illness, CPR might not be appropriate. Paramedic policies and protocols should include provisions for DNAR orders (6). Most states allow physicians to write DNAR orders on a Physicians Orders for Life-Sustaining Treatment (POLST) form or a computerized registry (40). A DNAR order should not automatically preclude other appropriate care, such as oxygen or transport to the hospital. Paramedics face dilemmas when a family member requests that CPR be withheld, but there is no formal DNAR order. Many family members report that they called 911 because they needed help with a frightening complication, wanted someone to confirm death, or did not know what else to do (41). Although it is compassionate to withhold CPR in this situation, it is also ethically problematic because the first responders cannot verify the patient's medical condition or rule out problems such as elder abuse (40).

Family Presence During Resuscitation Efforts

Many family members would like to be present during resuscitation efforts (5, 42). Studies show that the overwhelming majority of relatives who observe resuscitation attempts view it as important and helpful, for example, to accept the patient's death and prevent prolonged grief. In contrast, many physicians and nurses object to relatives being present during resuscitation, fearing that it will prove traumatic for laypeople, cause stress in caregivers, or even interfere with care. Because family members apparently find that the benefits of their presence outweigh the risks, hospitals should offer them the opportunity to be present (5). Hospitals should prepare the family for what they will see and provide emotional support.

SUMMARY

1. CPR is not appropriate for many patients, especially when cardiac arrest is expected.
2. Physicians should elicit patients' preferences about CPR and write DNAR orders in the medical record.

3. The question is not whether physicians should discuss DNAR orders with their patients, but how to do so with compassion and caring.

REFERENCES

1. Peberdy MA, Kaye W, Ornato JP, Larkin GL, Nadkarni V, Mancini ME, et al. Cardiopulmonary resuscitation of adults in the hospital: a report of 14720 cardiac arrests from the National Registry of Cardiopulmonary Resuscitation. *Resuscitation.* 2003;58:297–308.
2. Ebell MH, Afonso AM. Pre-arrest predictors of failure to survive after in-hospital cardiopulmonary resuscitation: a meta-analysis. *Fam Pract.* 2011;28:505–515.
3. Stub D, Bernard S, Duffy SJ, Kaye DM, et al. Post cardiac arrest syndrome: a review of therapeutic strategies. *Circulation.* 2011;123:1428–1435.
4. Guidelines 2000 for Cardiopulmonary Resuscitation and Emergency Cardiovascular Care. Part 2: ethical aspects of CPR and ECC. *Circulation.* 2000;102–I21.
5. Morrison LJ, Kierzek G, Diekema DS, Sayre MR, Silvers SM, Idris AH, et al. Part 3: ethics: 2010 American Heart Association Guidelines for Cardiopulmonary Resuscitation and Emergency Cardiovascular Care. *Circulation.* 2010;122:S665–S675.
6. Tomlinson T, Brody H. Futility and the ethics of resuscitation. *JAMA.* 1990;264:1276–1280.
7. Alpers A, Lo B. When is CPR futile? *JAMA.* 1995;273:156–158.
8. Ebell MH, Becker LA, Barry HC, Hagen M, et al. Survival analysis after in-hospital cardiopulmonary resuscitation. *J Gen Intern Med.* 1998;13:805–816.
9. Curtis JR, Park DR, Krone MR, Pearlman RA, et al. The use of the medical futility rationale in do not attempt resuscitation orders. *JAMA.* 1995;273:124–128.
10. Schneiderman LJ, Jecker NS, Jonsen AR. Medical futility: its meaning and ethical implications. *Ann Intern Med.* 1990;112:949–954.
11. Schneiderman LJ, Jecker NS, Jonsen AR. Medical futility: response to critiques. *Ann Intern Med.* 1996;125:669–674.
12. Teno JM, Hakim RB, Knaus WA, Wenger NS, Phillips RS, Wu AW, et al. Preferences for cardiopulmonary resuscitation: physican-patient agreement and hospital resource use. *J Gen Intern Med.* 1995;10:179–186.
13. Shmerling RH, Bedell SA, Lilienfeld A, Delbanco TLet al. Discussing cardiopulmonary resuscitation: a study of elderly outpatients. *J Gen Intern Med.* 1988;3:317–321.
14. Lo B, Mc Leod G, Saika G. Patient attitudes towards discussing life-sustaining treatment. *Arch Intern Med.* 1986;146:1613–1615.
15. Reilly BM, Magnussen CR, Ross J, et al. Can we talk? Inpatient discussions about advance directives in a community hospital. Attending physicians' attitudes, their inpatients' wishes, and reported experience. *Arch Intern Med.* 1994;154:2299–2308.
16. Hoffman JC, Wenger NS, Davis RH, et al. Patient preferences for communication with physicians about end-of-life decisions. *Ann Intern Med.* 1997;127:1–12.
17. Council on Ethical and Judicial Affairs AMA. Guidelines for the appropriate use of do-not-resuscitate orders. *JAMA.* 1991;265:1868–1871.
18. Fischer GS, Tulsky JA, Rose MR, et al. Patient knowledge and physician predications of treatment preferences after discussions of advance directives. *J Gen Intern Med.* 1998;13:447–454.
19. Diem SJ, Lantos JD, Tulsky JA. Cardiopulmonary resuscitation on television. Miracles and misinformation. *N Engl J Med.* 1996;334:1578–1582.
20. Murphy DJ, Burrows D, Santilli S, et al. The influence of the probability of survival on patients' preferences regarding cardiopulmonary resuscitation. *N Engl J Med.* 1994;330:545–549.
21. O'Brien LA, Grisso JA, Maislin G, et al. Nursing home residents' preferences for life-sustaining treatments. *JAMA.* 1995;254:1175–1179.
22. Lo B, Quill T, Tulsky J. Discussing palliative care with patients. *Ann Intern Med.* 1999;130:744–749.
23. Tulsky JA, Chesney MA, Lo B. How do medical residents discuss resuscitation with patients? *J Gen Intern Med.* 1995;10:436–442.
24. Tulsky JA, Chesney MA, Lo B. "See one, do one, teach one?" Housestaff experience discussing do-not-resuscitate orders. *Arch Intern Med.* 1996;156:1285–1289.
25. Back AL, Arnold RM, Quill TE. Hope for the best, and prepare for the worst. *Ann Intern Med.* 2003;138:439–443.
26. Lynn J, Teno J, Phillips RS, et al. Perceptions by family members of the dying experience of older and seriously ill patients. *Ann Intern Med.* 1997;126:97–106.
27. Mittelberger JA, Lo B, Martin D, et al. Impact of a procedure-specific do not resuscitate order form on documentation of do not resuscitate orders. *Arch Intern Med.* 1993;153:228–232.
28. O'Toole EE, Youngner SJ, Juknialis BW, et al. Evaluation of a treatment limitation policy with a specific treatment-limiting order page. *Arch Intern Med.* 1994;154:425–432.
29. Curtis JR, Cook DJ, Sinuff T, et al. Noninvasive positive pressure ventilation in critical and palliative care settings: understanding the goals of therapy. *Crit Care Med.* 2007;35:932–939.

30. Muller JH. Shades of blue: the negotiation of limited codes by medical residents. *Soc Sci Med*. 1992;34:885–898.
31. Gazelle G. The slow code—should anyone rush to its defense? *N Engl J Med*. 1998;338:467–469.
32. Frader J, Kodish E, Lantos JD. Ethics rounds. Symbolic resuscitation, medical futility, and parental rights. *Pediatrics*. 2010;126:769–772.
33. Cohen CB, Cohen PJ. Do-not-resuscitate orders in the operating room. *N Engl J Med*. 1991;325:1879–1882.
34. Truog RD. "Do not resuscitate" orders during anesthesia and surgery. *Anesthesiology*. 1991;74:606–608.
35. Walker RM. DNR in the OR: resuscitation as an operative risk. *JAMA*. 1991;266:2407–2412.
36. Olsson GL, Hall B. Cardiac arrest during anesthesia: a computer-aided study in 250, 543 anaesthetics. *Acta Anaes Scan*. 1988;32:653–664.
37. Jacobson JA, Gully JE, Mann H. "Do not resuscitate" orders in the radiology department: an interpretation. *Radiology*. 1996;198:21–24.
38. McDermott VG. Resuscitation and the radiologist. *Ann Intern Med*. 1998;129:831–833.
39. Heffner JE, Barbieri C. Compliance with do-not-resuscitate orders for hospitalized patients transported to radiology departments. *Ann Intern Med*. 1998;129:801–805.
40. Kellermann A, Lynn J. Withholding resuscitation in prehospital care. *Ann Intern Med*. 2006;144:692–693.
41. Feder S, Matheny RL, Loveless RS, Jr, et al. Withholding resuscitation: a new approach to prehospital end-of-life decisions. *Ann Intern Med*. 2006;144:634–640.
42. Tsai E. Should family members be present during cardiopulmonary resuscitation? *N Engl J Med*. 2002;346:1019–1021.

ANNOTATED BIBLIOGRAPHY

1. Tulsky JA, Chesney MA, Lo B. How do medical residents discuss resuscitation with patients? *J Gen Intern Med*. 1995;10:436–442.
   Shows how, in discussions with patients regarding CPR, residents failed to provide key information about CPR and missed opportunities to discuss the patient's values and goals.
2. Murphy DJ, Burrows D, Santilli S. The influence of the probability of survival on patients' preferences regarding cardiopulmonary resuscitation. *N Engl J Med*. 1994;330:545–549.
   Concludes that patients overestimate survival after CPR and that when such misunderstandings are corrected, patients are less likely to accept CPR.
3. Curtis JR, Park DR, Krone MR. The use of the medical futility rationale in do not attempt resuscitation orders. *JAMA*. 1995;273:124–128.
   Empirical study documenting problems and mistakes that occur when physicians claim that CPR would be futile.
4. Morrison LJ, Kierzek G, Diekema DS, et al. Part 3: ethics: 2010 American Heart Association Guidelines for Cardiopulmonary Resuscitation and Emergency Cardiovascular Care. *Circulation*. 2010;122:S665–S675.
   Consensus ethical guidelines presented in CPR certification courses.
5. Curtis JR, Cook DJ, Sinuff T, et al. Noninvasive positive pressure ventilation in critical and palliative care settings: understanding the goals of therapy. *Crit Care Med*. 2007;35:932–939.
   Use of NPPV in patients who have chosen to forego endotracheal intubation requires a discussion with the patient and family regarding the goals of care and parameters for success or failure to achieve those goals.

18

Tube Feedings

T ube and intravenous feedings can prolong life in patients who cannot take adequate nutrition by mouth. In conditions such as short bowel syndrome, parenteral hyperalimentation can allow patients to lead active lives for many years. However, in a severe, progressive illness such as advanced dementia or metastatic cancer, tube feedings might merely prolong death and subject patients to indignity. Eighty-six percent of patients with advanced dementia develop feeding problems, and 29% die within 6 months (1). More than one third of such patients have feeding tubes (2). Organizational, cultural, and fiscal features of the nursing home or hospital are related to rates of feeding tubes (2, 3).

CASE 18.1	Tube feedings in a patient with severe dementia (4)

A patient's daughter leaves a phone message: "My mother, Mrs. F, has eaten nothing all weekend. What should we do?" A 70-year-old woman with severe dementia, Mrs. F rarely speaks, is confined to a wheelchair, and requires diapers for incontinence. She has been kept out of a nursing home by the efforts of a devoted family and a geriatric day care center. During the past year, her social actions have decreased and her food intake has become increasingly erratic. First she stopped feeding herself. Now, although her family feeds her by hand, her intake continues to decline. Once she required overnight hospitalization for dehydration. During the past week, she has been clamping her mouth shut, pushing the spoon away with her hand, and spitting out food. Over the weekend, even coaxing with her favorite foods was unsuccessful. Those who care for her must now face a dreaded question: If hand feedings continue to fail, should she be fed through a feeding tube? The situation evokes strong and conflicting reactions. The patient's sister says, "We can't let her starve to death!" The daughter, however, says, "She's telling us to stop. We're just torturing her."

REASONS TO PROVIDE TUBE FEEDINGS

ALLOW REVERSAL OF CAUSES OF FEEDING PROBLEMS

Decreased oral intake might result from reversible medical problems, such as intercurrent illness, mouth lesions, side effects of medications, or psychosocial problems, such as a desire for more control, depression, or a change of caregivers. Sometimes, hand feedings can be made more acceptable to the patient, for example, by slowing the pace of feeding, offering smaller bites, altering the taste or consistency, reminding the demented patient to swallow, or gently touching her (4). Temporary use of tube or intravenous feedings might resolve the crisis and allow the underlying problem to be identified and treated.

PREVENT STARVATION

Everyone has temporarily experienced thirst or hunger and can imagine how agonizing it must be to starve to death. Similarly, everyone appreciates how upset infants become when they are not fed. By analogy, some people believe that adult patients with terminal illness or advanced dementia suffer when feeding tubes are withheld. In addition, tube feedings clearly prolong life for years in persons in persistent vegetative state (PVS). Finally, some physicians believe that discontinuing tube or intravenous feedings makes them the direct cause of the patient's death. A systematic critical review, however, concluded that feeding tubes in patients with dementia do not prolong life compared to attempts at hand feedings (5).

PROVIDE ORDINARY BASIC CARE

Many people regard tube feedings as basic humane care. In this view, feeding is an essential part of caring for the helpless, just like providing a warm, clean bed (6, 7). Recent Roman Catholic teaching considers artificial nutrition to be ordinary care in principle, although traditional Catholic doctrine allows tube feedings to be refused if excessively burdensome (7, 8).

REASONS TO WITHHOLD TUBE FEEDINGS

Those who would withhold tube feedings from patients with severe, progressive illness frame the issues differently. They agree that it is morally obligatory to give bottles to infants, provide groceries to homebound persons, and place spoonfuls of food in the mouth of a person with dementia. However, opponents offer several reasons for withholding tube feedings when patients such as Mrs. F refuse oral intake.

TUBE FEEDINGS MERELY PROLONG DYING

Many people believe that tube and intravenous feedings only prolong death for terminally ill patients. They consider it inhumane to force-feed people with severe dementia only to have them succumb to pneumonia or some other complication. Furthermore, it is problematic to say that withholding artificial feedings causes the patient's death. Determining *a single* cause of death when many factors are contributing to the patient's death is a controversial philosophical topic (9). Nonetheless, in such cases, death is legally attributed to the underlying dementia and not to foregoing medical interventions—provided that the reasons for withholding treatment are ethically acceptable. Chapter 14 discusses these distinctions in detail.

SUCH PATIENTS DO NOT SUFFER IF TUBE FEEDINGS ARE WITHHELD

Patients with severe dementia or metastatic cancer seldom experience thirst or hunger if they continue to refuse oral intake. In a study from a comfort care unit, almost all lucid, terminally ill patients reduced intake of food and fluids to less than their nutritional needs. About two thirds never experienced hunger, and about one third experienced hunger only initially. Symptoms of thirst or dry mouth were more common, with 36% experiencing them until death. In all patients, small intake of food and fluids, ice chips, and meticulous mouth care relieved symptoms of hunger and dry mouth (10). In another study, hospice nurses rated quality of death of patients who refused food and water as 8 on a 9-point scale, where 9 was a very good death (11). With reduced oral intake, symptoms such as nausea, vomiting, edema, cough, and incontinence are reduced (12). Furthermore, pain medications should be given if needed, just as they are provided to patients with respiratory failure who decline mechanical ventilation. Family members need to be reassured that any discomfort can and will be treated (13). A recent study suggests, however, that moderate parenteral hydration might reduce myoclonus and fatigue in patients with terminal cancer (14).

TUBE AND INTRAVENOUS FEEDINGS CANNOT BE CONSIDERED ORDINARY CARE

Labeling artificial feedings as "ordinary" care is questionable. Cessation of the desire for food and drink is part of the natural history of severe illnesses, such as severe dementia or metastatic cancer.

In other Western societies, such as the United Kingdom and Sweden, tube feedings are rarely administered to patients with severe dementia. In addition, long-term intravenous or nasogastric tube feedings have become technically possible only in the past 30 years. The Food and Drug Administration regulates artificial feedings as drugs and medical devices, not as foods. Furthermore, feeding gastrostomy or jejunostomy tubes require a surgical or endoscopic procedure for insertion.

More fundamentally, most writers on medical ethics and virtually all court decisions reject the distinction between "extraordinary" and "ordinary" care (*see* Chapter 14) (15–17). The issue is not whether an intervention can be considered "extraordinary" or "ordinary," but whether its benefits outweigh its burdens for the individual patient (15). As with other interventions, tube and intravenous feedings should not be provided simply because they are technically feasible.

TUBE AND INTRAVENOUS FEEDINGS HAVE BURDENS AND BENEFITS

Like all interventions, tube and intravenous feedings have burdens, as well as benefits. For patients with severe dementia or metastatic cancer, the benefits of tube feedings are limited (18). Treatable conditions are identified and corrected in few such patients (19). One cohort study found that 50% of patients with severe dementia who receive tube feedings died within 6 months (20). There is little evidence that tube feedings prolong life in patients with severe dementia, compared with continued offerings of food by hand (5).

The burden of tube feedings might be substantial. Complications of tube feedings in elderly patients include aspiration pneumonia in 46% of cases and agitation leading to self-extubation in 61% of cases (21). Tube feedings might not reduce the risk of aspiration pneumonia compared with oral intake (21). Aspiration pneumonia appears to be as common with gastrostomy tubes as with nasogastric tubes (22). Patients who pull out feeding tubes might be communicating refusal, expressing discomfort or anger, seeking attention or control, or acting in a purely reflexive manner.

Over one third of patients with dementia who have feeding tubes require physical or pharmacologic restraints (1). Restraining demented patients to prevent them from pulling out tubes compromises their independence and dignity, particularly because they cannot appreciate how the feeding tube will help them (4). Restraints also increase patient agitation. Sedation or "chemical restraint," which might appear to be more acceptable, also compromises patient dignity. Many patients would not want to be restrained. In a study of nursing home residents, 33% said they wanted tube feedings if they were unable to eat because of permanent brain damage that also left them unable to recognize people. However, after learning that physical restraints are sometimes applied to patients receiving tube feedings, 25% of residents who initially wanted tube feedings or were not sure changed their minds and preferred not to have them (23).

The President's Council on Bioethics, while emphasizing the inherent dignity of persons with disabilities such as severe dementia, stated that if treatment "would require sedation, physical restraint, frequent re-locations," "treatment itself adds to the un-consenting and un-comprehending patient's miseries, burdens, or degradations" (24).

> . . . In cases such as this where patient resistance makes the very activity of getting treated a great burden—not simply physically in terms of pain, but humanly in terms of the patient's overall well-being—the decision to cease treatment and accept an earlier death seems morally permissible once other alternatives fail, and it may even be the best choice among a range of imperfect options. (24)

CARING SHOULD BE PROVIDED DIRECTLY, NOT THROUGH SYMBOLS

If the goal of care is to provide comfort and compassion, then caregivers should do so directly rather than through symbolic actions (4), for example offering patients food and water by hand, moistening their mouth and lips, holding their hand, or giving a backrub.

Ironically, artificial feedings might be impersonal. With tube feedings, the caregiver might focus more attention on technical issues, such as positioning the feeding tube and checking the residual volume, than on the patient. If tube feedings proceed without complication, then social interaction between the caregiver and patient can be minimal. Moreover, the patient has no control over tube feedings except to pull out the tube. In contrast, with hand feedings patients determine the timing, pace, and even the content of feedings. Patients can turn away or clamp their mouths shut. Thus, hand feedings that provide inadequate nutrition might meet more of the patient's human needs than tube feedings that deliver adequate calories impersonally.

LEGAL ISSUES

According to court decisions, artificial feedings are similar to other medical interventions, which have benefits and burdens for the patient (17). The predominant judicial opinion is that artificial feedings are medical interventions that may be withheld under appropriate circumstances, not comfort measures that must always be given. In several states, courts have ruled that tube feedings may be withheld from a patient's PVS or minimally conscious state only if there is clear and convincing evidence that the patient would refuse. Some states set stricter standards for withholding or withdrawing tube feedings than for other medical interventions, when advance directives or surrogate decision-making is used (25).

CLINICAL RECOMMENDATIONS

When patients with conditions such as severe dementia stop eating and cannot be fed by hand, physicians and surrogates need to discuss the goals of care and the benefits and burdens of tube feedings. Decisions may be more difficult when patients have not provided advance directives. If there are reversible problems that impair oral intake, temporary intravenous or tube feedings are appropriate. Long-term tube feedings are appropriate if patients have no irreversible life-threatening problems and would consider their quality of life acceptable. Tube feedings, however, are not indicated if the patient has serious, progressive illness and a poor quality of life and if a caring surrogate agrees that the goal should be to provide comfort.

Decisions about feeding tubes in patients with advanced dementia often fail to follow guidelines for shared decision making between physicians and surrogates. When families of patients who died from dementia and had feeding tubes were interviewed, 14% said that there had been no discussion of feeding tubes, and 42% reported a discussion that was less than 15 minutes (1). Over one half believed that the health care provider strongly favored the use of a feeding tube, and 13% felt pressured to use a feeding tube. Other studies show that the prevalence of feeding tubes is strongly associated with characteristics of the nursing home.

CASE 18.1   *Continued*

Mrs. F's physician discussed with the family goals of care and the benefits and burdens of tube feedings. She asked about statements by the patient and about the family's concerns and emotions and addressed the sister's concerns. She discussed several options. One was offering food and fluids by hand but not inserting a feeding tube. The physician explained that patients like Mrs. F may live just as long with this "comfort feeding only" approach as with tube feedings and described how discomfort would be treated. The doctor said that many families choose this approach, giving them permission to do so. A second option was a time-limited trial of tube feedings, with reassessment in 2 weeks. If Mrs. F repeatedly pulls out the nasogastric tube, the goals of care would be reconsidered. The physician recommended against restraints or sedation to keep a tube in place. A third option was a feeding gastrostomy or jejunostomy, which is less obtrusive and more difficult to remove than a nasogasric tube. The physician emphasized that these decisions are very difficult, said that it was sad to see Mrs. F decline. No family could be more devoted, and they were a comfort to her. The doctor also promised to be there for them and Mrs. F. The physician suggested the family talk among themselves about what was best for Mrs. F and scheduled a time to continue discussions.

SUMMARY

1. Tube and intravenous feedings in patients with severe, progressive illness have burdens, as well as benefits.
2. Such interventions may be withheld or withdrawn from patients with advanced dementia if they do not serve the goal of relieving distress and discomfort.

REFERENCES

1. Teno JM, Mitchell SL, Kuo SK, et al. Decision-making and outcomes of feeding tube insertion: a five-state study. *J Am Geriatr Soc.* 2011;59:881–886.
2. Mitchell SL, Teno JM, Roy J, et al. Clinical and organizational factors associated with feeding tube use among nursing home residents with advanced cognitive impairment. *JAMA.* 2003;290:73–80.
3. Teno JM, Mitchell SL, Gozalo PL, et al. Hospital characteristics associated with feeding tube placement in nursing home residents with advanced cognitive impairment. *JAMA.* 2010;303:544–550.
4. Lo B, Dornbrand L. Guiding the hand that feeds: caring for the demented elderly. *N Engl J Med.*1984;311:402–404.
5. Candy B, Sampson EL, Jones L. Enteral tube feeding in older people with advanced dementia: findings from a Cochrane systematic review. *Int J Palliat Nurs.* 2009;15:396–404.
6. Pope John Paul II. On life-sustaining treatments and the vegetative state: scientific advances and ethical dilemmas. *Natl Cathol Bioeth Q.* 2004;4:573–576.
7. Sulmasy DP. Terri Schiavo and the Roman Catholic tradition of forgoing extraordinary means of care. *J Law Med Ethics.* 2005;33:359–362.
8. Bradley CT. Roman Catholic doctrine guiding end-of-life care: a summary of the recent discourse. *J Palliat Med.* 2009;12:373–377.
9. Brock D. Forgoing life-sustaining food and water: is it killing? In: Lynn J, ed. *By No Extraordinary Means.* Expanded edition ed. Bloomington, IN: Indiana University Press; 1989. 117–131.
10. McCann RM, Hall WJ, Groth-Juncker A. Comfort care for terminally ill patients: the appropriate use of nutrition and hydration. *JAMA.* 1994;272:1263–11266.
11. Ganzini L, Goy ER, Miller LL, et al. Nurses' experiences with hospice patients who refuse food and fluids to hasten death. *N Engl J Med.* 2003;349:359–365.
12. Billings JA. Comfort measures for the terminally ill: is dehydration painful? *J Am Geriatr Soc.* 1985;33:808–810.
13. Casarett D, Kapo J, Caplan A. Appropriate use of artificial nutrition and hydration—fundamental principles and recommendations. *N Engl J Med.* 2005;353:2607–2612.
14. Bruera E, Sala R, Rico MA, et al. Effects of parenteral hydration in terminally ill cancer patients: a preliminary study. *J Clin Oncol.* 2005;23:2366–2371.
15. President's Commission for the Study of Ethical Problems in Medicine and Biomedical and Behavioral Research. *Deciding to Forego Life-sustaining Treatment.* Washington, DC: U.S. Government Printing Office; 1983. 82–89.
16. Steinbrook R, Lo B. Artifical feedings: solid ground, not slippery slope. *N Engl J Med.* 1988;318:286–290.
17. Meisel A, Cerminara K. *The Right to Die: The Law of End of Life Decision Making.* 3rd ed. New York, NY: Aspen Publishers; 2004.
18. Ganzini L. Artificial nutrition and hydration at the end of life: ethics and evidence. *Palliat Support Care.* 2006;4:135–143.
19. Quill TE. Utilization of nasogastric feeding tubes in a group of chronically ill, elderly patients in a community hospital. *Arch Intern Med.* 1989;149:1937–1941.
20. Meier DE, Ahronheim JC, Morris J, et al. High short-term mortality in hospitalized patients with advanced dementia: lack of benefit of tube feeding. *Arch Intern Med.* 2001;161:594–599.
21. Ciocon JO, Sliverstone FA, Graver LM, et al. Tube feedings in elderly patients. *Arch Intern Med.* 1988;148:429–443.
22. Fiucane TE, Christmas C, Travis K. Tube feeding in patients with advanced dementia. *JAMA.* 1999;282:1365–1370.
23. O'Brien LA, Siegert EA, Grisso JA, et al. Tube feeding preferences among nursing home residents. *J Gen Intern Med.* 1997;12:364–371.
24. The President's Council on Bioethics. *Taking Care: Ethical Caregiving in Our Aging Society.* Washington, DC: U.S. Executive Office of the President; 2005.
25. Brody H, Hermer LD, Scott LD, et al. Artificial nutrition and hydration: the evolution of ethics, evidence, and policy. *J Gen Intern Med.* 2011;26:1053–1058.

ANNOTATED BIBLIOGRAPHY

1. Lo B, Dornbrand L. Guiding the hand that feeds: caring for the demented elderly. *N Engl J Med.* 1984;311:402–404. Argues that tube feedings might not be appropriate palliative care for severely demented patients who refuse feedings by hand, particularly if patients are tied down to prevent them from pulling out the tubes.

2. Gillick MR. Rethinking the role of tube feeding in patients with advanced dementia. *N Engl J Med.* 2000;342:206–210.

   Casarett D, Kapo J, Caplan A. Appropriate use of artificial nutrition and hydration—Fundamental principles and recommendations. *N Engl J Med.* 2005;353:2607–2612.

   Two articles that argue that tube feedings should be discouraged in patients with advanced dementia.
3. The President's Council on Bioethics. *Taking Care: Ethical Caregiving in Our Aging Society.* Washington, DC: U.S. Executive Office of the President; 2005.

   Emphasizes that when doctors and families must make hard choices for patients who lack decision-making capacity, they should try to benefit the life the patient still has, even when that life has been diminished by illness.

CHAPTER 19

Physician-Assisted Suicide and Active Euthanasia

Although traditional medical ethics prohibit assisted suicide and active euthanasia, public opinion and policies in the United States are divided. Active euthanasia is illegal throughout the United States, and most states prohibit physician-assisted suicide. The Supreme Court ruled that there is no constitutional right to physician-assisted suicide and that states may prohibit it (1). Two states, Oregon and Washington, permit physician-assisted suicide for patients with terminal illness. Despite legal bans on physician-assisted suicide and active euthanasia, studies document that are carried out (2). Two juries acquitted Jack Kevorkian, a nonpracticing pathologist who publicized numerous cases in which he assisted in a patient's suicide, before he was convicted of murder for administering a lethal dose to a patient.

DEFINING TERMS CLEARLY

Imprecise terminology and rhetorical slogans are common in discussions of assisted suicide and euthanasia. Several actions should be distinguished (*see* also Chapter 14).

ACTIVE VOLUNTARY EUTHANASIA

In active euthanasia, the physician administers a lethal dose of medication, such as potassium chloride. The physician supplies the means of death and is the final human agent in the events leading to the patient's death. Active euthanasia is sometimes called *mercy killing*. Euthanasia is called *voluntary* when the patient requests it, *involuntary* when the patient opposes it, and *nonvoluntary* when the patient lacks decision-making capacity and cannot express a preference. There is general agreement that involuntary euthanasia is wrong because it violates a patient's right not to be killed. Nonvoluntary euthanasia is also generally considered unacceptable because it might be applied selectively to the disadvantaged and the vulnerable. As we later discuss, some people believe voluntary euthanasia may be justified in some circumstances.

ASSISTED SUICIDE

In assisted suicide, the patient swallows a lethal dose of drugs or activates a device to administer the drugs. Physicians might assist in a variety of ways. They might refer the patient to the Hemlock Society for information, provide information directly, or provide the means for suicide.

Many people consider assisted suicide less ethically problematic than active euthanasia. Although the physician provides the means of death, the patient must carry out an independent act. This fact might have several important ethical implications. The patient's subsequent intervening action might lessen the physician's moral responsibility. Patients have free will and are morally responsible for their acts. Although other people might influence the patient, they are not regarded as the cause of the patient's actions unless there is coercion. Moreover, there might be less danger of abuse with assisted suicide than active euthanasia because patients can change their minds and not simply take the relevant pills.

Physicians, however, must not underestimate their moral responsibility if they assist a patient in committing suicide. The motive, intent, justification, and outcome are the same as in active euthanasia. In other situations, people may be held morally responsible for assisting or encouraging another person to commit an immoral act.

Some physicians who prescribe a lethal dose of medications might claim that they did not know that the patient planned to commit suicide. For example, some doctors might prescribe secobarbital on a patient's request without discussing suicide. It would be disingenuous to abjure responsibility in this situation. Doctors almost never prescribe secobarbital except as a means for suicide. Most important, discussions of the patient's interest in suicide present opportunities for the physician to improve palliative care, so that the patient feels that suicide is the best option.

Recently, the terms *physician-assisted death* or *physician aid in dying* have been used because they are more neutral and less emotionally charged. Opponents, however, argue that these terms cover over moral objections to these practices. This book uses the term *aid in dying* to refer to Oregon and Washington, which use them in state laws, but generally does not adopt it because it is used consistently to refer only to giving a prescription for a lethal dose of medication to a terminally ill patient. Indeed, in recent debates in Britain, the terms *assisted death*, *assisted dying*, and *medical assistance to die* were used to refer to both active euthanasia and physician-assisted suicide (3–5). Our concern is that a term that is used in inconsistent and ambiguous ways may worsen confusion over two ethically distinct actions.

WITHHOLDING OR WITHDRAWING MEDICAL INTERVENTIONS

Active euthanasia and assisted suicide are ethically different from withholding or withdrawing interventions, which are also termed *allowing to die* or *passive euthanasia*. Ethically and legally, medical interventions may be withheld or withdrawn if a competent patient or an appropriate surrogate refuses them (*see* Chapter 14). A patient's refusal of life-sustaining treatment is honored because patients have a right to be free of unwanted bodily invasions. Under such circumstances, the underlying illness, not the physician's action or inaction, is considered the cause of death. This is the case even though some patients who refuse life-prolonging interventions want to hasten their death, not just to be free of unwanted medical interventions. Therefore, objections to assisted suicide or active euthanasia should not lead physicians to impose interventions that the patient or surrogate does not want.

This distinction between killing and allowing to die may provide practical guidance, but it is logically problematic (6, 7). Many philosophers have rejected the distinction between acting and refraining from action, pointing out that withholding effective treatment would be condemned if done against the patient's wishes or for malicious motives.

ADMINISTERING APPROPRIATE DOSES OF OPIOIDS OR SEDATIVES

Active euthanasia and assisted suicide can be distinguished from high doses of opioids or sedatives to relieve severe pain in patients with terminal illness or to relieve dyspnea when patients forego mechanical ventilation (8). In these situations, the appropriate goal of care is to relieve suffering. In rare cases, the dose required to relieve refractory symptoms might hasten death. Concerns about active euthanasia and assisted suicide should not deter physicians from providing aggressive palliative care (8, 9). Indeed, fear that terminal symptoms will not be relieved leads some patients to seek assisted suicide or active euthanasia (10, 11).

REASONS IN FAVOR OF ASSISTED SUICIDE AND ACTIVE EUTHANASIA

RESPECT FOR PATIENT AUTONOMY

The prospect of a long, debilitating illness that would destroy their sense of identity and dignity horrifies many persons. People might fear increased dependence on others for basic needs such as feeding, bathing, and toilet use. They also might not want their family and friends to remember them as progressively debilitated. Proponents contend that competent patients with terminal illness should have control over the time and manner of their death. In this view, it is inconsistent to permit patients to end their lives by refusing medical interventions after a complication occurs but not to end it more directly beforehand.

COMPASSION FOR PATIENTS WHO ARE SUFFERING

Some argue that assisted suicide and active euthanasia show compassion for patients in the final stages of a terminal illness. Many people regard it as inhumane to require such patients to suffer a downhill course while waiting to die of complications. As one author puts it, "People who want an early peaceful death for themselves or their relatives are not rejecting or denigrating the sanctity of life; on the contrary, they believe that a quicker death shows more respect for life than a protracted one" (12). In some circumstances, terminally ill patients have refractory symptoms despite optimal palliative care. For example, some patients with cancer of the esophagus or head and neck cannot swallow their secretions and some cancer patients experience intractable bleeding. Such patients can be sedated so that they are no longer conscious of their symptoms, but they will not have dignified or peaceful deaths.

Proponents also argue that physicians cannot prevent people from killing themselves but only alter the means by which they do so. If lethal drugs are not available, patients might resort to hanging or guns. Such gruesome means of death distress family members and friends. Advocates contend that terminally ill patients should have a more humane means of ending their lives.

REASONS AGAINST ASSISTED SUICIDE AND ACTIVE EUTHANASIA

THE SANCTITY OF LIFE

Many people assert that these acts demean the sacredness of human life and violate fundamental moral prohibitions against killing human beings.

SUFFERING CAN ALMOST ALWAYS BE RELIEVED

Palliative care is often inadequate in terminally ill patients. Opponents fear that assisted suicide and active euthanasia will allow physicians to avoid the difficult task of providing physical and spiritual comfort to dying patients. Furthermore, some people suggest that suffering can be redemptive and that patients have a duty to endure it or cope courageously (13).

REQUESTS FOR ASSISTED SUICIDE ARE NOT AUTONOMOUS

Most terminally ill patients change their minds on suicide after receiving better palliative care or treatment for depression. Thus, their initial requests may not be truly autonomous. Even among patients with cancer, most suicidal individuals are clinically depressed, and major depression can be treated (14, 15).

FEARS OF ABUSE

A slippery slope might occur: if physician-assisted suicide is permitted for competent terminally ill patients, it would be inconsistent to deny it to patients who have previously requested it but have lost decision-making capacity (16). A patient with mild Alzheimer disease might not want to live if he or she could no longer recognize his or her family. At that stage, however, the patient would no longer be capable of making an informed request. Thus, if the patient is not permitted to request physician-assisted suicide or active euthanasia through an advance directive, the patient would face a cruel dilemma: to end life when it is still meaningful or to live in an unacceptably dehumanized condition. Furthermore, some patients with severe amyotrophic lateral sclerosis (ALS) might want to hasten their death to avoid further dependency and to relieve their suffering. However, such patients are not terminally ill and might lack the physical ability to ingest medication without assistance. Thus, respecting their wishes to hasten death might require active euthanasia.

A second type of slippery slope is empirical rather than logical (16). At first, physicians who participate in assisted suicide might carefully ensure that every case is appropriate, but over time they might become less diligent in providing palliative care or checking that the patient's request is voluntary. Eventually, assisted suicide might occur when palliative care was grossly inadequate or major depression was unaddressed. In Oregon, however, these concerns did not materialize (17).

Active euthanasia raises particular fears about abuse. Euthanasia for competent patients logically leads to euthanasia of patients who lack decision-making capacity. Furthermore, relief of unbearable suffering might be used to justify active euthanasia in mentally incapacitated patients who had never requested it. Another fear is that pressures to control health care costs will result in nonvoluntary euthanasia of persons whose care is regarded as too burdensome or too expensive (18). Patients with chronic illness or disability might feel pressured by family members or physicians into terminating their lives.

THE PHYSICIAN'S ROLE

Opponents argue that active euthanasia and assisted suicide are incompatible with the physician's role as healer. In this view, patients would lose trust in physicians if these practices were permitted. In one study, 19% of oncology patients said they would change physicians if their physician told them they had provided active euthanasia or physician-assisted suicide for other patients (19).

LEGALIZATION OF PHYSICIAN AID IN DYING IN OREGON

In Oregon and Washington, terminally ill, competent adults may request medication to end their life (17, 20). The patient must make a written request that is witnessed by two people who attest that the patient is competent, acting voluntarily, and not coerced. Fifteen days after this written request, the patient must repeat the request orally. An additional 48 hours must elapse before the prescription can be filled. The patient may rescind the request at any time. Physicians must ensure that patients are informed about their diagnosis, prognosis, and therapeutic alternatives, such as palliative care. A consultant must confirm that the patient has a terminal disease, is capable of making health care decisions, is informed, and is acting voluntarily. Patients with a psychiatric disorder that impairs judgment must be referred for counseling. Physicians who comply with the provisions of the law are granted legal immunity from criminal, civil, and professional disciplinary actions. Their actions are termed *physician aid in dying* because giving a patient a prescription for a dose of medication to end his life remains illegal in other circumstances. Physicians and other health care workers may refuse to participate. If a patient ingests a lethal dose of medication under this law, life insurance policies are not voided.

The law sets several important limits. The law specifically prohibits active euthanasia, mercy killing, and lethal injection. Physicians are not allowed to provide assistance to patients who are too incapacitated to take lethal medication themselves. Patients are excluded if they suffer from nonterminal illnesses, lack decision-making capacity, or are too sick to survive the waiting periods. Patients may not request aid in dying through advance directives or surrogate decision makers.

In Oregon, aid in dying accounts for slightly more than 1 in 1,000 deaths (21), a rate that has not increased over time (22). However, about 17% of family members report that the patient mentioned physician-assisted dying to them. Of these, about 10% asked their physicians for a lethal prescription. Those who make such a request are more concerned about independence and control over their lives than intractable physical suffering. About a third of patients who receive a lethal prescription from physicians do not use it.

Reported cases of aid in dying in Oregon do not confirm concerns that legalizing physician-assisted suicide would harm vulnerable patients or undermine palliative care (17, 23). Almost 90%

of patients receiving aid in dying were enrolled in hospice. Compared with other terminal patients, patients who died after ingesting a lethal dose of medication were younger and more highly educated. Only a few were not insured. Poverty, lack of education or health insurance, or poor quality of care did not play a major role in patients' requests (24). The number of reported deaths occurring through aid in dying has not increased over time, and patients from other states have not migrated to Oregon to request such assistance. However, screening for depression and referrals to psychiatrists may be suboptimal (17).

THE PRACTICE OF PHYSICIAN-ASSISTED SUICIDE AND ACTIVE EUTHANASIA

Despite legal prohibitions, physician-assisted suicide and active euthanasia are practiced in the United States.

REQUESTS ARE COMMON

In a national sample, 18% of physicians said that in their careers they had received a request for physician-assisted suicide, and 11% had received a request for active euthanasia (2). In another study, more than 50% of oncologists had received a request for physician-assisted suicide, and 38% had received a request for active euthanasia (25). Twelve percent of cancer patients said they had serious discussions about active euthanasia or physician-assisted suicide with their family or physician, and 3.4% said they hoarded drugs (25).

REQUESTS ARE MORE COMMON IN DEPRESSED PATIENTS

Nineteen percent of patients who received physician-assisted suicide and 39% of patients who received active euthanasia were depressed (2). In another study, cancer patients who were depressed were 4.6 times more likely to have discussed euthanasia drugs (25).

PHYSICIANS PROVIDE REQUESTED ASSISTANCE EVEN WHEN IT IS ILLEGAL

Despite prohibitions, 3.3% of physicians have written a prescription to be used to hasten death, and 4.7% have administered a lethal injection (2). Among oncologists, 13% have assisted suicide and 1.8% have performed active euthanasia (25). Approximately, 40% of patients who receive prescriptions for lethal doses of medication do not use them (2, 26).

PHYSICIANS ARE CONFUSED ABOUT THESE ACTIONS

In some cases that physicians characterized as physician-assisted suicide or active euthanasia, it would be accurate to describe the situation differently. For example, in 13% of cases, physicians actually provided high doses of opioids for pain relief; such palliation of symptoms is ethically distinct from assisted suicide or active euthanasia. In another 9% of cases, patients overdosed without asking the physician for a prescription for a lethal dose; this cannot be described as physician-assisted suicide or active euthanasia (19). Furthermore, 12% of physicians who said that they had assisted suicide actually ordered a nurse to inject medications to end the patient's life, an action that is actually active euthanasia (19).

PROPOSED SAFEGUARDS ARE OFTEN VIOLATED

When physicians prescribe a prescription for physician-assisted suicide, suggested safeguards, such as persistent requests and second opinions, are often not followed. In two studies, patients repeated their request in only 51% and 60% of cases, and doctors obtained a second opinion in only 1% and 40% of cases (2, 25). In 54% of cases of active euthanasia, a family member or partner rather than the patient made the request (2). A second opinion was obtained in only 32% of cases. In 94% of cases, immediate assistance was requested.

PHYSICIAN-ASSISTED SUICIDE HAS AN EMOTIONAL IMPACT ON THE PHYSICIAN

In one study, 18% of physicians who had assisted suicide were uncomfortable doing it (2). In another study, although 53% of respondents were comfortable assisting suicide or performing active euthanasia, 24% regretted performing those acts (19).

ASSISTED SUICIDE AND ACTIVE EUTHANASIA IN THE NETHERLANDS

In the Netherlands, active euthanasia and assisted suicide are legal in certain situations. A competent patient with a terminal illness must make a voluntary and persistent request for active euthanasia or assisted suicide, and two physicians must certify that the patient is terminally ill. In the Netherlands, active euthanasia occurs in 2.8% of deaths and assisted suicide occurs in 0.1% (27). These rates have slightly increased since legislation was enacted in 2002 to legalize these actions (27).

MOST PATIENTS WITHDRAW REQUESTS

Patients' requests for active euthanasia or assisted suicide usually do not last. When patients ask physicians to help them die, only one-third of requests are serious and persistent. Of these, only one-third actually receive active euthanasia or assisted suicide; most change their minds after obtaining better palliative care. Thus, only 11% of patients who initially request active euthanasia or assisted suicide later receive it (28).

PROCEDURAL SAFEGUARDS ARE SOMETIMES VIOLATED

In 0.2% of deaths, physicians ended the patient's life without the patient's explicit, concurrent request (27). In more than one-half of these cases, the patient had discussed these decisions previously with the physician. In about one-quarter of cases, however, the physician did not discuss these actions with anyone, including relatives or colleagues.

OUTCOMES FOR SURVIVORS

Family and friends of cancer patients who died by euthanasia had fewer symptoms of traumatic grief and fewer posttraumatic stress reactions than family and friends of patients who died of natural causes (29).

UNINTENDED COMPLICATIONS

When patients attempted physician-assisted suicide, technical problems occurred in 10% of cases, most commonly difficulty swallowing the pills. Adverse effects occurred in 7%, most commonly nausea and vomiting. In 18% of cases, a physician later administered a lethal drug, most commonly because the patient did not die or did not die as soon as expected. When physicians attempted active euthanasia, technical problems occurred in 5% of cases, most commonly difficulty finding a vein. Adverse effects occurred in 3% of cases, most commonly spasm and myoclonus. In 5% of cases, death did not occur or took longer than expected (30).

POLICY OPTIONS IN THE UNITED STATES

Several public policies are possible about physician-assisted suicide and active euthanasia. One option is to legalize these practices under certain conditions. A second option is to continue traditional prohibitions. However, these practices occur even though they are illegal. Abuses might be more likely to occur if decisions remain secret than if they are discussed openly and reported. This discrepancy between the law in the books and the law in practice also is problematic because enforcement might be inconsistent or biased (9). Another option is to keep active euthanasia and assisted suicide illegal but to acknowledge that in exceptional cases, such practices might be ethically justified and legally condoned and to clarify those circumstances (31). Prosecutors are reluctant to bring charges against physicians who convincingly assert that they were relieving the patient's suffering, and juries are reluctant to convict such doctors.

HOW SHOULD PHYSICIANS RESPOND TO REQUESTS FOR ASSISTED SUICIDE OR ACTIVE EUTHANASIA?

Physicians must be prepared for questions from patients on assisted suicide or active euthanasia. Like the general public, doctors disagree over the morality of these controversial actions (2). Regardless of their personal views, physicians can respond in certain ways (Table 19-1) (32–35).

FIND OUT THE REASONS FOR THE REQUEST

Why is the patient asking a question or making a request at this time? Because of improvements in palliative care, currently most requests are triggered not by unrelieved pain and physical symptoms, but by loss of dignity, independence, or a wish to control the timing and manner of their death (36). Requests might also result from psychosocial problems, a spiritual crisis, or a fear of abandonment (33, 37). Physicians need to screen patients for major depression, which can be treated even in terminally ill patients.

Fears that talking about assisted suicide or active euthanasia will encourage patients to carry out these acts are unfounded. Most terminally ill patients have already thought about these issues and feel relieved that physicians are willing to discuss them. Suicidal patients with terminal illness deserve the same careful evaluation and mobilization of resources as suicidal patients who are not terminally ill (38).

PROVIDE MORE INTENSIVE PALLIATIVE CARE

If their suffering or concerns are addressed, most patients find life worth living. Pain relief can be improved through using higher and more frequent doses of opioids, administering them on a regular schedule rather than as needed, and giving patients more control over dosage. In addition to alleviating physical suffering, physicians can help patients come to terms with their mortality and to find meaning in the final stage of their lives. Instead of trying to resolve problems or reassure patients, doctors should explore the patient's suffering using open-ended questions and empathic comments: "That sounds very distressing. Can you tell me more?" (39). Attentive listening validates the patient's emotions and shows the patient that he or she has been understood. The physician should consult with palliative care specialists, psychiatrists or psychologists, social workers, and chaplains as needed. Physicians also can arrange home hospice, mobilize family members and friends, and be available to patients.

REAFFIRM PATIENT CONTROL OVER TREATMENT DECISIONS

Some patients might seek to hasten death because they fear they will be subjected to unwanted life-prolonging interventions. Physicians need to reassure patients that decisions to forego life-sustaining interventions will be respected.

TABLE 19-1   Responding to Requests for Assisted Suicide or Active Euthanasia
Find out the reasons for the request.
Provide more intensive palliative care.
Reaffirm patient control over treatment decisions.
Do not impose your values on patients.
Consult a trusted and wise colleague.

DO NOT IMPOSE YOUR OWN VALUES ON PATIENTS

Proponents of assisted suicide should not write a lethal prescription on request without evaluating the patient for depression and inadequate palliative care. Conversely, opponents of these actions should not denigrate the patient's request, but rather communicate empathy and compassion for the patient's plight.

CONSULT A TRUSTED AND WISE COLLEAGUE

Most physicians find patient requests for assisted suicide or active euthanasia to be highly stressful. As with any other difficult case, a second opinion or discussion with a colleague is generally helpful. Often, a colleague can suggest how to improve palliative care or how to talk with the patient.

DECLINING TO GIVE ASSISTANCE

Physicians should not participate in assisted suicide or active euthanasia against their conscience or religious beliefs. When communicating their refusal, physicians need to address the patient's concerns and show empathy for the patient's plight. The physician might say, "I hear that you are deeply distressed by your illness. I'll try my best to relieve your suffering. But I can't help you kill yourself. My conscience won't allow me to do that." Such physicians need to emphasize their commitment to provide ongoing palliative care.

SITUATIONS IN WHICH ASSISTED SUICIDE MIGHT BE JUSTIFIED

Many physicians can conceive of a case in which they would consider assisted suicide morally permissible (40). The combination of all of the following circumstances would constitute the strongest case for agreeing to a patient's request (41, 42).

* *The patient has a terminal illness* or a progressive, incurable condition causing unrelenting suffering, such as ALS.
* *The patient is experiencing intractable symptoms* despite optimal palliative care. Even the best palliative care cannot relieve intractable bleeding or inability to swallow secretions. Actual distress is more compelling than anticipated future symptoms. Many physicians are more sympathetic to patients with physical distress than to patients with mental distress. The distinction between physical and mental suffering might be philosophically untenable, but it is helpful for pragmatic reasons because mistakes and abuse are less likely with physical distress.
* *The patient's request is voluntary, informed, and repeated.* Ideally, the patient raises the issue and is willing to discuss it with family members, friends, or clergy.
* *The physician has a long-term relationship with the patient* that started before the patient requested assistance with suicide.
* *The physician has consulted experts in* palliative care and depression.

In rare cases in which these conditions are present, it is not unethical for physicians to assist in suicide.

Active euthanasia is more problematic because it presents greater potential for abuse. Although requests by surrogates for active euthanasia are usually motivated by compassion, the risk of projection, misinterpretation, and abuse are great. Surrogates might interpret a gesture or a look as an unspoken request to hasten death, saying, for example, "I looked into his eyes and I just knew what he was asking me to do." Prohibiting active euthanasia for patients who lack decision-making capacity is sound public policy.

Physicians are sometimes confused as to whether they are providing palliative sedation, terminal sedation, or euthanasia (*see* Chapter 15). Doctors must be careful not to cross the line from palliative sedation to euthanasia (43).

SUMMARY

1. It should never be easy for a physician to respond to a request for assisted suicide from a patient who is dying in great suffering despite good palliative care.
2. Regardless of the physician's decision, patients deserve an honest answer to their questions or request.
3. Physicians should be dedicated to relieving suffering and to being with patients who are approaching death, regardless of their personal views on euthanasia or assisted suicide (43).

REFERENCES

1. Alpers A, Lo B. The Supreme Court addresses physician-assisted suicide: can its decisions improve palliative care. *Arch Fam Pract.* 1999;8:200–205.
2. Meier DE, Emmons CA, Wallenstein S, et al. Physician-assisted death in the United States: a national prevalence survey. *N Engl J Med.* 1998;338:1193–1201.
3. Harris D, Richard B, Khanna P. Assisted dying: the ongoing debate. *Postgrad Med J.* 2006;82:479–482.
4. Sommerville A. Changes in BMA policy on assisted dying. *BMJ.* 2005;331:686–688.
5. Branthwaite MA. Time for change. *BMJ.* 2005;331:681–683.
6. Brock D. Forgoing life-sustaining food and water: is it killing? In: Lynn J, editor. *By No Extraordinary Means.* Expanded edition ed. Bloomington, IN: Indiana University Press; 1989. 117–131.
7. Alpers A, Lo B. Does it make clinical sense to equate terminally ill patients who require life-sustaining interventions with those who do not? *JAMA.* 1997;277:1705–1708.
8. Lo B, Rubenfeld G. Palliative sedation in dying patients: "we turn to it when everything else hasn't worked." *JAMA.* 2005;294:1810–1816.
9. Alpers A. Criminal act or palliative care? Prosecutions involving the care of the dying. *J Law Med Ethics.* 1998;26:308–331.
10. Angell M. Euthanasia. *N Engl J Med.* 1988;319:1348–1350.
11. Foley KM. The relationship of pain and symptom management to patient requests for physician-assisted suicide. *J Pain Symptom Manage.* 1991;6:289–297.
12. Dworkin R. *Life's Dominion: An Argument about Abortion, Euthanasia and Individual Freedom.* New York, NY: Alfred A. Knopf; 1993.
13. Pellegrino ED. Doctors must not kill. *J Clin Ethics.* 1992;3:95–102.
14. Conwell Y, Caine ED. Rational suicide and the right to die: reality and myth. *N Engl J Med* 1991;325:1100–1102.
15. Block SD. Assessing and managing depression in the terminally ill patient. *Ann Intern Med.* 1999;132:209–218.
16. Lewis P. The empirical slippery slope from voluntary to involuntary euthanasia. 2007:197–210.
17. Steinbrook R. Physician-assisted death—from Oregon to Washington State. *N Engl J Med.* 2008;359:2513–2515.
18. Sulmasy DP. Managed care and managed death. *Arch Intern Med.* 1995;155:133–136.
19. Emanuel EJ, Daniels ER, Fairclough DL, et al. The practice of euthanasia and physician-assisted suicide in the United States: adherence to proposed safeguards and effects on physicians. *JAMA.* 1998;280:507–513.
20. Alpers A, Lo B. Physician-assisted suicide in Oregon: a bold experiment. *JAMA.* 1995;274:483–487.
21. Okie S. Physician-assisted suicide—Oregon and beyond. *N Engl J Med.* 2005;352:1627–1630.
22. Quill TE. Physician assisted death in vulnerable populations. *BMJ.* 2007;335:625–626.
23. Battin MP, van der Heide A, Ganzini L, et al. Legal physician-assisted dying in Oregon and the Netherlands: evidence concerning the impact on patients in "vulnerable" groups. *J Med Ethics.* 2007;33:591–597.
24. Sullivan AD, Hedberg K, Hopkins D. Legalized physician-assisted suicide in Oregon, 1998–2000. *N Engl J Med.* 2001;344:605–607.
25. Emanuel EJ, Fairclough DL, Daniels ER, et al. Euthanasia and physician-assisted suicide: attitudes and experiences among oncology patients, oncologists, and the general public. *Lancet.* 1996;347:1805–1810.
26. Back AL, Wallace JI, Starks HE, et al. Physician-assisted suicide and euthanasia in Washington state: patient requests and physician responses. *JAMA.* 1996;275:919–925.
27. Onwuteaka-Philipsen BD, Brinkman-Stoppelenburg A, Penning C, et al. Trends in end-of-life practices before and after the enactment of the euthanasia law in the Netherlands from 1990 to 2010: a repeated cross-sectional survey. *Lancet* 2012;Jul 10. [Epub ahead of print].
28. van der Maas PJ, van Delden JJM, Pijnenborg L, et al. Euthanasia and other medical decisions concerning the end of life. *Lancet.* 1991;338:669–674.
29. Swarte NB, van der Lee ML, van der Bom JG, et al. Effects of euthanasia on the bereaved family and friends: a cross sectional study. *BMJ.* 2003;327:189.
30. Groenewoud JH, van der Heide A, Onwuteaka Philipsen BD, et al. Clinical problems with the performance of euthanasia and physician-assisted suicide in The Netherlands. *N Engl J Med.* 2000;342:551–556.

31. Tulsky JA, Alpers A, Lo B. A middle ground on physician-assisted suicide. *Camb Q Healthc Ethics.* 1996;5:33–43.
32. Emanuel LL. Facing requests for physician-assisted suicide: toward a practical and principled clinical skill set. *JAMA.* 1998;280:643–647.
33. Quill TE. Doctor, I want to die. Will you help me? *JAMA.* 1993;270:870–873.
34. Block SD, Billings JA. Patient requests to hasten death: evalulation and management in terminal care. *Arch Intern Med.* 1994;154:2039–2047.
35. Bascom PB, Tolle SW. Responding to requests for physician-assisted suicide: "These are uncharted waters for both of us..." *JAMA.* 2002;288:91–98.
36. Quill TE. Legal regulation of physician-assisted death—the latest report cards. *N Engl J Med.* 2007;356:1911–1913.
37. Muskin PR. The request to die: role for a psychodynamic perspective on physician-assisted suicide. *JAMA.* 1998;279:323–328.
38. Hirschfeld RMA, Russell JM. Assessment and treatment of suicidal patients. *N Engl J Med.* 1997;337:910–915.
39. Lo B, Quill T, Tulsky J. Discussing palliative care with patients. *Ann Intern Med.* 1999;130:744–749.
40. Bachman JG, Alcser KH, Doukas DJ, et al. Attitudes of Michigan physicians and the public toward legalizing physician-assisted suicide and voluntary euthanasia. *N Engl J Med.* 1996;334:303–309.
41. Quill TE, Cassel CK, Meier DE. Care of the terminally ill: proposed clinical criteria for physician-assisted suicide. *N Engl J Med.* 1992;327:1380–1384.
42. Miller FG, Quill TE, Brody H, et al. Regulating physician-assisted death. *N Engl J Med.* 1994;331:119–123.
43. Lo B. Euthanasia in the Netherlands: what lessons for elsewhere? *Lancet* 2012;Jul 10. [Epub ahead of print].

ANNOTATED BIBLIOGRAPHY

1. Quill TE, Cassel CK, Meier DE. Care of the terminally ill: proposed clinical criteria for physician-assisted suicide. *N Engl J Med.* 1992;327:1380–1384.

   Proposes circumstances in which assisted suicide would be ethically permissible.
2. Pellegrino ED. Doctors must not kill. *J Clin Ethics.* 1992;3:95–102.

   Eloquent summary of reasons for opposing assisted suicide and active euthanasia.
3. Quill TE. Doctor, I want to die. Will you help me? *JAMA.* 1993;270:870–873.

   Emanuel LL. Facing requests for physician-assisted suicide: toward a practical and principled clinical skill set. *JAMA.* 1998;280:643–647.

   Bascom PB, Tolle SW. Responding to requests for physician-assisted suicide: "These are uncharted waters for both of us. . ." *JAMA.* 2002;288:91–98.

   Suggestions on how doctors can respond when terminally ill patients request physicians to hasten their death. The first two papers are by a proponent and an opponent of physician-assisted suicide, respectively.
4. Lo B. Euthanasia in the Netherlands: what lessons for elsewhere? *Lancet* 2012;Jul 10. [Epub ahead of print].

   The absence of widespread abuse of euthanasia the Netherlands is unlikely to settle controversies over euthanasia in other countries. However, cases that raise ethical concerns have important implications for other countries, particularly that physicians may be confused as to whether they are providing palliative sedation, terminal sedation, or euthanasia.

The Persistent Vegetative State

Patients in a vegetative state have no cortical function, but have preserved brainstem function (1, 2). Thus, they have spontaneous breathing and pulse, as well as wakefulness; however, they are not aware of their environment and cannot respond to other people or communicate with them. Although persistent vegetative state (PVS) is uncommon, the cases of Karen Ann Quinlan, Nancy Cruzan, and Theresa Schiavo (see Chapter 22), patients in PVS, dramatized fundamental questions about the goals of medicine and the definition of being a person.

This chapter describes the clinical features of PVS, discusses some of the philosophical quandaries it presents, and analyzes appropriate justifications for limiting life-prolonging interventions for patients in this condition.

CLINICAL FEATURES

DEFINITION OF VEGETATIVE STATE

As far as can be determined, patients in a vegetative state are unconscious, with no awareness of their environment (2). They show no purposeful activity and cannot obey verbal commands. The neurologic basis for this lack of consciousness or awareness is extensive damage to their cerebral cortex, thalami, or the connections between areas of the brain.

Patients in a vegetative state have wakefulness, with cycles of sleeping and waking. Thus, they are not comatose. While awake, they may have open eyes, blinking, roving eye movements, and unsustained visual pursuit. They may have facial movements and expressions and may grunt, grimace, smile, and produce tears. Patients might withdraw or posture in response to noxious stimuli and turn in the direction of sudden loud noises. Reflexes such as sucking, chewing, and swallowing might also be present. Pupillary, oculocephalic, and deep tendon reflexes are sometimes preserved. "Vegetative" functions, such as breathing and circulation, remain intact. Thus, patients in a vegetative state usually do not require mechanical ventilation.

Because of these preserved neurologic functions, some observers, particularly family members, believe that patients in a vegetative state are aware of surroundings or have responded to them. Some observers might claim that the patient watched them cross the room or cried when they talked to them. However, such alleged responses to external stimuli cannot be replicated in a consistent manner.

Patients in a vegetative state require tube feedings because they cannot swallow or protect their airway. They are incontinent and require total nursing care. Common complications are decubitus ulcers, aspiration pneumonia, and urosepsis.

The diagnosis of a vegetative state requires repeated and careful examinations by an experienced neurologist, with particular attention to behavioral assessment and oculomotor function. Errors in diagnosis are common.

Using functional magnetic resonance imaging (fMRI), researchers have found evidence of willfully modulated brain activity in some patients in PVS following traumatic brain injury. Twenty-three patients in PVS were asked to imagine doing tasks: swinging the arm back and forth as if playing tennis and visualizing walking through familiar surroundings. In two patients, fMRI activity in same brain areas was similar to activity in normal subjects imagining these tasks (3). In two other patients thought to be in PVS, similar fMRI findings led to clinical reevaluation that showed the patient was actually in a minimally conscious state (MCS) (3). Using a more clinically practical electroencephalography (EEG) technique, another study found that 3 of 16 patients (19%) who were clinically unresponsive and diagnosed as PVS could repeatedly and reliably generate appropriate EEG responses to commands to squeeze their right hand or to wriggle their toes (4). Thus, patients who are clinically unresponsive as judged by experts may show consistent evidence of responsiveness on further testing.

PROGNOSIS IN PERSISTENT VEGETATIVE STATE

A vegetative state is defined as *persistent* if it has lasted for 1 month (5). In the United States, about 10,000 to 25,000 adults and 4,000 to 10,000 children are in a PVS. A crucial issue is determining when a PVS has become permanent.

Prognosis for recovery of consciousness can be accurately established only after the patient has been in a vegetative state for some time (5). The required time of observation will depend on the etiology. Less than 1% of patients awaken from a vegetative state 3 months after nontraumatic injury, such as anoxic brain damage during a cardiac arrest. Similarly, less than 1% of trauma patients regain consciousness after 12 months in a vegetative state; all have moderate or severe residual neurologic impairments. There is no rigorous evidence that any specific intervention improves outcomes (2). Early intensive neurorehabilitation in a specialized unit may be beneficial. In light of these data, physicians should not say that it is "impossible" that patients in PVS will not regain consciousness. As in all clinical medicine, uncertainty must be acknowledged. The mean survival of patients in a PVS is 2 to 5 years. A few patients have been reported to survive longer than 15 years.

MINIMALLY CONSCIOUS STATE

Patients in an MCS have some awareness, which may be partial, fluctuating, and inconsistent, but reproducible. They might respond to a moving object with their eyes, respond yes or no to questions, follow simple commands, show purposeful behavior, or verbalize intelligibly. Their awareness might not be as impaired as their clinical limited responsiveness suggests. In one patient with MCS who could not communicate at the bedside, researchers found using fMRI that he could respond to yes/no autobiographical questions like "Do you have any brothers?" (3).

Patients in MCS have a better prognosis than those in PVS. Among patients who are in MCS after acute brain trauma, about 40% will regain consciousness within 3 months and about 50% will be living independently after 1 year. Long-term improvement is also possible. In one series, 13 of 35 patients who were in MCS a year after the onset of coma regained the ability to communicate with words or simple sentences. Most remained totally dependent on others (6).

PVS and MCS need to be distinguished from other catastrophic neurologic conditions. In brain death, there is neither cortical nor brainstem function (*see* Chapter 21). Patients are comatose, eyes are closed, and there is no spontaneous breathing. They have no facial expression and no vocalization. In the *locked-in syndrome,* patients are conscious but have no motor function. Such patients might be able to communicate by blinking their eyes. Patients with *severe dementia* might be virtually unresponsive, but they are conscious and might have some motor function.

WHAT TREATMENT IS APPROPRIATE?

Many persons would be horrified to be kept alive if there were virtually no likelihood of regaining consciousness. To them, life as a "vegetable" is a fate worse than death. They might interpret recent fMRI and EEG data as having awareness but being unable to express it except through sophisticated medical technology that is not practical for ordinary communication. Persons holding this view would reject tube feedings and other interventions.

A more radical and controversial position is that all medical interventions should be withheld or withdrawn from patients in a PVS because they have lost the essential characteristics of being a person, which include consciousness and the ability to have social interactions and to respond. In this view, it is not merely permissible to withdraw tube feedings from patients in a PVS but mandatory to do so (7).

In contrast, other people believe strongly that persons in a PVS should receive life-prolonging interventions. Some family members do not believe that the patient is unconscious, claiming that the patient responds to them. Recent fMRI and EEG data are consistent with this view. Other people reject the prognosis in medical studies, believing that the patient will improve despite unfavorable odds. Still others believe a life without consciousness remains sacred and should be sustained.

MEDICAL INTERVENTIONS MAY BE WITHHELD OR WITHDRAWN

As Chapter 13 discussed, when patients lack decision-making capacity, interventions ranging from cardiopulmonary resuscitation (CPR) to antibiotics for infection may be withheld on the basis of advance directives or decisions by appropriate surrogates (8).

Since the 1976 Karen Ann Quinlan case (*see* Chapter 22), a consensus has developed. In that case, the issue was whether to discontinue a ventilator (at the time, doctors did not know that patients in a PVS do not require ventilatory assistance). In recent cases, decisions to withhold CPR from patients in a PVS were not challenged. More recent controversies have focused on whether feeding tubes should be regarded differently from other medical interventions.

TUBE FEEDINGS ARE A MEDICAL INTERVENTION, WHICH MAY BE WITHHELD OR WITHDRAWN

Some people consider feeding tubes "ordinary" nursing care that must always be provided. Feeding tubes, however, have benefits and burdens that must be assessed for the individual patient. As discussed in Chapter 18, it is permissible to withhold or withdraw tube feedings from persons in a PVS, in accordance with the patient's prior directives or best interests (5, 9). In practice, many people are ambivalent about tube feedings in PVS.

Controversies over interventions in a PVS are not technical issues to be decided solely by physicians. Value judgments must be made regarding the definition of a human being and the level of uncertainty that is acceptable. Ultimately, these issues are not susceptible to logical proof or refutation. They can be resolved only by appealing to deeply personal or religious beliefs, which might lead people to strikingly different conclusions about appropriate care of patients in a PVS (10, 11).

SUMMARY

1. Although patients in PVS are awake and maintain some neurologic functions, they do not consistently respond to stimuli or commands.
2. Many ethical dilemmas regarding PVS can be resolved by applying guidelines for decisions in patients who lack decision-making capacity.
3. It is permissible to withdraw feeding tubes and other medical interventions in accordance with advance directives or decisions by appropriate surrogates.

REFERENCES

1. Monti MM, Laureys S, Owen AM. The vegetative state. *BMJ*. 2010;341:c3765.
2. Bernat JL. Current controversies in states of chronic unconsciousness. *Neurology*. 2010;75:S33–S38.
3. Monti MM, Vanhaudenhuyse A, Coleman MR, et al. Willful modulation of brain activity in disorders of consciousness. *N Engl J Med*. 2010;362:579–589.

4. Cruse D, Chennu S, Chatelle C, et al. Bedside detection of awareness in the vegetative state: a cohort study. *Lancet.* 2011;378:2088–2094.
5. The Multi-Society Task Force on PVS. Medical aspects of the persistent vegetative state. *N Engl J Med.* 1994;330:1499–1508, 1572–1579.
6. Luaute J, Maucort-Boulch D, Tell L, et al. Long-term outcomes of chronic minimally conscious and vegetative states. *Neurology.* 2010;75:246–252.
7. Schneiderman LJ, Jecker NS, Jonsen AR. Medical futility: response to critiques. *Ann Intern Med.* 1996;125:669–674.
8. Wade DT. Ethical issues in diagnosis and management of patients in the permanent vegetative state. *BMJ.* 2001;322:352–354.
9. Council on Scientific Affairs and Council on Ethical and Judicial Affairs. Persistent vegetative state and the decision to withdraw or withhold life support. *JAMA.* 1990;263:426–430.
10. Kritek PA, Slutsky AS, Hudson LD. Clinical decisions. Care of an unresponsive patient with a poor prognosis—polling results. *N Engl J Med.* 2009;360:e15.
11. Slutsky AS, Hudson LD. Clinical decisions. Care of an unresponsive patient with a poor prognosis. *N Engl J Med.* 2009;360:527–531.

ANNOTATED BIBLIOGRAPHY

1. Bernat JL. Chronic disorders of consciousness. *Lancet.* 2006;367:1181–1192.
    Monti MM, Laureys S, Owen AM. The vegetative state. *BMJ.* 2010;341:c3765.
    Larriviere D, Bonnie RJ. Terminating artificial nutrition and hydration in persistent vegetative state patients: current and proposed state laws. *Neurology.* 2006;66:1624–1628.
    Recent reviews of clinical, ethical, and legal issues regarding PVS and the MCS.
2. The Multi-Society Task Force on PVS. Medical aspects of the persistent vegetative state. *N Engl J Med.* 1994;330:1572–1579.
    Wade DT. Ethical issues in diagnosis and management of patients in the permanent vegetative state. *BMJ.* 2001;322:352–354.
    Comprehensive reviews of clinical features and prognosis.

21

Determination of Death

A ccurate and consistent determinations of death are essential because declaring a patient dead has profound consequences (1, 2); mourning begins, and funeral services, burial, or cremation are held. Spouses may remarry, pensions and health insurance coverage are terminated, properties pass on to heirs, and life insurance policies are paid.

Traditional cardiopulmonary criteria for death are problematic if a patient's breathing and circulation are sustained on life support after all cerebral functions have irreversibly ceased. Organ transplantation has raised unprecedented ethical issues about the declaration of death. Transplant teams want to retrieve organs as soon as possible. However, relatives and the public want assurance that organs are not harvested prematurely from persons who are not truly dead. Thus, surgeons who retrieve vital organs for transplantation may not cause or accelerate the patient's death. Thus, criteria for brain death have been developed.

Defining death is controversial because it involves cultural, social, and religious values, as well as scientific judgment. This chapter discusses ethical issues regarding cardiopulmonary, whole-brain, and higher brain criteria for death.

CARDIOPULMONARY CRITERIA FOR DEATH

Traditionally, physicians declare patients dead using cardiopulmonary criteria: the irreversible cessation of circulatory and respiratory functions. After cessation of heartbeat and breathing, brain functions cease permanently within minutes unless artificial life support is instituted. With the development of intensive care units, circulation and breathing can be sustained for months after the brain has irreversibly ceased to function. Disputes about cardiopulmonary criteria for death also arise when persons are killed by criminal acts. Some defendants in murder trials contended that the victim's death was caused by removal of vital organs for transplantation, not by their actions. Because of these problems with cardiopulmonary criteria for death, the definition of death was revised to include the irreversible cessation of brain function.

Determination of death using cardiopulmonary criteria has become more complicated with recent interest in retrieving organs for transplantation from persons declared dead by cardiopulmonary criteria (*see* Chapter 41) (3). Patients or surrogates decide that life-sustaining interventions will be withdrawn, resuscitation will not be initiated, and organs may be removed for transplantation. Generally, they are persons with serious brain injury who do not meet criteria for brain death or with other end-stage diseases. These donors are transported to the operating room, where life support is withdrawn, death is declared using cardiorespiratory criteria, and organs are promptly retrieved.

Several ethical concerns have been raised about this practice (3). First, are these donors really dead? The time from the development of asystole to declaration of death is typically about 2 to 5 minutes, beyond the period when circulation can spontaneously return. The longer the waiting period, however, the greater the risk that ischemia will compromise the donated organ. Second, cardiac transplantation presents several ethical concerns. Successful pediatric heart transplants have been carried out after only 75 seconds of asystole, shorter than the time that is believed to preclude autoresuscitation. Moreover, if the heart is transplanted and functions in the donor to provide circulation, has the determination of the donor's death been negated? Third, in order to achieve better outcomes after transplantation, some centers use extracorporeal membrane oxygenation to perfuse organs before organs are recovered. Large bore-catheters are inserted before death is declared. The care of the dying patient has been significantly modified with invasive procedures solely in order to benefit the transplant recipient. Finally, the family's experience of the patient's death may seem rushed and impersonal in the operating room. If organs cannot be retrieved because of prolonged hypotension, grieving might be more complicated for the survivors.

In response to these concerns, a consensus panel recommended that the term *donation* after cardiac death not be used, as the statutory standards for death by cardiopulmonary criteria require irreversible cessation of circulation, not death of the heart itself (3). This panel also argued that *permanent* cessation of circulatory and respiratory functions (because a decision has been made not to initiate resuscitation) is equivalent to *irreversible* loss of such function (it is impossible to be restored).

In rebuttal, other scholars have argued that this justification is a legal fiction that will confuse physicians, nurses, and the public and undermine trust in transplantation. In their view, it would be better to overturn the "dead donor rule" and say that these donors are not really dead but that it is morally acceptable to remove their organs for transplantation (4, 5).

BRAIN CRITERIA FOR DEATH

Patients who have irreversibly lost all brain function are considered dead, even though medical technology can support their circulation and breathing. Brain death in the United States is defined as irreversible loss of functioning in the entire brain, both the cortex and the brainstem. This is also called *whole-brain death*. Destruction of the brain generally leads to cessation of spontaneous cardiac function within a week.

Currently, the clinical tests for brain death include coma, absence of brainstem function, and apnea (6, 7). Potentially reversible causes of coma, such as drug overdose or hypothermia, must be ruled out. Circulation and spinal cord reflexes might be intact in brain death. Confirmatory testing with an electroencephalogram (EEG) and imaging studies of intracranial blood flow may be helpful but are not mandatory (6, 7). In children, the determination of brain death is more complicated because prognosis is more difficult to establish (8).

Recently, brain criteria for death have been questioned. In some patients declared dead by brain criteria, there might be persistence of some cerebral blood flow, oxygen and glucose metabolism, EEG activity, brainstem-evoked potentials, secretion of antidiuretic hormone, and temperature regulation (5, 9). Moreover, some patients diagnosed as dead by brain criteria mount a febrile response to infections and a stress response to surgical incisions. Thus, the body system continues to function as a whole organism.

In exceptional cases, there might be a substantial discrepancy between determinations of death using brain criteria and cardiopulmonary criteria. Several pregnant women meeting brain criteria had their vital functions sustained for months until the fetus could be delivered (5, 9).

The President's Council on Bioethics rejected integrated functioning as the key criterion characterizing a living organism and instead proposed that an organism is alive if it is receptive to its environment, is able to act upon the world to obtain what it needs, and has a drive to obtain what it needs, including air and nutrients. In their view, a person who has irreversibly lost consciousness and spontaneous breathing is dead (9).

Death determined by brain criteria needs to be carefully distinguished from the vegetative state. In death by brain criteria, there is no cortical or brainstem function. In contrast, patients in a vegetative state have intact brainstem function and spontaneous breathing and circulation.

MISUNDERSTANDINGS OVER BRAIN CRITERIA FOR DEATH

Only 35% of physicians who were responsible for declaring death were able to identify irreversible loss of all brain function as the criterion for determining death and apply it to simple case vignettes of death (10). Among other health care workers involved in the care of persons declared brain dead, more than 70% were unable to identify brain criteria for death. When asked to explain their personal opinions about two case vignettes, 58% of all respondents did not consistently use a coherent concept of death. Thirty-six percent believed that it is appropriate to retrieve organs from a patient in a vegetative state who does not meet whole-brain criteria for death. Moreover, hospital policies on brain criteria for death vary considerably and might be inconsistent with expert guidelines (11, 12).

HIGHER BRAIN CRITERIA FOR DEATH

Some writers argue that a person who has irreversible loss of higher brain function in the cerebral cortex, rather than loss of whole-brain function, should be considered dead, because consciousness, self-awareness, the potential for thought, and interactions with others are essential for being a person (13). In this view, persons in a persistent vegetative state (PVS) would be considered dead. However, a "higher brain" or neocortical definition of death has been rejected as public policy in the United States (14). The higher brain criteria for death confuse what it means to be a person with what it means to be alive. It might be appropriate to say that individuals without cortical function are no longer persons in the philosophic sense of having rights and interests. It does not follow logically, however, that they should be considered dead. Finally, burying or cremating individuals in PVS, who have spontaneous breathing and pulse, seems intuitively wrong.

DISAGREEMENT ON BRAIN CRITERIA FOR DEATH

Some persons reject the concept of brain criteria for death for religious or philosophic reasons (15, 16). For example, some orthodox Jews, Native Americans, and Japanese believe that a person is alive until he or she literally stops breathing (17, 18). No distinction is made between mechanical ventilation and spontaneous breathing. In this view, a person on a ventilator who meets the brain criteria for death is not dead.

LEGAL STATUS OF BRAIN CRITERIA FOR DEATH

Most states have adopted the Uniform Determination of Death Act, which declares, "Any individual who has sustained either (1) irreversible cessation of circulatory and respiratory functions, or (2) irreversible cessation of all functions of the entire brain, including the brainstem, is dead. A determination of death must be made in accordance with accepted medical standards" (3). Thus, a person may be declared dead if he or she meets either cardiopulmonary criteria (absence of breathing and pulse) or brain-death criteria. For most patients who are not on life support, these two criteria are equivalent. Courts have upheld determinations of death made by physicians according to brain criteria in accordance with state law (19).

Two states defer to the patient's beliefs about the definition of death. New Jersey authorizes the declaration of brain death, except in cases in which the physician has "reason to believe" that "such a declaration would violate the personal religious beliefs of the individual" (20). For such individuals, death must be declared according to traditional cardiorespiratory criteria. Similarly, New York requires "reasonable accommodation of the individual's religious or moral objection" to brain criteria for death (21). When such cases occur, the physician and staff should try to negotiate a compromise, respecting the patient's religious beliefs while allowing sufficient limitation of care to allow asystole to occur soon (15).

PRACTICAL SUGGESTIONS

An experienced neurologist should be consulted before a patient is declared brain dead. Explaining brain criteria for death to relatives requires sensitivity and patience. Some family members might believe the patient will regain consciousness, particularly if the death was sudden or unexpected. In almost all cases, compassionate explanations and emotional support from health care workers help the family accept the situation.

If organ transplantation is feasible, a physician not associated with the transplantation team should declare death to avoid any conflict of interest.

After a patient has been declared dead by brain-death criteria, all life-sustaining interventions should be discontinued, with certain exceptions. Maintaining life support might be appropriate until family members can come to the hospital, until organs for transplantation can be harvested or, under exceptional circumstances, until a fetus can be delivered.

SUMMARY

1. Patients may be declared dead using either whole brain or cardiopulmonary criteria.
2. Confusion over brain criteria for death is common; many physicians do not understand that irreversible loss of all brain function is required.

REFERENCES

1. Charo RA. Dusk, dawn, and defining death: legal classifications and biological categories. In: Youngner SJ, Arnold RM, Schapiro R, eds. *The Definition of Death*. Baltimore, MD: Johns Hopkins University Press; 1999:277–292.
2. Burt RA. Where do we go from here? In: Youngner SJ, Arnold RM, Schapiro R, eds. *The Definition of Death*. Baltimore, MD: Johns Hopkins University Press; 1999:332–339.
3. Bernat JL, Capron AM, Bleck TP, et al. The circulatory-respiratory determination of death in organ donation. *Crit Care Med*. 2010;38:963–970.
4. Shah SK, Truog RD, Miller FG. Death and legal fictions. *J Med Ethics*. 2011;37:719–722.
5. Miller FG, Truog RD. *Death, Dying, and Organ Transplantation*. New York, NY: Oxford University Press; 2012.
6. Wijdicks EF. The diagnosis of brain death. *N Engl J Med*. 2001;344:1215–1221.
7. Wijdicks EF, Varelas PN, Gronseth GS, et al. Evidence-based guideline update: determining brain death in adults: report of the Quality Standards Subcommittee of the American Academy of Neurology. *Neurology*. 2010;74:1911–1918.
8. Shemie SD, Pollack MM, Morioka M, et al. Diagnosis of brain death in children. *Lancet Neurol*. 2007;6:87–92.
9. President's Council on Bioethics. *Controversies in the Determination of Death*. Washington, DC: President's Council on Bioethics; 2008. http://bioethics.georgetown.edu/pcbe/reports/death/index.html. Accessed November 11, 2011.
10. Youngner SJ, Landefeld CS, Coulton CJ, et al. "Brain death" and organ retrieval: a cross-sectional survey of knowledge and concepts among health professionals. *JAMA*. 1989;261:2205–2210.
11. Powner DJ, Hernandez M, Rives TE. Variability among hospital policies for determining brain death in adults. *Crit Care Med*. 2004;32:1284–1288.
12. Oropello JM. Determination of brain death: theme, variations, and preventable errors. *Crit Care Med*. 2004;32:1417–1418.
13. Capron AM. Brain death—well settled yet still unresolved. *N Engl J Med*. 2001;344:1244–1246.
14. Bernat JL. The whole-brain concept of death remains optimum public policy. *J Law Med Ethics*. 2006;34:35–43, 3.
15. Inwald D, Jakobovits I, Petros A. Brain stem death: managing care when accepted medical guidelines and religious beliefs are in conflict. Consideration and compromise are possible. *BMJ*. 2000;320:1266–1267.
16. Olick RS. Brain death, religious freedom, and public policy: New Jersey's land ark legislative initiative. *Kennedy Inst Ethics J*. 1991;1:275–292.
17. Bagheri A. Individual choice in the definition of death. *J Med Ethics*. 2007;33:146–149.
18. Dorff EN. Applying traditional Jewish law to PVS. *NeuroRehabilitation*. 2004;19:277–283.
19. Burkle CM, Schipper AM, Wijdicks EF. Brain death and the courts. *Neurology*. 2011;76:837–841.
20. The New Jersey Declaration of Death Act. Revised statutes 1991 Title 26, Chapter 6A.
21. New York Codes 1987. §400.16(e)(3).

ANNOTATED BIBLIOGRAPHY

1. Wijdicks EF. The diagnosis of brain death. *N Engl J Med.* 2001;344:1215–1221.
   Clinical review of the diagnosis of death using brain-based criteria.
2. Capron AM. Brain death—Well settled yet still unresolved. *N Engl J Med.* 2001;344:1244–1246.
   President's Council on Bioethics. Controversies in the Determination of Death. Washington, DC: President's Council on Bioethics; 2008. http://bioethics.georgetown.edu/pcbe/reports/death/index.html. Accessed November 11, 2011.
   Miller FG, Truog RD. *Death, Dying, and Organ Transplantation.* New York, NY: Oxford University Press; 2012.
   Bernat JL, Capron AM, Bleck TP, et al. The circulatory-respiratory determination of death in organ donation. Crit Care Med. 2010;38:963–970.
   Analyses of philosophic debates over the cardiopulmonary and whole-brain criteria for determining death.

Legal Rulings on Life-Sustaining Interventions

ramatic legal cases regarding life-sustaining interventions have shaped clinical practice and motivated people to discuss their preferences for such interventions.

THE QUINLAN CASE

In 1976, the Karen Ann Quinlan case dramatized dilemmas regarding the withdrawal of life support when there is no hope of regaining consciousness (1).

THE CASE

Karen Ann Quinlan was a 22-year-old woman in a persistent vegetative state (PVS) because of an unknown illness. Her physicians agreed that she would never regain consciousness. She was on mechanical ventilation, and her physicians believed that she would die if the ventilator were withdrawn. Her father, after consulting with his priest and the hospital chaplain, asked that the ventilator be withdrawn. When the physicians refused, her father asked the courts to appoint him Karen's legal guardian with the authority to terminate the ventilator. The Catholic bishops of New Jersey supported his request.

THE COURT RULING

The New Jersey Supreme Court ruled that Karen Ann Quinlan's right to privacy included a right to decline medical treatment and that her father as guardian could exercise this right on her behalf, giving his "best judgment" as to whether she would have declined treatment herself.

The court held unanimously that if Karen's guardian and family, her attending physician, and a hospital "ethics committee" agreed that "there is no reasonable possibility" of recovering a "cognitive and sapient state," the ventilator may be withdrawn. In advocating hospital ethics committees, the court wrote, "In the real world and in relationship to the momentous decision contemplated, the value of additional views and diverse knowledge is apparent" (1). No party would face any civil or criminal liability for discontinuing the ventilator. The court also declared that generally such decisions need not be brought to court "not only because that would be a gratuitous encroachment upon the medical profession's field of competence, but because it would be impossibly cumbersome."

IMPLICATIONS OF THE CASE

As the first "right to die" case, the Quinlan case stimulated discussion about life-sustaining interventions. The ruling legitimized the idea that life-sustaining interventions might be inappropriate in some situations. The Quinlan court supported decision making by patients, families, and physicians without routine involvement of the courts. The Quinlan decision also encouraged the development of hospital ethics committees. In hindsight, the Quinlan case illustrates how medical prognostication is fallible. Although Ms. Quinlan's physicians expected her to die after the ventilator was discontinued, she survived for 10 years in PVS without ventilatory support. Physicians now realize that patients in PVS have intact brainstem function and breathe without assistance.

THE CRUZAN CASE

In the Cruzan case, the US Supreme Court issued its first decision on the "right to die" (2–5). The ruling sparked state and federal legislation to encourage the use of advance directives.

THE CASE

Nancy Cruzan was a 33-year-old woman who was in a PVS following an automobile accident in 1983. A month after the accident, a feeding gastrostomy tube was inserted. In 1986, realizing that her condition would not improve, her parents asked that the tube feedings be discontinued. Because the state hospital caring for Cruzan insisted on a court order, the case entered the legal system.

A year before her accident, Cruzan told her housemate that she "didn't want to live" as a "vegetable." If she "couldn't do for herself things alone even halfway, or not at all, she wouldn't want to live that way and she hoped that her family would know that" (6). Cruzan's parents asked that tube feedings be discontinued because they knew "in our hearts" that she would not want to continue living in her condition (6).

THE MISSOURI RULING

The 1988 Missouri Supreme Court ruling in the case severely restricted family decision making on behalf of incompetent patients (7). Life-sustaining interventions could be withheld only with "the most rigid of formalities," such as a living will or a clear and convincing statement that the patient would not want the specific intervention in that situation. The court found no reliable evidence that Nancy Cruzan would have specifically refused artificial feedings. It asserted that Missouri's "unqualified" interest in preserving life, regardless of the patient's prognosis, outweighed any rights an incompetent patient might have to refuse treatment.

THE US SUPREME COURT RULING

By a 5-to-4 vote, the US Supreme Court affirmed the Missouri ruling in 1990 (8). Although competent patients might have a "constitutionally protected liberty interest in refusing unwanted medical treatment," the Court declared that incompetent patients do not have the same right because they cannot exercise it directly. Thus, states may establish "procedural safeguards" governing medical decisions for incompetent patients that are more stringent than requirements for competent patients. The majority opinion declared that the individual's right to refuse treatment must be balanced against relevant state interests. The Court held that the Constitution allows states to assert an unqualified interest in "the protection and preservation of human life." It ruled that the Constitution also allows states to establish procedures to prevent abuses, to exclude quality of life as a consideration in treatment decisions, and to err on the side of continuing life-sustaining treatment. In short, states may require life-sustaining interventions when there is no clear and convincing evidence that the incompetent patient would refuse it. Although the Constitution permits states to rely on family decision making for incompetent patients, it does not mandate that they do so.

In dissent, Justice Brennan, joined by Justices Marshall and Blackmun, declared that being free of unwanted medical treatment is a fundamental constitutional right that extends to incompetent and competent patients and includes refusal of artificial fluid and nutrition. Families or patient-designated surrogates should generally make decisions for incompetent patients. In a separate dissent, Justice Stevens went further, declaring that the Constitution requires that the best interests of the incompetent patient be followed.

THE DEATH OF NANCY CRUZAN

After the Supreme Court ruling, the Cruzans petitioned the trial court in Missouri to rehear the case because new witnesses had come forward. One woman who worked with Cruzan testified that Cruzan had said that if she were a "vegetable," she would not want to be fed by force or kept alive by machines. Cruzan's attending physician changed his mind and was now in favor of stopping her feedings. The state of Missouri withdrew from further court proceedings, and in December 1990 the judge authorized removal of Cruzan's tube feedings (9).

IMPLICATIONS OF THE CRUZAN CASE

The Cruzan ruling spurred legislation to facilitate the use of advance directives. Many states adopted or revised laws specifically allowing patients to appoint health care proxies. The federal Patient Self Determination Act was enacted and took effect in December 1991. Under this law, virtually all hospitals, nursing homes, and health maintenance organizations must, at the time of admission, give patients written information about their right to provide advance directives.

THE PHYSICIAN-ASSISTED SUICIDE CASES

THE CASES

Competent, terminally ill patients who wanted to end their lives by taking a lethal dose of medications, along with physicians who were willing to write such a prescription, brought court cases in New York and Washington State. These patients had various terminal illnesses, such as cancer, AIDS, and emphysema. The plaintiffs asserted that New York and Washington's prohibitions on physician-assisted suicide were unconstitutional.

THE LOWER COURT RULINGS

Two federal appellate courts declared a constitutional right to physician-assisted suicide. The Second Circuit ruled that New York State violated the 14th Amendment's guarantee of equal protection by allowing some terminally ill patients to hasten death by foregoing life-sustaining treatments, while forbidding other terminally ill patients to hasten death using a prescription for a lethal dose of medication (10). In the Washington case, the Ninth Circuit declared that the 14th Amendment's guarantee of liberty included the right, to determine the time and manner of one's death through physician-assisted suicide (11).

THE US SUPREME COURT RULINGS

In 1997, the Supreme Court issued a pair of unanimous rulings that held that there is no constitutional right to physician-assisted suicide (12, 13). Thus, the Washington and New York laws prohibiting physician-assisted suicide did not violate the Constitution. The Supreme Court rejected the claim that terminally ill patients had a "fundamental liberty interest" in obtaining physician-assisted suicide. According to the Court, states have legitimate reasons for prohibiting assisted suicide (12), including preserving human life, preventing suicide, protecting vulnerable groups, protecting the integrity of the medical profession, and avoiding a slippery slope to euthanasia. The Court also ruled that under the Constitution states may permit patients to forego life-sustaining treatment while prohibiting physician-assisted suicide (13). The court declared that the distinction between physician-assisted suicide and withdrawal of life-sustaining treatment is important and logical. When physicians withdraw treatment, they intend only to respect the patient's wishes, not to end the patient's life. Moreover, the cause of death is the underlying fatal disease, not the physician's action.

The Court further declared that the Constitution allows states to prohibit physician-assisted suicide, which intentionally hastens death, while permitting palliative care that might hasten death, but is intended to relieve pain (13). According to the Court, the rationale of double effect distinguished the use of high-dose narcotics from euthanasia or assisted suicide. The Court noted that "painkilling drugs may hasten a patient's death, but the physician's purpose and intent is, or may be, only to ease his patient's pain.... The law has long used actors' intent or purpose to distinguish between two acts that may have the same result" (13).

IMPLICATIONS OF THE CASES

The majority opinion concluded that the double effect doctrine provides a rational and constitutional basis for states to allow high-dose narcotics for pain relief in terminally ill patients while prohibiting assisted suicide (14–16). Thus, the majority opinion offers a justification for aggressive palliative care. Three concurring justices went further, suggesting that the Constitution obligates states to permit physicians to provide adequate pain relief at the end of life, even if such care leads to unconsciousness or hastens death. The opinions might help lift legal barriers to palliative care.

THE SCHIAVO CASE

THE CASE

Theresa Schiavo, a 27-year-old woman, suffered a cardiac arrest in 1990 because of potassium abnormalities and never regained consciousness. In 1998, as the legally appointed guardian, her husband asked the court to discontinue tube feedings. Her parents opposed the withdrawal of tube feedings.

THE COURT RULINGS AND THE FLORIDA LAW

The trial court ruled that there was clear and convincing evidence that she would want the feedings discontinued. A long and complicated series of legal disputes ensued. The parents filed various appeals, contending that there was new evidence about her wishes that she was not in PVS and that her condition might improve. In 2002, the trial court held a new hearing on her current condition and on whether any new treatments might be effective. That court ruled "the credible evidence overwhelmingly supports that Terri Schiavo remains in a persistent vegetative state" (17). The court also held that the preponderance of the evidence was that no treatment would significantly improve her quality of life. The parents also claimed that new witnesses would testify that Terri's husband lied about her wishes. The court ruled that this new evidence, even if it were accepted as credible, would not meet the legal requirement that the original decision was "no longer equitable" (18). The state appellate court denied the parents' appeals in four separate rulings (19). The Florida Supreme Court declined to hear the case.

Prolife advocates, the Florida legislature, and Governor Jeb Bush then became involved in the case. In 2003, a law called "Terri's law" authorized the governor to issue a stay to prevent the withholding of nutrition and hydration from a patient in PVS who has no written advance directive when a member of the patient's family challenges the withholding of nutrition and hydration. In October 2003, Gov. Bush issued such a stay for Ms. Schiavo. In 2004, a Florida court ruled the law was unconstitutional, and the Florida Supreme Court affirmed that decision.

In 2005, Congress passed a law to give federal courts jurisdiction over this case. A federal district court refused to grant an injunction to halt the withdrawal of Ms. Schiavo's feeding tube, and a federal appeals court declared the law unconstitutional. The Supreme Court declined to hear the case.

IMPLICATIONS OF THE CASE
Disagreements Among Family Members

The Schiavo case illustrates how intractable and bitter disputes might arise among family members of patients who lack decision-making capacity. Both the husband and the parents accuse each other of acting in bad faith. The courts emphasized the desirability of having a final decision that closed the case. They urged the family to end the dispute and to move forward; however, this case shows how the legal system might not be able to resolve disputes when families are so sharply divided.

Involvement of Third Parties and the Courts

The Schiavo case is unique because of the involvement of prolife advocacy groups, the Florida legislature, and the governor. Also, the Internet has allowed considerable information about the case to be widely disseminated; however, such involvement of third parties raises several concerns. One is intrusion into the patient's privacy. Ordinarily, decisions about end-of-life care are delegated to families without interference by third parties who have no direct connection with the patient. In polls, the overwhelming majority of persons say that they would want decisions to be made by their families rather than by government officials; however, patients might not anticipate that their family might disagree over their care. Second, the public discussion of the case includes many assertions that contradict the court record. For instance, allegations continue to be made that Terri Schiavo is not in PVS and that new therapies might significantly improve her condition. Both a trial court and an appellate court have determined, however, that she is in PVS and that the preponderance of credible evidence indicates that no treatment would significantly improve her condition. In addition, allegations have been made that the patient's husband lied about statements she had allegedly made about her wishes for care.

Although society has designated the courts to resolve such difficult disputes, courts might not be able to provide a definitive answer or to resolve ongoing disagreements. The court challenges to "Terri's law" raise fundamental questions about the appropriate role of the legislative and executive branches of government in disputes that cannot be worked out among the family and physicians.

Importance of Advance Directives

Terri Schiavo did not complete an advance directive designating a proxy to make decisions for her; had she done so, the disputes between the parents and husband would likely have been resolved sooner. It is unrealistic to expect a young healthy woman to anticipate the situation that Terri Schiavo is now in and to have informed judgments about what she would want done in a catastrophic illness; however, it is not asking too much for a healthy person to appoint a proxy whom she trusts to make decisions for her.

SUMMARY

1. Landmark court cases have helped shape public policy regarding life-sustaining interventions.
2. Physicians need to know enough about these court rulings to correct misunderstandings by patients and colleagues.

REFERENCES

1. *In the Matter of Karen Quinlan*. 70 N.J. 10, 335 A. 2d 647 (1976).
2. Angell M. Prisoners of technology: the case of Nancy Cruzan. *N Engl J Med.* 1990;322:1226–1228.
3. Annas GJ. Nancy Cruzan and the right to die. *N Engl J Med.* 1990;323:670–673.
4. Orentlicher D. From the Office of the General Counsel. The right to die after Cruzan. *JAMA.* 1990;264:2444–2447.
5. Lo B, Steinbrook R. Beyond the Cruzan case: the U.S. Supreme Court and medical practice. *Ann Intern Med.* 1991;114:895–901.
6. Brief for petitioners. *Cruzan v. Missouri Department of Health* (No. 89-1503).
7. *Cruzan v. Harmon,* 760 S.W. 2d 408.
8. *Cruzan v. Missouri, Department of Health,* 497 U.S. 261, 110 S. Ct. 2841 (1990).
9. *Cruzan v. Harmon,* No. CV384-9P, Circuit court of Missouri (Mo. Cir. Ct. Jasper County Dec. 14, 1990) (Teel, J.).
10. *Quill v. Vacco,* 830 F3d 716 (2nd Cir. 1966).
11. *Compassion in Dying v. Washington,* 79 F3d 790 (9th Cir. 1966) (en banc).

12. *Washington v. Glucksberg,* 117 S. Ct. 2258 (1997).
13. *Vacco v. Quill,* 117 S. Ct. 2293 (1997).
14. Alpers A, Lo B. The Supreme Court addresses physician-assisted suicide: can its decisions improve palliative care? *Arch Fam Pract.* 1999;8:200–205.
15. Burt RA. The Supreme Court speaks: not assisted suicide but a constitutional right to palliative care. *N Engl J Med.* 1997;337:1234–1236.
16. Gostin LO. Deciding life and death in the courtroom. *JAMA.* 1997;278:1523–1528.
17. *In re Guardianship of Theresa Marie Schiavo,* No. 90-2908-GB-003 (Fla. Cir. Ct. 2002).
18. *In re Guardianship of Theresa Marie Schiavo,* 792 So. 2d 551 (Fla. 2001).
19. *In re Guardianship of Theresa Marie Schiavo,* 851 So. 2d 182 (Fla. 2003).

ANNOTATED BIBLIOGRAPHY

1. Burt RA. The Supreme Court speaks: not assisted suicide but a constitutional right to palliative care. *N Engl J Med.* 1997;337:1234–1236.
   Alpers A, Lo B. The Supreme Court addresses physician-assisted suicide: can its decisions improve palliative care? *Arch Fam Pract.* 1999;8:200–205.
   Two articles that discuss the important Supreme Court rulings in the two 1997 physician-assisted suicide cases.
2. Annas GJ. "Culture of life" politics at the bedside—The case of Terri Schiavo. *N Engl J Med.* 2005;352:1710–1715.
   Article on the Schiavo case.

The Doctor–Patient Relationship

IV

The Doctor-
Patient
Relationship

23

Overview of the Doctor–Patient Relationship

A strong doctor–patient relationship has many dimensions, as previous chapters have discussed. Physicians have a fiduciary obligation to act in their patients' best interests, which requires up-to-date knowledge and sound clinical judgment. Physicians should also help patients make informed decisions about their care, maintain confidentiality, avoid misrepresentation, and keep promises. Beyond that, patients also want caregivers who are compassionate and caring. In addition, patients want a physician who is available, coordinates care with specialists, and guides them through the complicated health care system.

DIFFERENT DOCTOR–PATIENT RELATIONSHIPS

In broad terms, several distinct types of doctor–patient relationships have been described. Such variation raises the question of what kind of doctor–patient relationship is most appropriate for a particular physician, patient, and clinical situation.

MODELS OF THE DOCTOR–PATIENT RELATIONSHIP

Several models of the doctor–patient relationship have been described: paternalism, informed choice, and shared decision making.

Paternalism

Physicians make treatment decisions with little input from the patient, based on what they believe to be the patient's best interests. Patients who prefer this decision-making style value the physician's expertise and believe that clear recommendations protect them from harm (1). Physicians' recommendations, however, might be unduly influenced by their personal values, which often differ from those of patients.

Informed Choice

Patients make the decisions about their own health care. Physicians provide relevant medical information but withhold their opinion. This is also known as the consumerist model. Physicians might decline to give a recommendation, even if a patient explicitly requests them to do so.

Shared Decision Making

Both the physician and patient play active roles (*see* also Chapter 3). The physician gives information to the patient on treatment benefits and risks, the patient gives information to the physician about his or her values, the patient and physician discuss treatment options, and both agree on a plan of care (2, 3). Shared decision making respects patients as persons and may have a positive impact on health outcomes (4). Shared decision making is commonly associated with a patient-centered approach to the medical interview, in which physicians ascertain and incorporate patients' expectations, feelings, and illness beliefs.

Several variations of shared decision making have been described. The physician may act as a teacher or friend: encouraging patients to think about health-related values, helping them deliberate about their options, and trying to persuade them to accept recommendations (5). This interaction requires more effort and engagement than simply giving a recommendation. In another variation, physicians serve as facilitators or coaches, helping the patient think through how her values apply to the decision at hand (6). In this approach, physicians go beyond the role of providing information, but do not make a recommendation.

WHAT DECISION-MAKING STYLE DO PATIENTS PREFER?

Patients prefer different decision-making styles. In one study, 62% of respondents preferred shared decision making, 28% preferred consumerism, and 9% preferred paternalism (4). Seventy percent usually experienced their preferred style of clinical decision making. In another survey, 96% of respondents preferred to be offered choices and to be asked their opinions, whereas 52% preferred to leave final decisions to their physicians and 44% preferred to rely on physicians for medical information rather than seeking out information themselves (7). Thus, although almost all patients wanted to be involved in decision making, many wanted the physician to make the final decision. Women, more educated people, and healthier people were more likely to prefer an active role in decision making. African American and Hispanic respondents and elderly respondents were more likely to prefer that physicians make the decisions. Patient preferences for decision making might vary across clinical scenarios. Patients who present with physical problems might prefer a more directive decision-making style. In contrast, for counseling and psychosocial problems, patients prefer shared decision making as often.

Looking at what decision-making style patients actually experience, physicians commonly used a more directive, or paternalistic, style with older, less educated, and sicker patients and used a more patient-centered style with younger, better educated, and more socioeconomically advantaged patients (4).

WHAT DECISION-MAKING STYLE SHOULD PHYSICIANS ADOPT?

Given this variation in preferred decision-making style, it makes sense to try to match patient preferences with the physician's actual style. Such matching respects patient autonomy and might enhance patient satisfaction with and trust in their doctors. Congruence might occur if patients choose physicians with compatible decision-making styles or if physicians modify their decision-making style to accommodate the patient's preferences. For example, physicians who generally refrain from giving explicit recommendations might do so for patients who prefer a directive style.

PHYSICIANS AND ENTREPRENEURISM

Modern medicine encourages physicians to adopt an entrepreneurial approach to their work. Many standard business practices, however, might conflict with the goals and ideals of medicine (8). Business people can greatly increase their net income through targeting profitable markets, dropping unprofitable services, and using advertising to increase the demand for their product (9). These practices are considered acceptable for people who are selling computers or running a restaurant. However, should physicians or health care organizations offer services only to well-insured patients (10); drop unprofitable services, such as primary care; or increase demand for profitable services that offer little or no benefit to patients? To the extent that health care is considered a basic need or a right rather than a commodity, a predominantly commercial approach is disturbing. Moreover, medicine as a profession defines itself as putting the patient's interests first (11).

RETAINER MEDICINE

In this arrangement, also called concierge medicine, physicians receive a monthly fee from each patient on their panel, in addition to payment from insurers. Patients have improved access, longer visits, and better continuity and coordination of care. Physicians have smaller panels, less stress, and higher income per hour of clinical practice. Critics charge that retainer medicine increases existing health disparities and poor access to primary care for patients who are not in such arrangements. Defenders argue that individual physicians, including those practicing retainer medicine, have no ethical obligation to supply any particular amount of primary care. In their view, the problem of access must be solved by legislators, government offcials, and insurers. But claiming, as individual physicians or as a profession, that access to care and health disparities are someone else's problem to fix presents a thin view of moral responsibility (12). Retainer medicine physicians, who especially know the value of better access to care and longer visits, should advocate for a health care system that provides them for all patients (12). Furthermore, all physicians should provide some medical care to those who have poor access to primary care—for example, by regularly volunteering to provide care for underserved patients.

ACCESS TO HEALTH CARE

More than 50 million Americans lack health insurance, and an additional 25 million are underinsured; these individuals lack reliable access to physicians and health care. A 2009 IOM report found compelling evidence that being uninsured causes "needless illness, suffering, and even death" (13). When people "acquire health insurance, many of the negative health effects of uninsurance are mitigated" (13).

The 2010 Patient Protection and Affordable Care Act was intended to extend health insurance to 31 million uninsured Americans. Furthermore, insurers may no longer deny coverage because of preexisting conditions, cancel coverage when illness occurs, or impose lifetime caps on coverage. To keep premiums affordable, the Act limits families' out-of-pocket medical expenses, creates insurance pools for small employers and for individuals, and subsidizes premiums for those who could otherwise not afford health insurance.

A controversial provision mandated individuals to obtain health insurance or employers to offer it or else pay a penalty (14). Proponents argue that this mandate would spread risk over a greater number of persons, keeping premiums more affordable and reducing adverse selection in insurance pools. Otherwise, many healthy people would choose not to purchase expensive health insurance, leaving sicker people in insurance pools, and creating a spiral of rising premiums and more people opting out. However, these voluntarily uninsured may be considered free riders: when they become sick, their emergency care may need to be paid for by taxpayers or subsidized by the insured. Opponents argue that this mandate is an unconstitutional federal interference with individual liberty, compelling people to purchase a product from a private company. In this perspective, such economic compulsion is unprecedented expansion of the power of the federal government and opens the door to other governmental violations of the individual's right to determine what to purchase in the free market.

The chapters in this section of the book discuss specific situations in which the doctor–patient relationship is problematic or difficult. Chapter 24 discusses situations in which physicians refuse to care for patients. Doctors might fear that their own health or safety is jeopardized or consider a patient difficult or obnoxious. Chapter 25 discusses the ethical issues that might arise when patients give gifts to their physicians. Chapter 26 analyzes sexual relationships between physicians and patients and discusses how such contact might harm patients. Chapter 27 suggests how physicians should respond when family members or friends provide unsolicited information about a patient and ask that it be kept secret. Chapter 28 analyzes how clinical research, which is essential for medical progress, presents risks to patients who participate in studies. The physician who is also a clinical investigator has additional responsibilities to ensure that the potential benefits of research are proportionate to the risks, to inform patients about the study, and to avoid conflicts of interest.

REFERENCES

1. Swenson SL, Zettler P, Lo B. 'She gave it her best shot right away': patient experiences of biomedical and patient-centered communication. *Patient Educ Couns.* 2006;61:200–211.
2. Murray E, Charles C, Gafni A. Shared decision-making in primary care: tailoring the Charles et al. model to fit the context of general practice. *Patient Educ Couns.* 2006;62:205–211.
3. Charles CA, Whelan T, Gafni A, et al. Shared treatment decision making: what does it mean to physicians? *J Clin Oncol.* 2003;21:932–936.
4. Murray E, Pollack L, White M, et al. Clinical decision-making: patients' preferences and experiences. *Patient Educ Couns.* 2007;65:189–196.
5. Emanuel EJ, Emanuel LL. Four models of the physician-patient relationship. *JAMA.* 1992;267:2221–2226.
6. White DB, Malvar G, Karr J, et al. Expanding the paradigm of the physician's role in surrogate decision-making: an empirically derived framework. *Crit Care Med.* 2010;38:743–750.
7. Levinson W, Kao A, Kuby A, et al. Not all patients want to participate in decision making. A national study of public preferences. *J Gen Intern Med.* 2005;20:531–535.
8. Kassirer JP. Managed care and the morality of the marketplace. *N Engl J Med.* 1995;333:50–52.
9. Jonsen AR. Ethics remain at the heart of medicine. Physicians and entrepreneurship. *West J Med.* 1986;144:480–483.
10. Brennan TA. Concierge care and the future of general internal medicine. *J Gen Intern Med.* 2005;20:1190.
11. ABIM Foundation, American Board of Internal Medicine, ACP-ASIM Foundation, et al. Medical professionalism in the new millennium: a physician charter. *Ann Intern Med.* 2002;136:243–246.
12. Lo B. Retainer medicine: why not for all? *Ann Intern Med.* 2011;155:641–642.
13. Committee on Health Insurance Status and Its Consequences. *America's Uninsured Crisis: Consequences for Health and Health Care.* Washington, DC: Institute of Medicine; 2009. http://www.iom.edu/Reports/2009/Americas-Uninsured-Crisis-Consequences-for-Health-and-Health-Care.aspx. Accessed November 16, 2011.
14. Hall MA. Clearing out the underbrush in constitutional challenges to health insurance reform. *N Engl J Med.* 2011;364:793–795.

Several variations of shared decision making have been described. The physician may act as a teacher or friend: encouraging patients to think about health-related values, helping them deliberate about their options, and trying to persuade them to accept recommendations (5). This interaction requires more effort and engagement than simply giving a recommendation. In another variation, physicians serve as facilitators or coaches, helping the patient think through how her values apply to the decision at hand (6). In this approach, physicians go beyond the role of providing information, but do not make a recommendation.

WHAT DECISION-MAKING STYLE DO PATIENTS PREFER?

Patients prefer different decision-making styles. In one study, 62% of respondents preferred shared decision making, 28% preferred consumerism, and 9% preferred paternalism (4). Seventy percent usually experienced their preferred style of clinical decision making. In another survey, 96% of respondents preferred to be offered choices and to be asked their opinions, whereas 52% preferred to leave final decisions to their physicians and 44% preferred to rely on physicians for medical information rather than seeking out information themselves (7). Thus, although almost all patients wanted to be involved in decision making, many wanted the physician to make the final decision. Women, more educated people, and healthier people were more likely to prefer an active role in decision making. African American and Hispanic respondents and elderly respondents were more likely to prefer that physicians make the decisions. Patient preferences for decision making might vary across clinical scenarios. Patients who present with physical problems might prefer a more directive decision-making style. In contrast, for counseling and psychosocial problems, patients prefer shared decision making as often.

Looking at what decision-making style patients actually experience, physicians commonly used a more directive, or paternalistic, style with older, less educated, and sicker patients and used a more patient-centered style with younger, better educated, and more socioeconomically advantaged patients (4).

WHAT DECISION-MAKING STYLE SHOULD PHYSICIANS ADOPT?

Given this variation in preferred decision-making style, it makes sense to try to match patient preferences with the physician's actual style. Such matching respects patient autonomy and might enhance patient satisfaction with and trust in their doctors. Congruence might occur if patients choose physicians with compatible decision-making styles or if physicians modify their decision-making style to accommodate the patient's preferences. For example, physicians who generally refrain from giving explicit recommendations might do so for patients who prefer a directive style.

PHYSICIANS AND ENTREPRENEURISM

Modern medicine encourages physicians to adopt an entrepreneurial approach to their work. Many standard business practices, however, might conflict with the goals and ideals of medicine (8). Business people can greatly increase their net income through targeting profitable markets, dropping unprofitable services, and using advertising to increase the demand for their product (9). These practices are considered acceptable for people who are selling computers or running a restaurant. However, should physicians or health care organizations offer services only to well-insured patients (10); drop unprofitable services, such as primary care; or increase demand for profitable services that offer little or no benefit to patients? To the extent that health care is considered a basic need or a right rather than a commodity, a predominantly commercial approach is disturbing. Moreover, medicine as a profession defines itself as putting the patient's interests first (11).

RETAINER MEDICINE

In this arrangement, also called concierge medicine, physicians receive a monthly fee from each patient on their panel, in addition to payment from insurers. Patients have improved access, longer visits, and better continuity and coordination of care. Physicians have smaller panels, less stress, higher income per hour of clinical practice. Critics charge that retainer medicine increases exi... health disparities and poor access to primary care for patients who are not in such arrangeme... Defenders argue that individual physicians, including those practicing retainer medicine, have... ethical obligation to supply any particular amount of primary care. In their view, the problem... access must be solved by legislators, government offcials, and insurers. But claiming, as individu... physicians or as a profession, that access to care and health disparities are someone else's problem to... fix presents a thin view of moral responsibility (12). Retainer medicine physicians, who especially know the value of better access to care and longer visits, should advocate for a health care system that provides them for all patients (12). Furthermore, all physicians should provide some medical care to those who have poor access to primary care—for example, by regularly volunteering to provide care for underserved patients.

ACCESS TO HEALTH CARE

More than 50 million Americans lack health insurance, and an additional 25 million are underinsured; these individuals lack reliable access to physicians and health care. A 2009 IOM report found compelling evidence that being uninsured causes "needless illness, suffering, and even death" (13). When people "acquire health insurance, many of the negative health effects of uninsurance are mitigated" (13).

The 2010 Patient Protection and Affordable Care Act was intended to extend health insurance to 31 million uninsured Americans. Furthermore, insurers may no longer deny coverage because of preexisting conditions, cancel coverage when illness occurs, or impose lifetime caps on coverage. To keep premiums affordable, the Act limits families' out-of-pocket medical expenses, creates insurance pools for small employers and for individuals, and subsidizes premiums for those who could otherwise not afford health insurance.

A controversial provision mandated individuals to obtain health insurance or employers to offer it or else pay a penalty (14). Proponents argue that this mandate would spread risk over a greater number of persons, keeping premiums more affordable and reducing adverse selection in insurance pools. Otherwise, many healthy people would choose not to purchase expensive health insurance, leaving sicker people in insurance pools, and creating a spiral of rising premiums and more people opting out. However, these voluntarily uninsured may be considered free riders: when they become sick, their emergency care may need to be paid for by taxpayers or subsidized by the insured. Opponents argue that this mandate is an unconstitutional federal interference with individual liberty, compelling people to purchase a product from a private company. In this perspective, such economic compulsion is unprecedented expansion of the power of the federal government and opens the door to other governmental violations of the individual's right to determine what to purchase in the free market.

The chapters in this section of the book discuss specific situations in which the doctor–patient relationship is problematic or difficult. Chapter 24 discusses situations in which physicians refuse to care for patients. Doctors might fear that their own health or safety is jeopardized or consider a patient difficult or obnoxious. Chapter 25 discusses the ethical issues that might arise when patients give gifts to their physicians. Chapter 26 analyzes sexual relationships between physicians and patients and discusses how such contact might harm patients. Chapter 27 suggests how physicians should respond when family members or friends provide unsolicited information about a patient and ask that it be kept secret. Chapter 28 analyzes how clinical research, which is essential for medical progress, presents risks to patients who participate in studies. The physician who is also a clinical investigator has additional responsibilities to ensure that the potential benefits of research are proportionate to the risks, to inform patients about the study, and to avoid conflicts of interest.

Refusal to Care for Patients

Physicians might refuse to care for persons for a variety of reasons, including an unacceptable threat to their personal safety, their personal moral objections to providing care, or a counterproductive or an adversarial doctor–patient relationship. Such refusal to provide care raises ethical dilemmas because the patient's medical needs and best interests might conflict with the physician's refusal. The following case illustrates such a refusal to care for a patient.

CASE 24.1   **Surgery in an HIV-infected patient**

Mr. N is a 43-year-old man with asymptomatic HIV infection. While crossing a street, he is struck by a car running a red light. He suffers a comminuted fracture of the proximal femoral shaft. The surgeons decline to operate because the patient's viral titer has not been checked recently, saying that this fracture can be managed without surgery. Moreover, in orthopedics operations, sharp bone fragments from seropositive patients may penetrate gloves and subject health care workers to an unacceptable risk of lethal illness.

In Case 24.1, the surgeon fears contracting a fatal blood-borne infection. Standard treatment for this fracture is operative fixation with an intramedullary rod. Closed treatment requires several months of traction and has poorer outcomes. Similarly, during the severe acute respiratory syndrome (SARS) epidemic of 2002 to 2003, some health care workers refused to work with infected patients. Although the law generally permits physicians to decide whether to accept new patients, it seems inhumane for physicians to refuse crucial medical care to sick persons in need. This chapter analyzes whether physicians have an ethical obligation to provide care for patients who present for needed treatment.

THE CONTEXT OF THE DOCTOR–PATIENT RELATIONSHIP

ETHICAL OBLIGATIONS TO CARE FOR PATIENTS

Physicians present themselves to the public as helpers of the sick and needy, who use their expertise for the benefit of patients. The ethical ideal is that patients will receive needed care, even in cases in which the physician might find it risky, difficult, or inconvenient. At the beginning of the HIV epidemic, the Surgeon General declared, "Health care in this country has always been predicated on the assumption that somehow, everyone will be cared for, and no one will be turned away. As a physician and an American, I'm proud to be part of a tradition of care that will not abandon the sick or disabled, whoever they are" (1).

In the doctor–patient relationship, the patient's best interests should take priority over the doctor's self-interest (*see* Chapter 4). The guideline of beneficence has several important implications for refusals to care for patients. Physicians should not refuse care to patients whom they personally dislike or whose actions, such as smoking, alcohol and substance abuse, or non-adherence to medications, make treatment more difficult. It would also be ethically objectionable for physicians to refuse care to patients on the basis of ethnic background, race, gender, or religious beliefs. The United States rejects discrimination based on these categories. Even in war, physicians are expected to attend to the sick and injured, regardless of which side they are on. Furthermore, physicians are exhorted to provide needed medical care even to patients whose actions are morally reprehensible. Doctors are expected to provide care to the perpetrator of a violent assault, as well as to the victim.

This ethical ideal of providing needed care, regardless of the patient's characteristics, has limits. In providing care, physicians are not expected to compromise their own moral or religious beliefs. For example, Catholic physicians are not required to perform abortions. Although physicians are urged to tolerate patient behavior they personally consider immoral, they are not obligated to carry out what they regard as an immoral action. One philosopher has cautioned physicians to distinguish deeply held moral objections from "personal distaste or prejudice" (2). Another acceptable limit is the physician's health and safety. In Case 24.1, the physicians claim that serious personal risks override their ethical obligation to provide care.

LEGAL DEFINITION OF THE DOCTOR–PATIENT RELATIONSHIP

Society as a whole and the medical profession have a moral obligation to care for sick persons, yet individual doctors generally have no legal duty to provide care. The law generally characterizes the doctor–patient relationship as a contract between autonomous individuals who are free to enter into or break off the relationship, provided that the patient is not abandoned (3). Courts have ruled that physicians have no legal duty to treat new patients who seek care in the absence of an agreement to provide medical care, such as a contract with a health maintenance organization (HMO). For example, it is legal for physicians to schedule new patient appointments only for people with adequate health insurance. Similarly, physicians may restrict the scope of their practice to a particular specialty or range of problems. Thus, an internist would not be expected to perform surgery, just as a psychiatrist would not be expected to treat meningitis.

The legal right to decline to care for patients, however, is limited in many important ways. Employment contracts, as with hospitals or HMOs, may oblige physicians to care for all qualified persons who seek treatment. Similarly, physicians who are on call for a hospital may be required as a condition of staff privileges to provide care to persons who present there. As discussed later in this chapter, emergency departments are required to provide indicated emergency care to patients who seek it.

The Americans with Disabilities Act also forbids physicians from declining to care for patients on the basis of race, sex, national origin, religion, or disability (4). Physicians and hospitals, however, are not required to provide care when an "individual poses a direct threat to the health or safety of others that cannot be eliminated or reduced by reasonable accommodation" (5). Direct threat refers to "a significant risk of substantial harm," not risks that are "slightly increased," "speculative," or "remote" (6). This determination of risk must be made according to objective, scientific evidence, not simply the health care worker's subjective judgment. Caring for HIV-infected persons is not considered a "direct threat" to health care workers (6).

OCCUPATIONAL RISKS TO PHYSICIANS

Some health care workers may refuse to care for patients from whom they might contract serious or fatal contagious diseases. Before the mid-20th century, physicians commonly contracted tuberculosis, polio, and other severe infections. After antibiotics and vaccines were developed, the risk of occupational infection dropped sharply. Recently, however, physicians have again contracted fatal occupational infections.

SERIOUS OCCUPATIONAL RISKS

Early in the HIV epidemic, many physicians feared occupational HIV infection and refused to care for seropositive persons. The risk of seroconversion after a percutaneous exposure to the blood of a seropositive patient is 0.3%, and after mucocutaneous exposure the risk is 0.09% (7). Surgeons and operating room staff are at higher risk for occupational HIV infection than office-based physicians. Almost all surgical residents have suffered a needlestick injury, more than one half of which involved a patient with a blood-borne infection or who was at risk for such an infection (8). Postexposure pro- phylaxis with antiretrovirals reduces transmission by 80% (9), and preexposure prophylaxis might also be effective. In addition, the laparoscopic techniques for many operations further reduce risks to surgeons and operating room staff.

More recently, during the SARS epidemic of 2002 to 2003, a disproportionate percentage of cases and deaths occurred among physicians and nurses caring for hospitalized patients with SARS. Most doctors and nurses cared for patients with SARS despite knowing they were at risk for a poten- tially fatal disease. The magnitude of a risk is only one component of the perception of risk. The risk of occupational HIV infection and SARS seems especially ominous because there were no effective preventive measures or treatment and these fatal diseases can be transmitted to family members.

Other serious infections that can be acquired through occupational exposure are hepatitis C and multidrug-resistant tuberculosis. In addition, angry or psychotic patients might physically threaten or harm health care workers. In one survey, 20% of residents said that they had been physically assaulted during their training (10). Because of these serious occupational risks, physicians might be reluctant to provide care to patients they regard as contagious or violent. Avoiding such patients, however, might conflict with providing care to patients in need.

RESPONDING TO OCCUPATIONAL RISKS
Acknowledge and Address Fears

Physicians must acknowledge their human fears and limitations; only then are reflection, discussion, and constructive action possible. Fears about safety need to be acknowledged as an understandable human reaction, rather than condemned as hysteria (11). In previous epidemics, many physicians, including Galen and Sydenham, fled from patients with fatal contagious diseases (12). Health care workers need their concerns addressed in a nonjudgmental way.

Some techniques for encouraging health care workers to accept occupational risks are usually ineffective. Moral exhortations to provide care might go unheeded. Indeed, health care workers might be outraged at the suggestion that it is unethical to worry about their safety. Reassurance that a risk is low or comparable to other risks generally is counterproductive (13). People reject the suggestion that because they accept risks of greater magnitude, such as the risk of automobile accidents, they should also accept the risk in question (13).

Reduce the Occupational Risks

Hospitals and clinics must provide a safe working environment, which includes protective equip- ment such as masks, gowns, and gloves; however, at the onset of an epidemic, the best protective measures might not be known and protective measures may be ineffective. New equipment might need to be developed and made available, such as retractable needles to prevent blood-borne infections. Health care institutions also should have security guards readily available when care is provided to violent patients.

Balance Risks to Health Care Workers and Benefits to Patients

Health care workers should provide care if the medical benefit to the patient is clearly established, substantial, and highly probable, provided that appropriate precautions have been taken to reduce risk. On the other hand, severe risks to health care workers might justify delaying or postponing interventions whose benefits are unproved, uncertain, or marginal.

Judgments about the benefits and risks of treatment need to be scientifically sound. In Case 24.1, it would be misleading for physicians to say that operative reduction for this condition is not indicated in seropositive persons. Such surgery is routinely performed for this indication in patients who have other diseases, such as cancer, with poor prognoses. If physicians bias their medical judgments to avoid caring for seropositive persons, patients and the public will justifiably question their recommendations on other issues.

CONSCIENTIOUS OBJECTION BY PHYSICIANS

Some health care workers have conscientious objections to providing certain types of care, such as contraception and abortion. Moreover, they might believe that they would be complicit with an immoral action if they even discuss these options with patients or refer them to other physicians. Most obstetricians, however, are willing to help patients obtain an abortion even if they have moral objections to it in that situation (14).

There are several strong reasons to honor such conscientious objection (15). Physicians and other health care professionals should be free to exercise their independent judgment. They should not be asked to forsake their moral beliefs as a condition of practice. The right to refuse to act in ways that conflict with personal moral beliefs is an essential component of religious freedom. Many physicians also have conscientious objections to providing information about an intervention or referring patients to a provider who would provide it.

There are also strong countervailing reasons to ensure that patients receive medically appropriate care. When patients present for care, they should be informed of the medically feasible options for care and have access to medically appropriate care delivered in a timely manner. Under the doctrine of informed consent, physicians may not withhold information about accepted options for care even if they personally disagree. If a standard intervention is beyond the scope of the physician's or institution's practice, the patient should be referred to a provider who can provide the care. The case of emergency contraception raises particular concerns about access because there is a limited window of time when it should be administered.

These conflicting ethical positions may be reconciled by placing the duty to provide care that a patient needs on the health care institution, rather than on the individual health care professional (16–18). The medical clinic, hospital, or pharmacy should have a collective obligation to assure that patients receive needed care. Institutions should make reasonable attempts to accommodate their employees' personal beliefs by arranging staffing so that another professional will provide the service (15). Health care workers who raise a conscientious objection should not obstruct the patient from receiving care from others or provide misinformation to the patient (17).

If a health care professional or institution decides that for reasons of conscience they cannot provide certain services, they should inform patients in advance. Many patients have to select a provider for insurance purposes, and it would be highly burdensome for them to switch providers when they need the specific service.

Similar dilemmas arise if a health care organization declares that certain services violate their mission. For example, Catholic hospitals do not provide family planning or abortion services. Although there are strong reasons to respect an institutional policy that is based on religious beliefs, it is also important to inform patients when they select a provider, establish care, schedule appointments, or present for care that such interventions will not be provided. Further dilemmas arise when hospitals forbid individual physicians from providing information to patients about family planning or abortion or referring patients for such services. Individual physicians should have the scope to discuss and recommend interventions that they judge medically appropriate. Restricting such communication on the basis of an organization's policies or religious mission denies important medical information to patients and imposes the institution's views on patients and health care providers. Many patients who seek care at an institution do not accept the moral beliefs that animate the institution. Because of geography, insurance restrictions, or ambulance policies, patients may have no alternative provider.

Although conscientious objections should be reasonably accommodated, there are important limits. First, refraining from providing an intervention must be distinguished from insisting on providing interventions that an informed patient has refused. As Chapter 5 discusses, patients have a right to be free of unwanted medical interventions. Thus, a provider may not insist that patients receive CPR, tube feedings, or other life-sustaining interventions over their objections, even if that insistence is based on deeply held moral values. Second, claims of conscience may not justify refusing needed treatment to patients because of their race, ethnicity, national origin, gender, or religion. Such discrimination is illegal and violates the physician's ethical duty to respect patients as persons.

DIFFICULT DOCTOR–PATIENT RELATIONSHIPS

Ideally, the doctor–patient relationship is a partnership whose goal is the patient's well-being. In some cases, however, the relationship might be unproductive or adversarial and the physician might consider the patient a "problem" or "difficult" patient (19), as in the following case (20).

CASE 24.2   Disruptive and uncooperative patient

Ms. W is a 35-year-old woman with end-stage renal disease who repeatedly misses dialysis appointments and requires emergency dialysis. She also does not take her medications regularly or follow her diet, is frequently intoxicated, and disrupts the dialysis unit with her obscene and insulting language and attempts to strike health care workers who are connecting her to the dialysis machine. Other patients request to change the time of their dialysis, and nurses try to avoid shifts when she is scheduled. When she presents to the emergency department with shortness of breath and is found to have congestive heart failure and hyperkalemia, the nephrologist considers refusing dialysis.

In Case 24.2, Ms. W repeatedly misses appointments, fails to take her medications, and requires emergency care after missing scheduled appointments. Furthermore, she is disruptive, angry, and violent. Physicians commonly view such patients as "bad" patients who have broken the implicit rules of the doctor–patient relationship (19). Health care workers are understandably frustrated when the patient's own actions bring about or exacerbate medical problems. Some patient behaviors go beyond undermining their own health. Missing scheduled dialysis times disrupts the dialysis team's schedules and inconveniences staff. The patient may provoke such strong negative reactions in health care workers that a therapeutic relationship no longer exists (19). Doctors resent spending so much time and energy on such a patient that the care of other patients is compromised. Finally, physical threats or actual violence make it impossible for the dialysis staff to provide care and for other patients to receive care (21). Health care workers and other patients have a right to be free of abuse, threats, and violence.

RESPONDING TO DIFFICULT DOCTOR–PATIENT RELATIONSHIPS

In most cases, physicians can find ways to improve a difficult doctor–patient relationship (Table 24-1).

TABLE 24-1   Improving Difficult Doctor–Patient Relationships

Acknowledge that problems exist.

Try to understand the patient's perspective.

Try to understand your own responses.

Try to negotiate mutually acceptable grounds for continued care.

Acknowledge That Problems Exist

The first step is for physicians and patients alike to acknowledge problems. The physician might say, "I sense that both of us are disappointed with how your care is turning out."

Try to Understand the Patient's Perspective

Physicians might feel that some patients intentionally vex them, making their work more difficult. From the patient's perspective, however, there might be sound reasons for missing appointments, such as difficulties with insurance coverage, transportation, or childcare. Illness might cause patients to feel angry, frustrated, helpless, or out of control. Also, patients might not have control over some behaviors because of psychiatric conditions.

Physicians can elicit patients' perspectives through open-ended questions about the impact of their illness, competing demands in their life, and barriers to care. Acknowledging a patient's emotions also encourages further discussion. Once their problems and frustration are acknowledged, patients might be better able to appreciate how their behavior is disrupting their care or the care of other patients.

Try to Understand Your Own Responses

Health care workers need to understand how their actions might exacerbate the patient's behavior. Physicians and nurses who are frustrated and angry might vent their anger on the patient or treat her curtly. Differences in ethnic background, social class, and lifestyle might exacerbate tensions.

Try to Negotiate Mutually Acceptable Plans for Continued Care

Physicians can try to set limits on disruptive behaviors and find mutually acceptable conditions for the doctor–patient relationship (22). A psychiatric or social work consultation can often be helpful. Physicians can give patients notice that certain behaviors will lead to termination of the doctor–patient relationship. Doctors can negotiate a formal "contract" that explicitly sets conditions under which the patient and physician will continue the relationship.

CASE 24.2   *Continued*

In response to the physician's open-ended questions, Ms. W said she was frustrated at having to come to dialysis on a rigid schedule and admitted that when she drank heavily she missed sessions. Her physician said, "We're trying our best to help you, but it's hard for us if you take a swing at us and don't keep appointments." To set limits on her abusive and violent behavior, the doctor might say, "I'm willing to try to find a way that we can work together. But if you want to get care here, you cannot make obscene or abusive comments or swing at anyone." The doctor negotiated an agreement that the unit would continue to provide dialysis provided that a family member would accompany Ms. W to dialysis sessions and that she accept treatment for substance abuse and counseling (20). Ms. W and several relative signed the contract.

When Ms. W did not change her behavior, her doctor notified her that he will no longer provide chronic dialysis and gave her a list of nephrologists in the area. However, she continued to present to the emergency department with congestive heart failure and uremia.

TERMINATING THE DOCTOR–PATIENT RELATIONSHIP

The patient and physician may agree to transfer the care of the patient to another physician. Physicians may also terminate the doctor–patient relationship in certain situations—for example, when a patient breaks her agreement about subsequent behavior and continues to be disruptive and violent. Because termination is a drastic measure, it should be used only as a last resort after attempts to find common ground for ongoing care have failed.

Patient Abandonment

Legally and ethically, physicians may not abandon patients with whom they have established a doctor–patient relationship (20). When terminating a relationship, physicians need to give patients reasonable written notice, so that they can find a new physician and obtain needed timely care for ongoing medical problems. To help patients find another physician, doctors can give patients a list of other qualified physicians in the area or refer them to the county medical society.

Obligation to Provide Emergency Care

An emergency department must provide emergency care to patients who seek it. The public relies on emergency departments and physicians to provide proper emergency treatment and expects them to do so. Delays in emergency care might seriously harm patients.

The federal Emergency Medical Treatment and Labor Act (EMTLA) prohibits emergency departments from transferring patients in unstable condition who need emergency care, as well as pregnant women in active labor. Every person seeking treatment in an emergency department must receive a screening examination. If the patient is found to have an emergency condition, the hospital must provide treatment to stabilize the patient's condition, within the constraints of the available staff and facilities.

CASE 24.2   *Continued*

When Ms. W presents to the emergency department with life-threatening uremia and congestive heart failure, emergency dialysis must be provided (21), and a nephrologist and dialysis nurse must be called in. Therefore, the health care workers who have terminated her from providing chronic dialysis might still have to perform emergency dialysis. Sometimes, it is possible to make arrangements for different individuals or institutions to share the emergency care of such patients.

SUMMARY

1. Physicians have an ethical obligation to care for patients even at some personal risk or inconvenience.
2. Before unilaterally terminating a difficult doctor–patient relationship, physicians should try to understand the patient's perspective and to find some mutually acceptable arrangement for continuing care.

REFERENCES

1. Koop CE. Testimony before Presidential Commission on AIDS. 1987 September 8.
2. Jonsen A, Siegler M, Winslade W. Clinical Ethics. 3rd ed. New York, NY: Macmillan Publishing Co.; 1991:73–74.
3. Annas GJ. Not saints, but healers: the legal duties of health care professionals in the AIDS epidemic. Am J Public Health. 1988;78:844–849.
4. Americans with Disabilities Act of 1990. 42 USC §§12181, 12182.
5. Americans with Disabilities Act Public Accommodation Regulations. 28 CFR § 36.201.
6. Gostin LO, Feldbaum C, Webber DW. Disability discrimination in America: HIV/AIDS and other health conditions. JAMA. 1999;281:745–752.
7. Panlilio AL, Cardo DM, Grohskopf LA, et al. Updated U.S. Public Health Service guidelines for the management of occupational exposures to HIV and recommendations for postexposure prophylaxis. MMWR Recomm Rep. 2005;54:1–17.
8. Makary MA, Al-Attar A, Holzmueller CG, et al. Needlestick injuries among surgeons in training. N Engl J Med. 2007;356:2693–2699.
9. Centers for Disease Control and Prevention (CDC). Case-control study of HIV seroconversion in health-care workers after exposures to HIV-infected blood—France, United Kingdom and United States, January 1988–August 1994. MMWR Morb Mortal Wkly Rep. 1995;44:929–933.

10. Cook DJ, Liutkus JF, Risdon CL, et al. Residents' experiences of abuse, discrimination and sexual harassment during residency training. McMaster University Residency Training Programs. CMAJ. 1996;154:1657–1665.
11. Gerbert B, Maguire B, Badmer V, et al. Why fear persists: health care professionals and AIDS. JAMA. 1988;260:3481–3483.
12. Zuger A, Miles SH. Physicians, AIDS, and occupational risk. Historic traditions and ethical obligations. JAMA. 1987;258:1924–1928.
13. National Research Council. Improving Risk Communication. Washington, DC: National Academy Press; 1989.
14. Harris LH, Cooper A, Rasinski KA, et al. Obstetrician-gynecologists' objections to and willingness to help patients obtain an abortion. Obstet Gynecol. 2011;118:905–912.
15. Cantor J, Baum K. The limits of conscientious objection—May pharmacists refuse to fill prescriptions for emergency contraception? N Engl J Med. 2004;351:2008–2012.
16. Charo RA. The celestial fire of conscience—Refusing to deliver medical care. N Engl J Med. 2005;352:2471–2473.
17. Greenberger MD, Vogelstein R. Public health. Pharmacist refusals: a threat to women's health. Science. 2005;308:1557–1558.
18. Manasse HR Jr. Public health. Conscientious objection and the pharmacist. Science. 2005;308:1558–1559.
19. Stokes T, Dixon-Woods M, McKinley RK. Breaking up is never easy: GPs' accounts of removing patients from their lists. Fam Pract. 2003;20:628–634.
20. Orentlicher D. Denying treatment to the noncompliant patient. JAMA. 1991;265:1579–1582.
21. Friedman EA. Must we treat noncompliant ESRD patients? Semin Dial. 2001;14:23–27.
22. Quill TE. Partnerships in patient care: a contractual approach. Ann Intern Med. 1983;98:228–234.

ANNOTATED BIBLIOGRAPHY

1. Annas GJ. Not saints, but healers: the legal duties of health care professionals in the AIDS epidemic. *Am J Public Health.* 1988;78:844–849.
   Discusses how physicians have no legal duty to treat patients in most situations, despite a strong moral duty to do so.
2. Cantor J, Baum K. The limits of conscientious objection—May pharmacists refuse to fill prescriptions for emergency contraception? *N Engl J Med.* 2004;351:2008–2012.
   Charo RA. The celestial fire of conscience—Refusing to deliver medical care. *N Engl J Med.* 2005;352:2471–2473.
   Articles on health care workers' refusals to provide care based on conscience, arguing that patients should be referred to other facilities that will provide needed care.
3. Friedman EA. Must we treat noncompliant ESRD patients? *Semin Dial.* 2001;14:23–27.
   Discusses legal, ethical, and clinical aspects of denying treatment to noncompliant, abusive, violent dialysis patients.
4. Gostin LO, Feldbaum C, Webber DW. Disability discrimination in America: HIV/AIDS and other health conditions. *JAMA.* 1999;281:745–752.
   Summary of disability law that explains that physicians may decline to care for infectious patients only if there is a significant risk of substantial harm.

Gifts From Patients to Physicians

Modest gifts from patients, such as cookies, candy, flowers, and toys for children, gratify physicians and allow patients to express their appreciation. Other gifts, however, are problematic. Expensive gifts might compromise the physician's judgment. Very personal gifts imply more than a professional relationship. Physicians who feel uncomfortable about a gift might be uncertain how to respond.

Gifts from patients are often considered simply matters of social convention and etiquette, not ethics. This chapter points out how gifts from patients might raise ethical issues because they might change the doctor–patient relationship, impair clinical judgment, or erode public trust. Because physicians often find it embarrassing to discuss gifts, this chapter also suggests how to respond to problematic gifts from patients.

REASONS PATIENTS GIVE GIFTS TO PHYSICIANS

Because gifts may have multiple meanings, physicians should consider why a patient is giving a specific gift at a particular time (1).

TO THANK PHYSICIANS

Patients commonly send gifts to express appreciation to physicians for their care. Patients who have recovered from serious illness are understandably grateful to their physicians, particularly if the diagnosis was difficult, the treatment was complicated, or the physician was particularly supportive or involved. The gift is similar to a tip for outstanding service.

TO SATISFY THEIR OWN NEEDS

Gifts might also reflect the patient's psychological needs.

CASE 25.1	Cookies from a lonely elderly patient

A 74-year-old widow has hypertension, osteoarthritis, and mild depression. She has no surviving relatives, few friends, and few social activities. A new resident takes over her care. She talks about her sadness and emptiness, and he encourages her to attend a senior center. On the next visit she brings him a box of home-baked cookies.

TO ENHANCE FUTURE CARE

Gifts might represent expectations for future care rather than thanks for past efforts. Patients might believe that a gift will gain them special consideration. For instance, some patients might want to have the last appointment of the day because of difficulties getting off from work. Other patients might hope that gifts will gain them more timely appointments or faster responses to phone calls. In rare cases, patients who give gifts might subsequently ask physicians to do something that is ethically questionable.

CASE 25.2   **Request for disability certification**

A patient with mild asthma gives his physician a toy for his son at Christmas. The next month he asks the physician to complete a form for a disability parking sticker. The patient does not meet the objective criteria for hypoxemia or dyspnea listed on the form.

In Case 25.2, the timing of the gift and the request are disturbing. The physician might feel manipulated because an apparently thoughtful gift probably had strings attached. Deceiving third parties about a patient's condition is ethically problematic (*see* Chapter 6). To do so after receiving a gift would appear like accepting a bribe.

TO MEET CULTURAL EXPECTATIONS

In some cultures, gifts to physicians or other healers are routinely expected. Such gifts might show respect or be considered an essential aspect of the healing process. In some societies, bribery might be necessary to ensure access to care. Physicians need to consider whether gifts might have special cultural significance for patients and correct any misconceptions about the US medical care system.

PROBLEMS WITH GIFTS

It is human nature for patients who have given gifts to expect some consideration in return, either consciously or unconsciously (2); however, some gifts might lead to inappropriate expectations by patients.

EXPECTATIONS FOR SPECIAL TREATMENT

Some patients might believe that gifts entitle them to special treatment, such as the following:

Beyond more convenient or prompter appointments, some patients might feel entitled to call the physician at home for routine issues. Even apparently small gifts are problematic if such expectations become burdensome to physicians. For example, physicians want to limit add-on appointments and after-hours phone calls to reduce personal stress and to protect their family life, yet they might find it difficult to refuse a request from a patient who has given a gift.

CHANGES IN THE DOCTOR–PATIENT RELATIONSHIP

Some gifts might change the doctor–patient relationship inappropriately.

CASE 25.1   *Continued. Focus on the physician's problems rather than the patient's*

The lonely, elderly patient starts to bring gifts of food at every visit. Moreover, visits now focus on the physician rather than on the patient. The patient inquires about what foods the physician likes so that she can plan her next gift. She also expresses concern about whether he is getting enough sleep and has enough time off.

In Case 25.1, an overworked and underappreciated house officer might be delighted that someone takes a personal interest in him, but it is problematic if the physician assumes the role of a surrogate grandchild. Patient visits should focus on the patient's problems, not the physician's. The physician might miss opportunities to encourage and reinforce the patient's efforts to become more socially active in the community. In the long run, it is problematic for lonely patients to depend on the medical system for their emotional and social needs.

Other gifts violate the boundaries of the professional relationship. An extreme example might be the gift of lingerie or other intimate apparel, which implies a romantic relationship, not a professional one. Patients who overstep the boundaries of a professional relationship are acting out their own needs or fantasies. Not only should such gifts be refused, but also appropriate boundaries need to be promptly and firmly reestablished. After such a gift, a physician might need to transfer care to another physician.

For isolated patients, their physician might listen or pay attention to them more than anyone else. Bringing a gift might give them a sense of purpose or alleviate their loneliness. Taking initiative and showing concern for other people might be therapeutic. For other patients, giving physicians small gifts provides a personal connection to an impersonal medical system.

IMPAIRMENT OF CLINICAL JUDGMENT

Gifts can create or strengthen personal ties, but too close a relationship might be undesirable. It is difficult to provide care to a close relative because emotional ties might cloud clinical judgment (2). In a similar way, gifts that establish or imply a very close personal relationship might compromise the physician's judgment. Expectations of special treatment might compromise care, as when a patient expects the physician to manage a complicated problem on the basis of a telephone call rather than an office visit. Psychologically, it may be difficult to say no to patients who have given gifts, even if they request interventions that are unsound medical practice. Similarly, a gift from a seriously ill patient might be problematic if it leads the physician to misrepresent bad news or causes the patient to develop unrealistic expectations.

EROSION OF PUBLIC TRUST

The doctor–patient relationship might be weakened if other patients believe that they will receive second-class care unless they offer gifts. Physicians serve as gatekeepers, allocating appointments, their time and attention, and health care resources. Generally, phone calls or appointments are allocated primarily on the basis of patient need. It would damage both the individual physician and the profession as a whole if patients believed that the best way to get the physician's attention is through a gift. Even a perception that physicians are allocating their efforts on the basis of favoritism might erode public trust.

SOLICITING GIFTS

Although this chapter has focused on gifts that patients offer to physicians, solicitation of gifts by physicians also merits attention. It is unethical for physicians to solicit personal gifts in return for services rendered because physicians' fees should be adequate compensation for their services. It might also be problematic for physicians to solicit contributions for some cause, such as a hospital or a political movement. Such solicitations might seem a natural way for physicians to work for causes they believe in, but patients might not feel free to decline the solicitation if their physician solicits it personally and knows whether they have responded. They might fear that the physician will not render prompt or meticulous care in the future if they refuse.

HOW TO RESPOND TO GIFTS FROM PATIENTS

In responding to gifts, physicians need to take into account the nature of the gift and the circumstances.

ACCEPT APPROPRIATE GIFTS GRACIOUSLY

Most small gifts from patients are well intentioned and appropriate and should be accepted graciously. Indeed, many patients would feel insulted if physicians did not accept homemade cookies, toys for

Christmas, or clothes for a new baby. Similarly, it would be unfeeling not to accept a small gift after the physician has devoted a great deal of effort in helping a patient recover from a difficult illness.

DO NOT LET GIFTS GO TO YOUR HEAD

Physicians should not allow gifts from patients to give them an exaggerated sense of their importance or their skill. Many patients, because they are sick and dependent, are extremely grateful for competent, humane care. It is gratifying that such qualities in physicians are recognized and reinforced, but physicians should appreciate that they might simply have provided the kind of care that every patient deserves.

APPRECIATE THAT SOME GIFTS ARE PROBLEMATIC

Some gifts might seem disproportionate to the services rendered (3).

CASE 25.3	Tickets to an opera

A 52-year-old businessman establishes care with a new physician. At the first visit, they discuss preventive measures such as exercise and diet. The next week the businessman offers the physician orchestra tickets to the opera opening night gala.

Intuitively, some gifts seem out of proportion to what the physician has done. Most physicians would feel comfortable accepting gifts worth less than $50, but many would feel uncomfortable accepting opening night opera tickets as in Case 25.3 after a routine new patient visit. Even if a wealthy patient considers this a small gift, it might give the wrong impression to other patients. Furthermore, the physician might wonder whether such a lavish gift reflects unrealistic expectations for care. Finally, many physicians feel uncomfortable accepting cash gifts because they seem associated with commerce and profits.

GET ADVICE ABOUT THE GIFT

Most physicians, even if they are uncomfortable about gifts, hesitate to discuss them with colleagues. Physicians might not appreciate that many colleagues also feel awkward and uncertain about gifts. Other people, however, can help the physician interpret the significance of gifts and understand the patient's possible expectations. In judging a gift's appropriateness, physicians can apply a practical rule of thumb: How would colleagues and other patients react if they knew about the gift? If others would question the gift, it is best not to accept it.

DECLINE GIFTS WITHOUT REJECTING THE PATIENT

Even when physicians believe that declining a gift is appropriate, they might find it awkward to do so. Several strategies might allow the physician to decline the gift, while respecting the patient's feelings. Physicians should start by saying that they are grateful and touched. One approach is to explain that accepting such a gift might compromise the physician's ability to give high-quality care in the future. Although this approach is straightforward, patients often protest that they would never ask for special consideration. A second approach is to decline the gift politely but firmly without giving more specific reasons. Physicians might simply say that they could not possibly accept the gift and that their policy is not to accept such gifts, even though they are touched by the thoughtfulness. Alternatively, the physician can resolve concerns about a large gift, as in Case 25.3, by sharing it with others, for example, donating it to house staff.

If the physician suspects that gifts reflect the patient's social isolation or other needs, as in Case 25.1, these issues should be addressed separately during patient visits.

WHAT IF THE PATIENT LATER REQUESTS SPECIAL TREATMENT?

After a gift, the patient might later request special treatment. A practical guideline is for physicians to do what they would have done if the same request had come from a patient who had not given a gift (3).

SUMMARY

1. Usually, gifts are thoughtful gestures of appreciation that should be accepted graciously.
2. Some gifts may be ethically problematic.
3. Discussing gifts with colleagues and considering how other patients would react might help physicians respond to them appropriately.

REFERENCES

1. Spence SA. Patients bearing gifts: are there strings attached? *BMJ*. 2005;331:1527–1529.
2. Murray TH. Gifts of the body and the needs of strangers. *Hastings Cent Rep*. 1987;17:30–38.
3. Lyckholm LJ. Should physicians accept gifts from patients? *JAMA*. 1998;280:1944–1946.

ANNOTATED BIBLIOGRAPHY

1. Lyckholm LJ. Should physicians accept gifts from patients? *JAMA*. 1998;280:1944–1946.
   Brief, thoughtful review of the topic.
2. Spence SA. Patients bearing gifts: are there strings attached? *BMJ*. 2005;331:1527–1529.
   Emphasizes that gifts may have multiple meanings and encourages physicians to reflect on why the patient is giving a specific gift at a particular time.

26

Sexual Contact Between Physicians and Patients

T he Hippocratic Oath forbids sexual relationships between physicians and patients. Some people, however, believe that this prohibition is no longer appropriate because sexual mores have changed and sex between consenting adults should be private. This chapter argues that sexual contacts between physicians and patients are unethical if they take advantage of patients' trust, dependency, and vulnerability.

In a national survey, 9% of physicians reported at least one sexual contact with a patient or former patient (1). Most cases involved male physicians and female patients. This study excluded cases in which the sexual relationship preceded the medical care, such as the provision of medical care to a spouse. Twenty-three percent of respondents said that one or more of their patients had revealed sexual contact with a previous physician. In other studies, between 5% and 10% of mental health professionals admitted to sexual contact with patients (2).

JUSTIFICATIONS FOR SEXUAL CONTACT

Several justifications are commonly offered for relaxing the traditional prohibition on sexual contacts between physicians and patients (3).

RESPECT FOR PRIVACY

Generally, sexual relationships between consenting adults are considered private matters with which other people and society have no right to interfere. In this view, it is demeaning and unrealistic to view patients as so vulnerable that they cannot make their own decisions about their private lives. Restricting freedom to enter into sexual relationships would be paternalistic and intrusive.

LACK OF HARM TO PATIENTS

Many people believe that patients are no more likely to be harmed in sexual relationships with their physicians than they are in other sexual relationships. In the United States, short-term relationships and divorces are common. Anecdotally, many people know of happy marriages between physicians and former patients. In this view, even if some sexual relationships with physicians harm patients, there is no reason to prohibit all such relationships.

LACK OF SOCIAL OPPORTUNITIES FOR PHYSICIANS

In small towns and rural areas, a physician might care for a large proportion of the community. Social opportunities for physicians would be very limited if romantic and sexual relationships with patients were barred.

OBJECTIONS TO SEXUAL CONTACT WITH CURRENT PATIENTS

Professional codes of ethics consider sexual relationships with current patients unethical. The American Medical Association (AMA) declared, "Sexual conduct or a romantic relationship with a patient concurrent with the physician–patient relationship is unethical" (2). Patients might feel "angry, abandoned, humiliated, mistreated, or exploited by their physicians. Victims have been reported to experience guilt, severe mistrust of their own judgment, and mistrust of both men and physicians" (2). There are several reasons for such role-specific restrictions on physicians (Table 26-1).

TABLE 26-1   Objections to Sexual Relationships With Current Patients
Physicians should not take advantage of the doctor–patient relationship.
Physicians have power over patients.
Trust in the profession will be undermined.
Some patients are particularly vulnerable.

PHYSICIANS SHOULD NOT TAKE ADVANTAGE OF THE DOCTOR–PATIENT RELATIONSHIP

It might be difficult for patients to make truly autonomous decisions on sexual relationships with physicians. The physician–patient relationship commonly arises during the patient's illness, which can cause patients to be vulnerable and dependent (4). Patients usually place great weight on their physicians' advice and judgment and naturally develop feelings of trust, gratitude, and admiration toward physicians. Unconsciously, the patient might mistake such feelings for romantic or sexual attraction. Patients, as well as physicians, might not appreciate how such positive feelings result from the doctor's role as well as the doctor's personal attributes. Although such transference has been most clearly described in patients undergoing psychotherapy, similar feelings might occur in all physician–patient relationships. Physicians might also misinterpret their own feelings of caring and concern for patients, which are a natural part of the doctor–patient relationship, as romantic or sexual attraction.

During their care, patients make intimate revelations to physicians.

CASE 26.1   Current patient receiving active therapy
A 45-year-old male physician is treating a 32-year-old woman for depression and peptic ulcer disease. The woman reveals that she was sexually abused as a child. The physician, who is going through a divorce, finds her attractive and considers initiating a romantic and sexual relationship with her.

In Case 26.1, a depressed patient discloses intimate personal information, which she might not have told anyone else. Physicians may take a detailed sexual or mental health history. Patients may reveal their innermost fantasies and fears. Patients undress for examinations and allow physicians to touch them and even invade their bodies during medical or surgical procedures. Such intimacy within the doctor–patient relationship is one-sided. Physicians do not reveal their personal feelings, thoughts, or bodies to patients. Thus, physicians know much more personal information about patients than patients know about them. Physicians might betray the patient's trust if they take advantage of such intimate information, consciously or unconsciously, in pursuing sexual relationships with patients.

PHYSICIANS HAVE POWER OVER PATIENTS

The power that physicians have over patients might make it difficult for patients to decline sexual relationships with them. In Case 26.1, the very framing of the issues implies unequal power: the physician considers initiating a sexual liaison, as if it were inconceivable that the patient would refuse. Because physicians order tests and treatments and schedule appointments, they control patients' access to medical care. There might be an implied or inferred threat that if the patient does not agree to sexual contact, the her care will suffer (5). Some physicians might falsely reassure patients that an effective therapeutic relationship can continue after a sexual liaison (5). In egregious cases, the physician might portray a sexual liaison as part of medical therapy.

TRUST IN THE PROFESSION WILL BE UNDERMINED

If the medical profession were to condone sexual relationships with patients, the public might begin to believe that physicians are motivated by self-interest and are willing to take advantage of patients. Patients might become reluctant to visit physicians or discuss intimate matters, particularly psychiatric or gynecological problems.

SOME PATIENTS ARE PARTICULARLY VULNERABLE

In Case 26.1, the patient's depression might compromise her ability to consent freely to a sexual relationship. Patients who have suffered incest or rape might find it difficult to refuse sexual relationships with authority figures and might feel particularly betrayed if the current relationship repeats previous traumatic experiences. Such persons might not even be aware that they are repeating a previous pattern of behavior.

THE PATIENT'S MEDICAL CARE MIGHT BE COMPROMISED

When physicians provide care to a spouse, they might not be thorough in taking a history, conducting an examination, or ordering diagnostic tests (6). When physicians are providing medical care to a sexual partner, their clinical judgment is likely to be compromised (7).

LEGAL ISSUES

Sexual relationships between physicians and current patients might lead to criminal charges or to disciplinary action by licensing boards (8). Physicians might also face civil suits for malpractice. Malpractice insurers might exclude coverage for civil claims relating to sexual misconduct, because such behavior is not part of providing medical care.

COMPARISONS WITH OTHER PROFESSIONS

In other professions, sexual relationships with clients are also condemned. Churches are strongly criticized for covering up sexual relationships between clergy and parishioners and transferring offending priests or ministers without appropriate disciplinary action. Similarly, lawyers have been criticized for sexual relationships with clients, particularly in divorce cases. As in medicine, the concern is abuse of trust and power by professionals.

SEXUAL RELATIONSHIPS WITH FORMER PATIENTS

Although sexual relationships with current patients are generally considered inappropriate, there is less agreement about relationships with previous patients. In the previously cited survey, although 94% of physicians considered it unethical to have sexual relationships with current patients, only 36% of physicians considered it unethical to have sexual relationships with former patients (1).

CASE 26.2   **Former patient, with no ongoing relationship**

A female emergency physician treats a 28-year-old man who requires a tetanus shot for a foot injury. Several years later they meet again as single parents whose children attend the same school. They discover that they share many interests. The physician wonders if a romantic relationship would be unacceptable because of their previous professional relationship.

In Case 26.2, it is unlikely that the former patient feels dependent on the physician. Furthermore, the patient revealed little personal information during the doctor–patient relationship and is not particularly vulnerable on that basis. A relationship between equals seems as possible for them as for any other couple.

Feelings of dependency, however, might persist after care is terminated, as in the following case.

CASE 26.3   **Recent surgical patient**

A male surgeon performs an emergency laparotomy on a woman with appendicitis. During postoperative visits, he finds himself spending much more time with her than he usually does with patients. She is appreciative of his attention and solicitous about his long hours and fatigue. A month after her final postoperative visit, he invites her to dinner.

In Case 26.3, the patient might have strong feelings of gratitude and dependency soon after emergency surgery. Unlike Case 26.2, it might be more difficult for the patient to make an independent judgment about a relationship or to decline invitations from the surgeon, compared with other men she knows.

The AMA states, "Sexual or romantic relationships with former patients are also unethical if the physician uses or exploits trust, knowledge, emotions, or influence derived from the previous professional relationship" (2). Thus, it is important to identify situations in which dependency in doctor–patient relationship continues (9). Several factors should be considered.

TERMINATION OF MEDICAL CARE

Termination of care and absence of contact should be complete, including cessation of office visits, telephone consultations, prescriptions, and reminder postcards about appointments or screening tests. In addition, a new physician should be identified so that the patient no longer regards the partner as his or her physician. The purpose of terminating care should not be the initiation of a sexual relationship.

NATURE OF THE DOCTOR–PATIENT RELATIONSHIP

Some types of medical care are so intimate that the doctor–patient relationship might never be completely ended. After counseling and therapy, patients might feel dependency and gratitude toward physicians years after therapy has been terminated. The American Psychiatric Association considers any sexual contact with a former psychiatric patient as unethical. Some patients might be particularly vulnerable because of past victimization. In specialties that involve unique and intimate physical touching, such as surgery or gynecology, the patient might still regard the physician as being in that role years later. In contrast, in Case 26.2, a tetanus immunization is so routine that the patient's dependence on the physician might be similar to dependence on a librarian.

TIME SINCE LAST MEDICAL CARE

In Case 26.3, during the immediate postoperative period the patient's feelings of vulnerability and dependency undoubtedly continue. Amorous advances by the physician might take advantage of these feelings in the patient. The passage of time helps extinguish feelings of dependency toward physicians and reduces the risk that physicians will abuse their power in initiating sexual relationships with patients (5). The crucial issue, however, is not simply the amount of time but rather the lack of a continuous relationship and the "potential for misuse of emotions derived from the former professional relationship" (2).

CIRCUMSTANCES OF RENEWAL OF CONTACT

If the doctor and former patient renew their acquaintance in a medical context, the patient might resume his or her previous role as dependent patient. However, if the physician and former patient meet again in a nonmedical context, as in Case 26.2, it is less likely that the previous doctor–patient relationship has an impact.

SUGGESTIONS

Physicians who are considering sexual relationships with current or former patients might consider the following suggestions.

RECOGNIZE EARLY SIGNS OF ROMANTIC INTEREST

Rarely are sexual or romantic feelings so overwhelming that the physician is swept away by uncontrollable passion. Physicians should be alert to early signs of romantic feelings for a patient. For example, they might look forward to the next visit or pay particular attention to their appearance on the day of the patient's visit. Sexual misconduct often begins with seemingly minor violations of the boundaries of the doctor–patient relationship, such as talking about the physician's problems rather than the patient's or scheduling appointments outside office hours (7). Recognizing these early symptoms gives physicians time to act thoughtfully and to consider the potential problems (10).

SEEK ADVICE

It is hard to think critically about romantic or sexual interests. The AMA recommends that "it would be advisable for a physician to seek consultation with a colleague before initiating a relationship with a former patient" (2). Confidential advice can provide an honest appraisal of the potential harm to the patient, the physician, and the medical profession. Such counsel might be a safeguard for physicians who might otherwise act impulsively. Although discussing such an intimate decision with other people might seem intrusive, sexual relationships are not completely private if they harm patients or undermine public trust in the medical profession.

RESPONDING TO ADVANCES BY PATIENTS

In some cases, the patient takes the initiative in pursuing a romantic or sexual liaison. Physicians, however, may still be considered responsible because they are in a better position than patients to recognize the potential harms of such relationships. In medical decisions, physicians do not simply accede to a patient's requests or demands. Physicians have an ethical duty to act in patients' best interests, even if it clashes with their own self-interest.

SUMMARY

1. Patients naturally feel trust, dependency, and gratitude toward their physicians.
2. Sexual relationships with current patients exploit such feelings and are unethical.
3. Sexual relationships with former patients are also unethical if the physician takes advantage of emotions and influence deriving from the doctor–patient relationship.

REFERENCES

1. Gartrell NG, Milliken N, Goodson WH III, et al. Physician–patient sexual contact: prevalence and problems. *West J Med.* 1992;157:139–143.
2. Council on Ethical and Judicial Affairs of the American Medical Association. Sexual misconduct and the practice of medicine. *JAMA.* 1991;266:2741–2745.
3. Appelbaum PS, Jorgenson LM, Sutherland PK. Sexual contact between physicians and patients. *Arch Intern Med.* 1994;154:2561–2565.
4. Pellegrino ED, Thomasma DG. *For the Patient's Good: The Restoration of Beneficence in Health Care.* New York, NY: Oxford University Press; 1988.
5. Appelbaum PS, Jorgenson L. Psychotherapist–patient sexual contact after termination of treatment: an analysis and proposal. *Am J Psychiatry.* 1991;148:1466–1473.
6. LaPuma J, Stocking CB, LaVoie D, et al. When physicians treat members of their own families. *N Engl J Med.* 1991;325:1290–1294.
7. Gabbard GO, Nadelson C. Professional boundaries in the physician–patient relationship. *JAMA.* 1995;273:1445–1449.
8. Dehlendorf CE, Wolfe SM. Physicians disciplined for sex-related offenses. *JAMA.* 1998;279:1883–1888.
9. Malmquist CP, Notman MT. Psychiatrist–patient boundary issues following treatment termination. *Am J Psychiatry.* 2001;158:1010–1018.
10. Gutheil TG, Gabbard GO. Misuses and misunderstandings of boundary theory in clinical and regulatory settings. *Am J Psychiatry.* 1998;155:409–414.

ANNOTATED BIBLIOGRAPHY

1. Council on Ethical and Judicial Affairs of the American Medical Association. Sexual misconduct and the practice of medicine. *JAMA.* 1991;266:2741–2745.
   Thoughtful discussion of the topic, proposing that all sexual contact during the physician–patient relationship is unethical.
2. Gabbard GO, Nadelson C. Professional boundaries in the physician–patient relationship. *JAMA.* 1995;273:1445–1449.
   Discusses how sexual misconduct with patients usually begins with apparently minor violations of the therapeutic relationship.

CHAPTER 27

Secret Information About Patients

P hysicians might receive information about a patient from family members or friends who ask that their role be kept secret (1). Doctors find such unsolicited information disconcerting. Telling the patient the secret or recording it in the medical record might pass on inaccurate or unhelpful information, while keeping the secret might involve the physician in deception. This chapter discusses the ethical issues posed by such secret information and how physicians can respond. The related issue of secrets that patients disclose confidentially to doctors is discussed in Chapter 5.

TYPES OF SECRETS FROM RELATIVES

Most commonly, a family member tells the doctor about the patient's deleterious personal habits, such as alcohol use or smoking (1). The family member often tells a member of the physician's staff, rather than the physician directly. The informer hopes that the physician will make the patient stop these unhealthy behaviors. Another type of secret involves mental or physical incapacity. The family member might tell the physician that the patient is demented, depressed, or psychotic. Similarly, the family might be concerned that an elderly patient can no longer drive safely or live independently. The confider also might seek to draw the physician into family disputes over money, marital problems, or the lifestyles of grown children. Finally, family members might alert the physician to hidden physical symptoms, such as chest pain, that the patient might choose not to discuss.

ETHICAL PROBLEMS WITH SUCH SECRETS

Secret information can be problematic in many ways. The information might be inaccurate. The informer might have ulterior motives, such as gaining an advantage in a family dispute. Secrets are disrespectful to the patient because they involve deception rather than open discussions. Finally, such secret disclosures trap the physician in a bind because both disclosing and keeping the secret are ethically objectionable.

APPROACHES TO SECRETS

When presented with such a secret by the patient's family, the physician has several options, some of which involve deception or undermine patient trust.

REVEAL THE SECRET TO THE PATIENT

There are several ethical objections to keeping such a secret. Patients might consider it a violation of trust and privacy if physicians talk to other people about them behind their backs (2). Patients might question the physician's allegiance. It is also deceptive for physicians to base their recommendations and plans on secret information from third parties rather than on the history obtained from the patient. Chapter 6 discusses why deception is ethically problematic for physicians.

Keeping secrets from patients is also impractical. Like all forms of deception, it might require additional, increasingly elaborate deception. Patients might ask why the physician is posing a particular question or ordering a particular test, in which case physicians will have to either reveal the secret information or deceive the patient.

DO NOT DISCLOSE TO THE PATIENT

One physician who was philosophically opposed to keeping such secrets found that in about one half of cases he did not tell the patient (1). First, there may be no point in doing so because the information is obvious or trivial. For example, a family member's report that the patient was a heavy smoker provides no new information if the patient smells of cigarettes. Second, the physician does not disclose the information because it is not relevant to the patient's medical care. For example, few physicians want to get involved in a parent's concerns about an adult patient's marriage. Third, disclosure might do more harm than good in the short run. Revealing the mother's objections to the patient's marriage might well precipitate or intensify a family argument. Fourth, the physician might intend to tell the patient, but finds no opportunity to bring it up naturally in the conversation. The right moment to disclose the secret may never occur.

In some cases, the physician might promise to keep the secret. The physician might later be caught between conflicting obligations to be forthright with patients and to keep promises. Physicians can avoid this dilemma and maintain their primary obligation to the patient by rejecting the informer's initial request to keep the information secret. Family members often preface their revelations with phrases such as, "I don't want my husband to know I told you, but...." It would be prudent for physicians to interrupt at this point, before the information is revealed, and explain their policy of disclosing such information and its source to patients.

ASK INFORMERS TO DISCLOSE THEIR ROLE

Ethically, the best approach is for the physician to convince the informer to tell the patient about the information presented to the physician or to allow the physician to disclose the source of the information. If this is done, the physician can discuss the issue freely with the patient.

SUMMARY

1. Physicians face dilemmas when family members or friends give information about patients that they ask to be kept secret.
2. Acquiescence with such secrets, even if well intentioned, might undermine the patient's trust.
3. Telling the family member or friend that the information needs to be shared with the patient is the most effective way to prevent such an outcome.

REFERENCES

1. Burnum JF. Secrets about patients. *N Engl J Med.* 1991;324:1130–1133.
2. Bok S. *Secrets: On the Ethics of Concealment and Revelation.* New York, NY: Pantheon Books; 1982.

ANNOTATED BIBLIOGRAPHY

1. Burnham JF. Secrets about patients. *N Engl J Med.* 1991;324:1130–1133.
   Thoughtful discussion of the topic based on the author's clinical experience.

28

Clinical Research

R esearch with human participants is essential to better understand the pathophysiology of illness and to improve clinical care. Participants in research accept risks and inconvenience primarily to advance scientific knowledge and to benefit others. Thus, there is an unavoidable ethical tension between protecting the well-being of research participants and gaining new knowledge to benefit society. Although clinical care also involves benefits and risks, the patient who undergoes the risks also derives the clinical benefits.

Physicians can be involved in research in various roles. Treating physicians may help refer and recruit participants in research. When patients consider entering a research project, they may ask their treating physician for advice. Furthermore, when researchers identify eligible participants from medical records, many institutional review boards (IRBs) require researchers to obtain the treating physician's permission before contacting patients with whom they have no previous relationship. Finally, treating physicians can also serve as investigators in research. Because clinical research might benefit society and future patients, physicians generally should encourage their patients to participate in well-designed studies, while protecting the individual patient's interests.

This chapter takes the perspective of the physician in clinical practice. References at the end of the chapter take the perspective of the investigator.

ETHICAL PRINCIPLES FOR RESEARCH

Three ethical principles should guide research with human participants (1). The principle of **respect for persons** requires investigators to obtain informed and voluntary consent from research participants, to protect participants with impaired decision-making capacity, and to maintain confidentiality.

The principle of **beneficence** requires that the research design be scientifically sound and that the risks of the research be acceptable in relation to the likely benefits. Risks to participants include both physical harm from research interventions and also psychosocial harm, such as breaches of confidentiality, stigma, and discrimination. If the research question has already been settled or is trivial, or if the design of the study is so weak that valid conclusions are impossible, no risk to participants can be justified. The risks of participating in the study must be minimized, for example, by screening potential participants to exclude those very likely to suffer adverse effects and by monitoring participants for adverse effects.

Traditionally, clinical research has been regarded as risky, and potential participants were considered guinea pigs who needed to be protected from dangerous interventions. Increasingly, however, clinical research is regarded as beneficial rather than risky because it provides access to potentially life-saving new therapies in such conditions as cancer, HIV infection, and organ transplantation. Patients with such conditions might want increased access to clinical research, not greater protection.

The principle of **justice** requires that the benefits and burdens of research be distributed fairly. Vulnerable populations lack the capacity to make informed and free choices about participating in a research project or are at increased risk for adverse events from the study. Vulnerable groups should be neither overrepresented in dangerous studies nor underrepresented in trials of promising new therapies. Justice also requires equitable access to the benefits of research. Rather than excluding from research vulnerable populations such as children and pregnant women, appropriate measures should be put in place to protect them and allow rigorous studies on the safety and efficacy of therapies in these groups to be carried out.

OVERVIEW OF RESEARCH ETHICS

Federal regulations require that many types of research with human participants be approved by an IRB. The IRB must ensure that the risks of the research are appropriate in light of the prospective benefits, that the risks of research are minimized, and that participants give informed consent.

Clinical research, which is intended to produce generalizable knowledge, must be distinguished from innovative clinical practice, in which a physician goes beyond usual practice to try to benefit a particular patient. For example, an internist might use a drug for an indication not approved by the Food and Drug Administration.

RISKS AND BENEFITS OF RESEARCH

Even though a research study has been approved by an IRB, the balance of risks and benefits may not be appropriate for an individual patient.

CASE 28.1	Osteoporosis clinical trial

Mrs. L is a 70-year-old woman with a family history of osteoporosis. She is interested in entering a randomized placebo-controlled phase III clinical trial of a new preventive agent that is given intravenously once a year. Currently approved drugs that are effective in preventing osteoporotic fractures need to be taken by pill once daily.

The use of placebo controls in clinical trials about osteoporosis is controversial (2). Measures to prevent osteoporotic fractures are only partially effective. Between 12 and 160 women need to be treated for a year to prevent a fracture (2). Many fractures will be clinically silent, diagnosed only by x-ray studies. To be adequately powered, a randomized trial will need at least 30 excess fractures in one arm. Some ethicists argue that the risk of foregoing standard preventive measures is small and that, therefore, a placebo control is acceptable. For some patients, however, the risks are higher and are unacceptable. For example, if Mrs. L has a very low bone density, previous compression fractures, or a history of falls, her risk of fracture is greater. She therefore would be at increased risk if she foregoes standard drugs. Her personal physician should ensure that Mrs. L understands these risks and recommend that she receive a drug that is known to be effective, rather than enrolling in the clinical trial and receive placebo or an unproven intervention. In other cases, a patient may be at unacceptable risk in a trial because she is more susceptible to adverse effects of a drug being tested—for example, because of preexisting impairment in an organ system in which adverse effects commonly occur.

In a randomized double-blind clinical trial, it sometimes becomes necessary to break the blinding to provide appropriate care to a patient. For example, in a serious emergency, the treating physician needs to know the patient's medications. In this situation, the individual patient's well-being is paramount, and the scientific goals of the research should be secondary.

INFORMED AND VOLUNTARY CONSENT

The ethical guideline of respect for persons and their autonomy requires that adult participants give informed and free consent to participate in research. The treating physician can play an important ethical and clinical role in helping the patient make an informed decision.

Table 28-1 lists pertinent issues that the prospective participant needs to be told and understand to give informed consent.

TABLE 28-1	Informed Consent in Research Projects

The nature of the research project
The procedures of the study
The potential harms and benefits of the study
Assurances that participation in the research is voluntary
Misconceptions about research

The Nature of the Research Project and Study Procedures

The prospective participant should understand that research is being conducted, what its purpose is, how it differs from standard care, and how the participants are being recruited. Participants need to know what they will be asked to do in the research project. On a practical level, they should be told how much time will be required and how often. Procedures that are not standard care should be identified as such. Alternative procedures or treatments that might be available outside the study should be discussed. If the study involves blinding or randomization, these concepts should be explained in terms that the patient can understand. Any financial interest of the investigators in the study intervention should be disclosed (3).

Risks and Potential Benefits of the Study

Medical, psychosocial, and economic risks and benefits should be described in lay terms. Economic risks might also be important. Participants should appreciate that insurance companies may deny reimbursement for procedures that are not standard clinical care.

Assurances That Participation in the Research Is Voluntary

Participants must appreciate that they may decline to participate in research, that declining will not compromise their medical care, and that they may withdraw from the project at any time.

Misconceptions About Research

A common misconception is that research will provide direct therapeutic benefits to the participants. This has been termed as the *therapeutic misconception* (4–6). Participants often do not understand how research differs from clinical care, often incorrectly believing that the study is designed to provide them a personal benefit and that the choice of interventions will be based on their needs. Moreover, they may not appreciate that the intervention is unproven and that they may not benefit and may, in fact, be harmed by the study intervention. Most promising new interventions, despite encouraging preclinical results, fail to show significant advantages over standard therapy in rigorously designed clinical trials (7, 8). In a randomized trial, participants may not receive the study intervention. Research participants commonly downplay the risks and are unrealistically optimistic about the benefits.

Prospective participants in clinical trials should also not underestimate the potential benefits. In clinical trials of cancer chemotherapy, patients randomized to the control group have better outcomes overall than patients who are eligible to participate, but choose not to (9). This may be due to collateral benefits, such as more intensive monitoring for adverse effects, greater attention to protocol details, and coordination of interventions by the research nurse.

The treating physician can often play a crucial role in helping the patient make an informed decision by eliciting and correcting any misunderstandings and encouraging the patient to ask questions. In some cases, the treating doctor may make a recommendation about participating in the research project.

SELECTION OF PARTICIPANTS IN RESEARCH

CASE 28.2   Research on patients with dementia

A new urinary catheter has been developed. A clinical trial is proposed to evaluate whether it is more effective and safer than the conventional catheter. Nursing home residents with Alzheimer disease and incontinence will be recruited as participants because enrollment and follow-up will be easier than in ambulatory patients.

Patients Who Lack Decision-Making Capacity

As in Case 28.2, patients who lack decision-making capacity cannot give informed consent to research studies and might not be able to protect themselves from harm. Research is essential, however, to improve therapies for their conditions. When prospective research participants lack such decision-making capacity, surrogates may give permission for them to participate in research. Ethical controversy occurs because surrogate decisions regarding research with mentally incapacitated persons often are not based on the patients' wishes or best interests. In one study, 31% of surrogates who believed that the patient would refuse to participate nonetheless gave consent, apparently contradicting the patient's preferences (11). Furthermore, 20% of surrogates who would not enroll in the study themselves nevertheless allowed the patient to participate in the research, perhaps acting contrary to the patient's best interests. Treating physicians can help assure the participation in research by persons who lack decision-making capacity is appropriate.

Patients Whose Consent Might Not Be Free

Some potential participants in research are vulnerable because their consent might be constrained. Participants might depend on physician-researchers for ongoing medical care, as in nursing homes, Veterans Affairs hospitals, or public hospitals and clinics. As in Case 28.2, such dependent populations are sometimes recruited as research participants because recruitment and follow-up are easier than with more autonomous individuals. Such patients, however, might not feel free to refuse to participate.

Fairness requires that vulnerable populations not be targeted as participants primarily for the convenience of investigators, if other populations would also be suitable participants for the study. In addition, researchers need to justify why they are not studying persons with unimpaired decision-making capacity, such as patients with spinal cord injury who require catheters. The use of vulnerable participants for research is more justifiable if the research addresses the condition that makes the participants vulnerable, if it offers the prospect of direct therapeutic benefit, and if advocates for the vulnerable population have approved the project.

CONFLICTS OF INTEREST

CONFLICTING INTERESTS FOR TREATING PHYSICIANS

Finder's Fees

Finder's fees are payments to clinicians for referring patients to a research project.

CASE 28.3   Finder's fees

To encourage enrollment in a clinical trial of a new antibiotic, physicians are offered $350 for referring patients who subsequently enroll in the study. The referring physician needs to make a phone call to the coordinating research nurse, who will explain the study to the patient.

Enrollment is often the rate-limiting step in clinical trials, and finder's fees facilitate their timely completion. Finder's fees, however, give the appearance that physicians refer patients to clinical trials for their own interest, rather than the patient's (12). Critics of finder's fees point out that the analogous situation of kickbacks for referring patients to another physician for clinical care is considered unethical. Furthermore, the physician's reward might seem excessive for the services rendered.

Dual Roles for Clinician-Investigators

If an investigator is also the treating physician. eligible research participants may find it difficult to decline to participate in research. What is best for a particular patient's care might not be what is best for the research project. In some situations, it might be better for the patient to drop out of the study and receive individualized care. An investigator, however, wants study participants to enroll and continue in the trial so that the research question can be answered. Moreover, in some clinical trials physicians receive payments for each enrolled patient and study visit, with payments exceeding actual expense. The role of personal physician should take priority over the role of clinical researcher.

RESPONDING TO A CONFLICT OF INTEREST

Treating physicians must address conflicts of interest regarding clinical research. Chapter 29 provides a broader discussion of conflicts of interest.

Disclose Conflicting Interests

Treating physicians should disclose to patients any financial interest in a research project they discuss (3). In one study, however, most participants in cancer clinical trials were not highly concerned about investigators' financial conflicts of interest (13). More than 70% of respondents would still have enrolled in the clinical trial even if the researcher had financial ties to the drug company sponsoring the trial or had received royalty payments. Only 31% wanted disclosure of the researcher's financial interests. The respondents in this study, however, did not receive any information about the risk of financial incentives to enroll.

Manage Conflicts of Interest

Although disclosure is necessary to protect participants, in some situations treating physicians need to go further to manage or eliminate conflicts of interest. Finder's fees and payments for enrolling participants and study visits should be commensurate with the services provided.

Ban Certain Unacceptable Conflicts of Interest

If an investigator holds a patent on the experimental intervention or has a management position or stock options in the company manufacturing it, he stands to gain or lose money personally depending on whether the study yields a positive or negative result. Such an investigator should not serve as principal investigator or other roles where the possibility of undue influence is high, such as determining endpoints, analyzing the data, or writing the first draft of a manuscript.

SUMMARY

1. Rigorous clinical research is essential to evaluate promising new therapies.
2. Treating physicians should also help assure that participants appreciate the key features of the research study and that there are no special considerations that would make it unduly risky for the patient to participate in the research.
3. Conflicts of interest might impair objectivity and erode public trust in research.

REFERENCES

1. National Commission for the Protection of Human Subjects of Biomedical and Behavioral Research. The Belmont Report: Ethical Principles and Guidelines for the Protection of Human Subjects of Biomedical and Behavioral Research. Washington, DC: U.S. Government Printing Office; 1979.
2. Brody BA, Dickey N, Ellenberg SS, et al. Is the use of placebo controls ethically permissible in clinical trials of agents intended to reduce fractures in osteoporosis? *J Bone Miner Res.* 2003;18:1105–1109.
3. Moore v. Regents of University of California, 51 Cal. 3d 120; Cal. Rptr. 146, 793 P.2d 479 (1990).
4. Lidz CW, Appelbaum PS. The therapeutic misconception: problems and solutions. *Med Care.* 2002;40:V55–V63.
5. Appelbaum PS, Lidz CW. Re-evaluating the therapeutic misconception: response to Miller and Joffe. *Kennedy Inst Ethics J.* 2006;16:367–373.
6. Miller FG, Joffe S. Evaluating the therapeutic misconception. *Kennedy Inst Ethics J.* 2006;16:353–366.
7. Horstmann E, McCabe MS, Grochow L, et al. Risks and benefits of phase I oncology trials, 1991 through 2002. *N Engl J Med.* 2005;352:895–904.
8. Joffe S, Miller FG. Rethinking risk-benefit assessment for phase I cancer trials. *J Clin Oncol.* 2006;24:2987–2990.
9. Gross CP, Krumholz HM, Van Wye G, et al. Does random treatment assignment cause harm to research participants? *PLoS Med.* 2006;3:e188.
10. Vist GE, Hagen KB, Devereaux PJ, et al. Outcomes of patients who participate in randomised controlled trials compared to similar patients receiving similar interventions who do not participate. *Cochrane Database Syst Rev.* 2007;(2):MR000009.
11. Warren JW, Sobal J, Tenney JH, et al. Informed consent by proxy. An issue in research with elderly patients. *N Engl J Med.* 1986;315:1124–1128.
12. Lind SE. Finder's fees for research subjects. *N Engl J Med.* 1990;323:192–195.
13. Hampson LA, Agrawal M, Joffe S, et al. Patients' views on financial conflicts of interest in cancer research trials. *N Engl J Med.* 2006;355:2330–2337.

ANNOTATED BIBLIOGRAPHY

1. Lo B. *Ethical Issues in Clinical Research: A Practical Guide.* Philadelphia, PA: Lippincott Williams & Wilkins; 2009.
   Comprehensive textbook of ethical issues in clinical research, with case discussions.
2. Lidz CW, Appelbaum PS. The therapeutic misconception: problems and solutions. *Med Care.* 2002;40:V55–V63.
   Explains that research subjects commonly believe that research is designed to provide them therapeutic benefits, when, in fact, the goal of research is to advance scientific knowledge.
3. Federman DD, Hanna KE, Rodriguez LL, eds. *Responsible Research: A Systems Approach to Protecting Research Participants.* Washington, DC: National Academies Press; 2003.
   Report from the Institute of Medicine on the oversight of research with human participants, discussing how to improve the IRB system.
4. Field MJ, Behrman RE, eds. *The Ethical Conduct of Clinical Research Involving Children.* Washington, DC: National Academies Press; 2004.
   Report from the Institute of Medicine on the special ethical issues concerning research with children.
5. Emanuel E, Grady C, Crouch R, et al., eds. *The Oxford Textbook of Clinical Research Ethics.* New York, NY: Oxford University Press; 2008.
   Multiauthored book providing in-depth discussion of particular issues in research ethics.

Conflicts of Interest

Overview of Conflicts of Interest

I n *The Doctor's Dilemma,* George Bernard Shaw questioned whether people can be impartial when they have strong financial interests in a decision. He wrote, "Nobody supposes that doctors are less virtuous than judges; but a judge whose salary and reputation depended on whether the verdict was for plaintiff or defendant, prosecutor or prisoner, should be as little trusted as a general in the pay of the enemy. To offer me a doctor as my judge, and then weight his decision with a bribe of a large sum of money . . . is to go wildly beyond . . . [what] human nature will bear" (1). Shaw's words have particular relevance to contemporary US medicine because of increasing concerns over conflicts of interest in medicine.

A conflict of interest is a situation in which a person entrusted with the interests of a client, dependent, or the public tends to be unduly influenced by a secondary interest (2). A conflict of interest does not mean unethical, unprofessional, or illegal behavior. For physicians in clinical practice, the patient's health should be their primary interest and take precedence over their own financial self-interest or the interests of a third party, such as a hospital. Financial conflicts may result from reimbursement incentives, personal investments in medical facilities, or gifts from drug companies. Other secondary interests include physician's personal or professional self-interest, which might be salient when physicians respond to mistakes, deal with impaired colleagues, or need to learn invasive procedures. Conflicts of interest also occur when physicians conduct research or teach. When carrying out research, the physician's primary interest should be to obtain and present valid information. In teaching, the physician's primary interest should be the accurate presentation of knowledge and a critical appraisal of the pertinent evidence.

Conflicts of interest might be ethically problematic for physicians for several reasons. Patients might suffer physical harm. Even though the patient suffers no clinical harm, the integrity of medical judgment might be compromised. Furthermore, conflicts of interest undermine patients' trust that physicians are acting on their behalf.

Chapters 30 to 36 analyze specific conflicts of interest. This chapter discusses how to define conflicts of interest, who should decide what constitutes an unacceptable conflict of interest, and how physicians can manage conflicts of interest.

WHAT IS A CONFLICT OF INTEREST?

CONFLICTS OF INTEREST IN NONMEDICAL SITUATIONS

Conflicts of interest occur in all professions and in public service. A public official is entrusted with acting in the public interest. Her role-specific primary interest is to serve the interests of the public; other interests, such as her self-interest or the interest of a business that contributed to her campaign, should be secondary. She would violate that trust by allowing those secondary interests to unduly influence her official decisions. In another example, a trustee has a role-specific primary interest in the welfare of the elderly person or child she represents. In the private sector, an employee responsible for purchasing for a company has a primary interest in fiscal responsibility and obtaining value when making purchases. In these situations, the primary interest would be subverted by accepting gifts, entertainment, or kickbacks from a company that the official oversees, a financial institution that a trustee works with, or a potential supplier to the company. The following case illustrates conflicts of interest in a nonmedical profession.

CASE 29.1   **Conflicts of interest for a judge**

A judge is assigned to preside over several cases in which she has a personal connection:
A landlord–tenant case in which the landlord is her uncle.
A divorce case involving a former law partner.
A breach of contract dispute involving a company in which she owns stock.

A judge takes on the responsibility of deciding and managing cases fairly and respecting the law. This primary interest would be undermined if the judge presides over a case in which she has a personal stake in the outcome (3). The judge's self-interest, or the interest of friends or colleagues, must be secondary. In Case 29.1, there are several concerns. The judge might decide the case in favor of the relative, the former partner, or her self-interest, even though the evidence did not support such a ruling. Even if the ruling is fair, the process by which the trial was conducted might be biased. For instance, the judge might take into account inappropriate factors or make rulings about motions and objections that no impartial decision maker would make. These procedural errors would be disturbing even if the final ruling was appropriate. Moreover, conflicts of interest undermine public trust in the judicial system. This is an important consideration even if there is no indication that the particular case was managed improperly.

The judge facing a conflict of interest might honestly believe that she will be impartial and might even consciously try to compensate for having ties to a litigant. Nonetheless, the opposing party and the public might still suspect that another judge would have decided or managed the case differently. Thus, the judge is required to withdraw from cases that pose a conflict of interest. Society sets rules that determine when judges or public officials must recuse themselves (3). The decision to withdraw is not up to the individual judge or official. There is no implication that the judge facing a conflict of interest is immoral or unprofessional. Simply put, it would be untenable to place any human being in such a situation, and the possibility that the primary interest will be compromised requires the judge to withdraw.

HOW ARE CONFLICTS OF INTEREST DEFINED?

People often use the term *conflict of interest* without defining it clearly.

Compromise of Physicians' Primary Interest

In clinical care, the narrowest definition of conflict of interest is that the patient's outcome is worse because the physician subordinated the patient's best interests. The physician might do so either intentionally or subconsciously.

Compromise of Physicians' Judgment or the Decision-Making Process

More broadly, the physician's judgment or decision-making process might be compromised because of secondary interests, even though clinical outcomes are not impaired. The physician might fail to order an indicated test or therapy or order an unnecessary test. It is difficult to determine whether this error results from a conflict of interest or from poor judgment, incompetence, or a lapse of attention.

Potential for Detrimental Outcomes or Compromised Judgment

A still broader definition of conflict of interest, which we adopt, includes situations in which there is an unacceptable probability for secondary interests to unduly influence the primary interest. This definition does not require evidence of *actual* harm to patients or compromised judgment in the particular situation (2). Several arguments support this broader definition. First, it is usually impractical or impossible to determine whether harm occurred or decision procedures were inappropriate in any given case. To make such a determination would require extensive data collection. As a matter of public policy, it would be prudent to ask physicians to avoid situations that offer a significant possibility of compromising patient care or research, even if no misbehavior can be proven in a particular case. Avoiding such situations also more effectively prevents the occurrence of harm, which is preferable to determining after the fact whether harm occurred. This broader definition is consistent with how conflicts of interest are handled in other professions, as we discussed with judges and government officials.

The determination of an unacceptable probability of undue influence should be made by independent, reasonable observers, not by the physician in the situation. This determination should take into account many factors, including the nature of the relationship and the likelihood and seriousness of the potential compromise of the primary interest (2). Furthermore, individual patients generally are not in position to determine whether clinical judgment and decision-making process were sound. However, patient advocacy groups or public interest groups play an important role in setting rules regarding conflicts of interest.

MISCONCEPTIONS ABOUT CONFLICTS OF INTEREST

Perceived or Apparent Conflicts of Interest

Certain situations sometimes are described as only *perceived* or *apparent* conflicts of interest, with the implication that there is no harm and even no potential for harm. For example, many physicians believe that accepting small gifts from drug companies, such as pens and writing pads, is harmless (*see* Chapter 33). The perception of a conflict of interest, however, might be damaging, even though the actual or potential harm to patients is small. If the public believes that physicians are serving the interests of drug companies rather than those of their patients, trust in the individual doctor or the profession as a whole might be undermined. Recent commentators have argued that the concept of perceived or apparent conflicts of interest is misguided because all conflicts of interest represent a tendency for a secondary interest to unduly influence the primary interest (2); no actual bias or unacceptable consequences need to be demonstrated in any particular situation. Furthermore, not any perception that a conflict of interest exists should be given equal weight. A conflict of interest should be judged by a reasonable person in light of past experience and available facts about the situation. Thus, a situation is not a conflict of interest if a person has no decision-making authority or if the secondary interest is unrelated to primary interest. For example, it is not conflict of interest if a physician's receptionist owns stock in a drug company, because he exercises no discretion over prescribing decisions. Nor is it conflict of interest for a physician to invest in a mutual fund involving drug companies, as the doctor has no control over the purchase or sale of stocks in the fund.

Competing Versus Conflicting Interests

The interests of the patient and physician never coincide completely. *Conflicting* interests, as we have defined them, should be prioritized in a certain way. The well-being of the patient should be regarded as primary, and the self-interest of the physician should be secondary. In contrast, in *competing* interests, both have claims to priority. For example, time devoted to patient care cannot be spent on the physician's important competing interests in continuing medical education, teaching, clinical research, or family activities. Such competing interests need to be accommodated.

Implications About Unethical Behavior

Some physicians might be offended because concerns about potential or perceived conflicts of interest apparently impugn their integrity and imply they are acting unethically. Doctors need to understand that the public is not singling them out for censure, but simply treating them as human and, therefore, fallible. It is the situation that is problematic, not the person.

Situations That Are Not Conflicts of Interest

The term *conflict of interest* is often used loosely. A conflict of interest, in the senses defined previously, needs to be distinguished from conflicts between ethical guidelines, disagreements among health care professionals, or disagreements between patients and physicians.

FINANCIAL CONFLICTS OF INTEREST

Medicine is regarded as an altruistic profession because its primary goal is to benefit the patient, not to maximize physicians' income; however, no one expects physicians to work for free or begrudges them a comfortable income. Helping the sick is difficult work and requires extensive training. This tension between altruism and self-interest is unavoidable in medicine (4). Financial rewards to the doctor should ideally be secondary to fostering patients' well-being.

Any reimbursement system can offer incentives to physicians to act contrary to patients' best interests. Fee-for-service reimbursement provides incentives to increase services and to give services of little or no benefit, thereby raising the cost of health care (*see* Chapter 31). Incentives to control costs might lead physicians to withhold beneficial care (*see* Chapter 32).

The concern about financial incentives is not simply that unscrupulous physicians will deliberately subordinate the patient's interests to their own self-interest or the interests of hospitals or insurance plans (5). Incentives also exert unconscious influence on physician decisions. When several management options are plausible, as often occurs in clinical practice, "financial incentives may influence even the best, most highly principled doctors to overlook subtle clues that suggest an optimal approach" (5).

Conflict of interest policies often focus on financial relationships. Financial conflicts of interest may not be more serious or more common than nonfinancial conflicts of interest, but because they are within the experience of the public, easier to quantify, and more feasible to manage than nonfinancial relationships.

HOW SHOULD CONFLICTS OF INTEREST BE ADDRESSED?

When physicians face a conflict of interest, they should take the following steps (Table 29-1), which are discussed in detail in subsequent chapters that address specific conflicts of interest.

TABLE 29-1   Managing Conflicts of Interest
Reaffirm that the patient's interests are paramount.
Disclose conflicts of interest.
Manage the situation to protect patients.
Prohibit certain actions and situations.

REAFFIRM THAT THE PATIENT'S INTERESTS ARE PARAMOUNT

Individual physicians and the medical profession need to reaffirm their fiduciary responsibility to their patients. The doctor's primary responsibility is to foster the well-being of patients.

To check whether they are acting in the patient's best interest, doctors might ask what they would recommend if they were working under the opposite reimbursement system. Physicians paid by salary might ask whether they would recommend the intervention under fee-for-service. Similarly, fee-for-service physicians might ask what they would recommend if they or the hospital would lose money doing the procedure. The answer is simple: Physicians should recommend care that is in the patient's best interests, no more and no less. The goal of economic incentives should be to "prompt the physician to consider costs appropriately—to remind him pointedly that economics really does matter—but not to distort his reasoning. A well-designed incentive should prompt the physician to consider more carefully what he does with clinical uncertainties and borderline options; it should not induce him to forego what he believes is clearly in the patient's interest" (6).

Although reaffirming fiduciary responsibilities to the patient is a necessary first step, other steps might also be needed.

DISCLOSE CONFLICTS OF INTEREST

Disclosure is essential for several reasons. First, the requirement to disclose incentives to patients, health care institutions, or the public might prevent physicians and organizations from making unacceptable arrangements. If the physician would find it hard or awkward to justify a situation, it probably presents an unacceptable conflict of interest. Second, patients who know about a conflict of interest might make more informed decisions by placing the physician's recommendations in context and compensating for any bias. However, it is generally unrealistic to expect patients to assess whether a situation has biased the physician's judgment. Indeed some behavioral science research suggests disclosure may be counterproductive (2). Finally, unless conflicts of interest are disclosed, society and health care institutions cannot judge whether they need to be managed or prohibited.

MANAGE THE SITUATION TO PROTECT PATIENTS

In some circumstances, society may determine that additional steps beyond disclosure must be taken to safeguard patients or the public. Physicians' actions may be regulated and their discretion limited. In clinical care, patients should be able to appeal denials of coverage and have a prompt response (*see* Chapter 32). In clinical research, review by an institutional review board is required (*see* Chapter 28).

PROHIBIT CERTAIN ACTIONS AND SITUATIONS

Although disclosure and precautions are necessary steps, they might still be insufficient to protect patients. Some actions and situations present such strong and direct conflicts of interest that they should be prohibited. Because "it is difficult if not impossible to distinguish cases in which financial gain does have improper influence from those in which it does not," it might be prudent to prohibit certain actions and situations (7). For example, drug companies that sponsor continuing medical education may not attempt to influence the choice of topics or speakers (*see* Chapter 33).

SUMMARY

1. Conflicts of interest might harm patients, impair physician judgment, and undermine trust in the medical profession.
2. The patients' interests should be primary, and the physician's self-interest or the interests of third parties should be secondary.

REFERENCES

1. Shaw GB. *The Doctor's Dilemma*. London, UK: Penguin Books; 1946.
2. Lo B, Field MJ, eds. *Conflict of Interest in Medical Research, Education, and Practice*. Washington, DC: The National Academies Press; 2009. http://www.iom.edu/Reports/2009/Conflict-of-Interest-in-Medical-Research-Education-and-Practice.aspx. Accessed November 16, 2011.
3. Gillers S. *Regulation of Lawyers: Problems of Law and Ethics*. New York, NY: Aspen Publishers; 2005.
4. Jonsen AR. Watching the doctor. *N Engl J Med*. 1983;308:1531–1535.
5. Hillman AL. Health maintenance organizations, financial incentives, and physicians' judgments. *Ann Intern Med*. 1990;112:891–893.
6. Morreim EH. *Balancing Act: The New Medical Ethics of Medicine's New Economics*. Boston: Kluwer Academic Publishers; 1991:124.
7. Thompson DF. Understanding financial conflicts of interest. *N Engl J Med*. 1993;329:573–576.

30

Bedside Rationing of Health Care

Physicians are ethically obligated to act in patients' best interests (*see* Chapter 4). Acting in the best interests of one patient, however, might sometimes preclude physicians from acting on behalf of another patient who is much more likely to benefit from care. Dilemmas arise because resources, such as physician time and intensive care beds, are in limited supply and people have different priorities for limited resources (1, 2).

CASE 30.1   Limited coronary care beds

Mr. H presents to the emergency department with substernal chest pain. An electrocardiogram (ECG) shows an acute anterior myocardial infarction, multifocal ventricular premature beats, and some couplets. The cardiac care unit (CCU) and intensive care unit (ICU) are full. One of the patients in the CCU is a 73-year-old man who had an emergency operation for a ruptured aortic aneurysm. A week after the operation, he is comatose, septic, in respiratory and renal failure, and has hypotension despite vasopressors. Another patient in the CCU experienced chest pain after an angioplasty earlier in the day but has no persistent ECG changes and has normal cardiac enzymes. The physicians consider whether to transfer one of these patients out of the CCU to free a bed for Mr. H.

In Case 30.1, the patient with multisystem failure is so sick that he is highly unlikely to survive even if CCU care is continued. The postangioplasty patient is receiving only monitoring, not active treatment, and is highly likely to have a good outcome even if he is transferred out of the unit. In contrast, Mr. H might benefit greatly from thrombolytic and antiarrhythmic therapy, which can be administered only in an ICU. If CCU beds were allocated on a strictly first-come, first-served basis, Mr. H would be denied substantial benefits.

This chapter discusses the ethical considerations that arise when one patient's interests conflict with other patients' interests. In addition, this chapter analyzes whether the scarcity of financial resources justifies limiting the care of an individual patient. Other chapters deal with conflicts of interest between the health care provider and the patient, rather than conflicts of interest between patients.

The terms used to discuss these issues are often used inconsistently and commonly evoke strong emotions (3–5). In this book, *allocation* refers to decisions that set levels of funding for programs rather than determine care for individual patients. For example, funds must be allocated between Medicaid and other social programs, such as education and transportation, and, within Medicaid, between inpatient services and prenatal care. Sometimes these policy-level choices are termed *macroallocation*. In contrast, this book uses the term *rationing* to refer to decisions at the bedside or in the office to limit care for individual patients because of limited resources. The term rationing often connotes limiting beneficial care because it is too expensive. The term *microallocation* is also used in this context. The term rationing excludes clinical decisions that are a straightforward implementation of macroallocation policies, such as health plans' decisions not to cover cosmetic surgery.

BEDSIDE RATIONING

Unlike other countries, such as Great Britain, the United States has not developed coherent societal allocation policies (6, 7). The ethical issue is whether, in the absence of a fair societal agreement on allocation, physicians can ethically carry out rationing at the bedside.

ARGUMENTS AGAINST BEDSIDE RATIONING

Traditionally, bedside rationing by physicians has been considered unethical (8, 9). Its opponents argue that doctors should act as fiduciaries and patient advocates, helping patients receive all the beneficial care that the system allows. One eminent physician wrote, "Physicians are required to do everything that they believe may benefit each patient without regard to costs or other societal considerations. In caring for an individual patient, the doctor must act solely as the patient's advocate, against the apparent interests of society as a whole" (10). This fiduciary role maintains patient trust. In their other roles as citizens and civic leaders, physicians should help determine how resources should be allocated. At the bedside, however, physicians should not limit care to one patient primarily to benefit other patients or to save money for society.

ARGUMENTS IN FAVOR OF BEDSIDE RATIONING

In recent years, as the rise in medical care costs continues to exceed inflation, it has become clear that physicians cannot avoid choices among interventions that vary in cost-effectiveness. An absolute prohibition against bedside rationing, therefore, is ethically problematic (Table 30-1).

Beneficence Is Not An Absolute Duty

An absolutist view of patient advocacy would not serve patients well in the long run because health care would become unaffordable to all but the most wealthy. Although the physician's primary goal is the well-being of patients, an important secondary objective is to control the cost of care to increase access to health care (11). The physician's ethical obligation to act in an individual patient's best interests is not absolute. In several circumstances, physicians are ethically or legally required to act against the patient's best interests to benefit third parties. For example, although maintaining confidentiality of medical information is in a patient's best interest, it is overridden when infectious diseases or threats of physical violence might harm third parties (see Chapter 5). Furthermore, the guideline of beneficence is limited. The physician is not obliged to do literally everything that might benefit the patient. The traditional ethic of advocacy needs to be redefined to "proportional advocacy": the advocate "argues not for 'everything possible' but for everything 'probably beneficial'" (12). Similarly, the American Medical Association declares that "physicians must advocate for any care they believe will materially benefit their patients" (13). Other advocates of the fiduciary role enjoin physicians to practice "parsimonious" or "efficient" medicine, without defining those terms (8, 9). These views acknowledge that if physicians ordered all tests and drugs that provided any benefit, costs would soar. All these views allow some forms of rationing, without calling it such. It is more honest to acknowledge that such limits occur and to consider when it is justified.

Microallocation Without Physicians Harms Patients

If physicians were not involved in microallocation, then clinical decisions would be made according to utilization review guidelines or by health care administrators. Such decisions fail to take

TABLE 30-1	Arguments in Favor of Bedside Rationing
Acting in the patient's best interests is not an absolute duty.	
Leaving physicians out of microallocation decisions will harm patients.	
Other patients might be seriously harmed if resources are not rationed.	

into account meaningful differences in individual patient circumstances that are too complex to be captured in simple guidelines or rules (14, 15). Physicians can often bring to bear pertinent clinical information to justify an exception to a general rule (16, 17).

Other Patients Might Be Seriously Harmed

Providing care to one patient might deny care to another patient who would receive much greater medical benefit from limited resources, including physician time. In these situations, informal rationing is the standard medical practice that has strong ethical justification.

CASE 30.2	Limited physician time

Mr. M, a 48-year-old man, comes to the physician's office after 40 minutes of crushing substernal chest pain and shortness of breath. At the same time, a 21-year-old woman with asthma comes to the office with worsening shortness of breath for the past day, despite increasing use of inhaled bronchodilators. These patients do not have appointments, and the physician's schedule is already full.

Because their time is limited, physicians must decide which patients deserve higher priority. In a life-threatening situation such as a probable myocardial infarction in Case 30.2, an emergency case in which delay of care might cause grave harm, takes priority over other cases. Mr. M needs to be stabilized and transported to the emergency department. Regularly scheduled patients presumably would agree to wait because they would want similar priority if they should find themselves in a serious emergency. However, how is an emergency defined? If care is promptly instituted for the woman with a severe asthma attack, then her symptoms will be relieved more rapidly and hospitalization might be avoided; however, it is a value judgment how much benefit or potential harm to the asthma patient justifies asking regularly scheduled patients to wait. Referring the asthma patient to the emergency department only pushes the dilemma back a step, since patients presenting for care there are routinely triaged.

Patients and society expect physicians to allocate their time. It is difficult to imagine that anyone other than a physician or nurse would decide who should wait. General rules can be set—for example, patients with serious emergencies should take priority and patients with minor or self-limited illnesses should wait. Physicians, however, need to interpret those general rules in a particular case—for example, deciding whether a patient's asthma attack warrants asking other patients to wait.

In Case 30.1, essential medical resources—CCU beds—are in short supply. In clinical practice, physicians frequently transfer patients to allow others to receive intensive care. When the CCU or ICU is full, physicians identify patients who are too sick to benefit from continued intensive care and set more restrictive standards for admission to the unit. Increasing the supply of CCU beds will not resolve the problem of rationing but only postpone the dilemma of the last bed. Transferring patients to other hospitals with open CCU beds is also not a solution because Mr. H needs immediate treatment.

In Case 30.1, an identified patient would be seriously harmed if care were not rationed. In the following case, a future patient will predictably be harmed unless care is rationed.

CASE 30.3	Shortage of blood products

A 36-year-old man with alcoholic cirrhosis is admitted for severe variceal bleeding and encephalopathy. He is not a candidate for liver transplantation because of active alcohol and amphetamine use. The surgeons do not believe he will survive a portacaval shunt operation. After 3 days, he has consumed 42 units of blood and continues to bleed briskly despite endoscopic sclerotherapy and percutaneous placement of a therapeutic portal-systemic shunt (TIPS). The regional blood bank has only three more units of his type despite appeals for donations. It is New Year's Eve, when automobile accident victims will need transfusions.

In Case 30.3, there is no identified individual who will be harmed if blood products are not rationed, but the existence of such an individual is virtually certain. Many persons with trauma can recover completely with vigorous emergency care. Thus, a future patient is likely to be seriously harmed if all available blood were given to the patient in Case 30.3, who has not improved despite maximal care.

Physicians might be reluctant to ration interventions to patients who are already receiving care because of loyalty or fidelity—that is, doctors might believe that they have implicitly promised to provide ongoing care and not to curtail it to benefit other patients. The position's emotional appeal is clear, and keeping promises is an important ethical guideline. However, maintaining fidelity should refer to appropriate ongoing care, not to unlimited care regardless of the benefits to the patient or the harms to others.

Although limitations on transfusions are justified in Case 30.3, there are problems in implementing such limits in a fair manner. Various physicians might set different limits in practice. Some physicians might stop after 40 units, others after 60 units. More specific practice standards would make such decisions more consistent and, therefore, fairer.

RATIONING ON THE BASIS OF COST

In some situations, compelling ethical arguments exist for limiting care to one patient to provide much more beneficial clinical services to other patients. When rationing is done primarily to save money rather than to benefit other patients directly, however, the reasons are generally weaker. The following case illustrates these issues.

CASE 30.4   Expensive care for a patient with poor prognosis and quality of life

Mrs. D is a 76-year-old nursing home resident with severe dementia. She recognizes her family only occasionally and does not respond to health care workers' questions or requests. She develops chronic renal failure and symptoms of uremia. While competent, she had never expressed her preferences about renal dialysis. Although her primary physician and nephrologist recommend that renal dialysis not be performed, her family insists on it. They believe that as long as she recognizes them and smiles, her life should be prolonged. They understand that dialysis likely cause a sharp decline in her functioning and that most patients like her do not survive a year after initiating dialysis (18).

At the time, the public hospital is considering closing obstetrical and substance abuse services because of budget deficits. The physicians feel they are accomplices to an unjust health care system if they use resources on this patient when more pressing health needs are unmet. A vascular surgery consultant writes in the medical record, "In the current climate of out-of-control medical costs, it is unconscionable to provide expensive care for this patient."

As discussed in Chapter 14, it would be appropriate to provide renal dialysis to Mrs. D because it would achieve the family's goal of prolonging her life at a quality they consider acceptable. The physicians, however, believe that Mrs. D's quality of life is so poor that the cost of dialysis is not justified.

OBJECTIONS TO BEDSIDE RATIONING ON THE BASIS OF COSTS

Physicians should support more enlightened policies regarding allocation, but in most circumstances attempts by physicians to ration care on the basis of costs at the level of the individual patient, although well intentioned, are not justified.

No Public Policy Authorizes Physicians to Ration on the Basis of Costs

Although the physicians caring for Mrs. D felt partly responsible for the soaring cost of health care, no public policy authorizes physicians to limit the care of patients on renal dialysis to save resources for other patients. On the contrary, U.S. public policy pays for dialysis to all patients with end-stage renal failure. In the 1960s, selecting patients for a limited number of renal dialysis machines on the basis of prognosis or quality of life proved so controversial that Congress singled out end-stage renal disease for universal coverage under the Medicare program.

Bedside Rationing Based on Costs Would Be Unfair

It would be inconsistent and, therefore, unfair if one physician or hospital withheld dialysis from Mrs. D, but another might provide it. Indeed, the public nursing home in the area provided chronic dialysis to numerous patients with severe Alzheimer disease. It violates the ethical guideline of justice to treat similar patients unequally. Whether or not Mrs. D receives dialysis should not be based on the choice of physician or hospital.

Bedside rationing might also be unfair if only certain patients or certain interventions are singled out for review. It makes little sense to limit one health care intervention as not cost-effective without looking at the cost-effectiveness of other interventions as well. Many people would object to limiting dialysis for Mrs. D if other interventions, such as intensive care for patients with extremely poor prognoses, were not similarly scrutinized.

Money Saved by Rationing Cannot Be Reallocated

Physicians in the United States who save money on the care of an individual patient generally cannot redirect those resources to patients or projects with higher priority (19). If physicians withheld dialysis from Mrs. D, they could not redirect funds to more pressing medical or social needs, such as prenatal care or childhood immunizations. Furthermore, in managed care organizations savings from limiting care to patients might be directed toward higher salaries for administrators or greater profits for investors rather than to more cost-effective interventions. In the absence of broader health care reform, attempts to limit health care costs at the bedside are ineffective gestures.

Limiting care for one patient to make resources available to other patients is more strongly justified if several conditions are met (20). First, saved resources would be reallocated to interventions that provide greater benefits for the population of patients receiving care. Second, the physicians would not benefit directly from saving resources. Third, the limitations in care are applied to all similar patients with no exceptions based on privileged social status.

Opponents of bedside rationing would argue that physicians in Case 30.4 fulfilled their ethical obligations to use limited resources prudently by discussing with Mrs. D's family her limited life expectancy on dialysis and making a strong recommendation against it.

TIERED FORMULARY BENEFITS

It is ethically acceptable for physicians to limit services to one patient to conserve a pool of money for services to a population of patients. Formulary restrictions are one common example. Because drug expenditures are the fastest growing of all health care costs, most insurance plans have established restricted formularies and tiered copayments. For example, patients might have a US$20 copayment for preferred drugs on the formulary, a US$30 copayment for nonpreferred formulary drugs, and a still higher copayment for nonformulary drugs. Preferred drugs are usually cheaper than other drugs in the same class because a discount from the manufacturer has been negotiated.

There might be no meaningful clinical differences among drugs in a class but significant differences in cost—for example, different angiotensin-converting enzyme inhibitors for congestive heart failure. It is ethical for the physician to start with the presumption that preferred formulary drugs are appropriate. Hence, the physician can recommend that the patient try a preferred drug. The risk to the patient is small, provided there is close follow-up care.

TABLE 30-2	Suggestions for Physicians Considering Bedside Rationing

Try to get more resources for the patient within the system.

Make decisions openly.

Get a second opinion.

Notify patients or surrogates when care is rationed.

This presumption in favor of a preferred drug may be overridden if a patient later develops unacceptable side effects or has an unsatisfactory clinical outcome. Furthermore, a patient might have poor adherence to a formulary drug that requires more than one dose a day. Physicians need to judge whether it is warranted to use a nonformulary drug to provide a clinically meaningful benefit to an individual patient (11).

The physician should provide guidance to patients as to whether a nonpreferred drug is worth the higher out-of-pocket cost. In addition, physicians also need to help patients when their drug coverage does not allow them access to all the prescriptions they need at an affordable cost.

SUGGESTIONS FOR PHYSICIANS

Physicians who are considering rationing life-sustaining interventions at the bedside should take several actions (Table 30-2).

TRY TO GET MORE RESOURCES FOR THE PATIENT WITHIN THE SYSTEM

Physicians should try to obtain more resources within the system. For example, in Case 30.1, beds in the postoperative recovery room might be used as temporary ICU beds. Such efforts, however, might lead to other problems, such as disrupting operating room schedules.

MAKE DECISIONS OPENLY

Discussing rationing dilemmas explicitly can identify unquestioned assumptions and hidden value judgments. When people must make their arguments and values explicit, others can present rebuttals or disagreements or suggest ways to resolve the problem.

GET A SECOND OPINION

Eliciting a second opinion from another attending physician or from a hospital ethics committee or consultant might improve decision making. For example, such a review might suggest other options or point out unwarranted value judgments.

NOTIFY PATIENTS OR SURROGATES WHEN CARE IS RATIONED

Patients or their surrogates should be notified when beneficial care is rationed. It is disrespectful to transfer patients out of intensive care or stop transfusions without explaining to them or their families what is happening. If possible, it is preferable to make such explanations before a clinical crisis occurs.

SUMMARY

1. Bedside rationing may be ethically appropriate if restricting services that provide only limited benefit to one patient would allow another patient to receive much greater medical benefits.
2. Decisions to ration to save money are problematic, if funds cannot be redirected to patients or projects with higher priority.
3. Physicians facing bedside rationing decisions should take steps to help ensure that these decisions are consistent and fair.

REFERENCES

1. Thurow LC. Learning to say "no". *N Engl J Med*. 1984;311:1569–1572.
2. Fuchs VR. The "rationing" of medical care. *N Engl J Med*. 1984;311:1572–1573.
3. Eddy DM. Clinical decision making: from theory to practice. Rationing by patient choice. *JAMA*. 1991;265:105–108.
4. Asch DA, Ubel PA. Rationing by any other name. *N Engl J Med*. 1997;336:1668–1671.
5. Ubel PA, Goold S. Recognizing bedside rationing: clear cases and tough calls. *Ann Intern Med*. 1997;126:74–80.
6. Schwartz WB. The inevitable failure of current cost-containment strategies. Why they can provide only temporary relief. *JAMA*. 1987;257:220–224.
7. Boren SD. I had a tough day today, Hillary. *N Engl J Med*. 1994;330:500–502.
8. Pellegrino ED, Thomasma DG. *For the Patient's Good: The Restoration of Beneficence in Health Care*. New York, NY: Oxford University Press; 1988.
9. Kassirer JP. Managing care—should we adopt a new ethic? *N Engl J Med*. 1998;339:397–398.
10. Levinsky NG. The doctor's master. *N Engl J Med*. 1984;311:1573–1575.
11. Brennan TA, Lee TH. Allergic to generics. *Ann Intern Med*. 2004;141:126–130.
12. Jonsen AR. *The New Medicine and the Old Ethics*. Cambridge, MA: Harvard University Press; 1990:59.
13. Council on Ethical and Judicial Affairs. *Code of Medical Ethics: Current Opinions with Annotations*. Chicago, IL: American Medical Association; 1998:143.
14. Hall MA, Berenson RA. Ethical practice in managed care: a dose of realism. *Ann Intern Med*. 1998;128:395–402.
15. Hillman AL. Managing the physician: rules versus incentives. *Health Aff (Millwood)*. 1991;10:138–146.
16. Kmetik KS, O'Toole MF, Bossley H, et al. Exceptions to outpatient quality measures for coronary artery disease in electronic health records. *Ann Intern Med*. 2011;154:227–234.
17. Ellrodt AG, Conner L, Riedinger M, et al. Measuring and improving physician compliance with clinical practice guidelines. *Ann Intern Mec*. 1995;122:277–282.
18. Kurella Tamura M, Covinsky KE, Chertow GM, et al. Functional status of elderly adults before and after initiation of dialysis. *N Engl J Med*. 2009;361:1539–1547.
19. Daniels N. Why saying no to patients in the United States is so hard. *N Engl J Med*. 1986;314:1380–1383.
20. Pearson SD. Caring and cost: the challenge for physician advocacy. *Ann Intern Med*. 2000;133:148–153.

ANNOTATED BIBLIOGRAPHY

1. Daniels N. Why saying no to patients in the United States is so hard. *N Engl J Med*. 1986;314:1380–1383.
   Points out that in the US system there is no way to direct money saved on one patient to more cost-effective purposes.
2. Boren SD. I had a tough day today, Hillary. *N Engl J Med*. 1994;330:500–502.
   This is a first-person account by a medical director of a managed care plan, describing the types of expensive interventions that insurers are asked to cover.
3. Asch DA, Ubel PA. Rationing by any other name. *N Engl J Med*. 1997;336:1668–1671.
   Clarifies the range of situations in which physicians may limit beneficial services because they are too costly.
4. Pearson SD. Caring and cost: the challenge for physician advocacy. *Ann Intern Med*. 2000;133:148–153.
   Suggests criteria for ethically appropriate bedside rationing.
5. Brennan TA, Lee TH. Allergic to generics. *Ann Intern Med*. 2004;141:126–130.
   Analyzes how physicians should balance their obligations to individual patients with a just allocation program that serves a population of patients.

31

Incentives for Physicians to Increase Services

U nder fee-for-service reimbursement, physicians and health care institutions can increase their revenue by providing more services—for example, seeing more patients, seeing them more frequently, or performing more interventions.

PROBLEMS WITH FEE-FOR-SERVICE REIMBURSEMENT

Fee-for-service reimbursement offers incentives to increase all services, not just those that are effective. Patients who receive interventions that are unnecessary or only marginally beneficial are exposed to unwarranted risks. In two recent examples, physicians, many of whom believed their reimbursement was unfairly low, adjusted their practice to increase their revenue, even though many patients may have received harm rather than benefit.

Medicare reimbursed oncologists for intravenous chemotherapy drugs at much higher levels than the cost at which doctors could purchase them. Many oncologists, however, believed that this reimbursement did not cover office for administering the drugs. Medicare reduced reimbursement for specific drugs that offered high profit margins but did not offer patients clear clinical advantages over other drugs. Oncologists responded by switching from drugs that experienced the largest cuts in reimbursement to other high-margin drugs (1). Moreover, some doctors switched from oral to intravenous chemotherapy despite inconvenience to patients.

Fee-for-service incentives also greatly influenced the care of renal dialysis patients. Basic payments for dialysis have not kept pace with inflation. Providers reimbursed separately for injectable drugs, such as erythropoietin-stimulating agents and vitamin D, and use of these drugs soared (2) despite lack of evidence that they are effective. In fact, randomized clinical trials found no benefit to higher target levels of hemoglobin and higher doses of erythropoietin-stimulating agents and probable harm from increased overall mortality and cardiovascular events (3). Medicare now includes injectable drugs in a bundled payment rate. With this reversal of financial incentives, the use of these injectable drugs is expected to sharply decrease (4).

Fee-for-service reimbursement schedules also encourage physicians to carry out invasive procedures rather than talk with patients about decisions or counsel them about preventive care (5). For example, Medicare reimburses a cardiologist a professional fee of $445 for inserting a temporary pacemaker, a procedure that takes about 30 minutes. In contrast, Medicare reimbursement for a 1-hour family meeting about withdrawing life-sustaining procedures is $100.

SELF-REFERRAL BY PHYSICIANS

Physician self-referral can occur in several ways. Many physicians carry out clinical laboratory testing, electrocardiograms, and chest x-rays in their own offices. Also many doctors invest in freestanding imaging centers or ambulatory surgery centers, to which they refer patients (6). Other physicians purchase time at an imaging facility at discounted rates and bill insurers at a higher rate (6). A substantial percentage of providers who bill for magnetic resonance imaging (MRI), computed tomography (CT), and positron emission tomography (PET) scans use these arrangements (7). Such self-referral raises ethical concerns about overuse of services and conflicts of interest.

Physicians who self-refer order significantly more imaging studies and generate higher radiology costs and total costs than other physicians (8, 9). After physicians acquire a financial interest in MRI scanners, they order significantly more scans (10). It is believed that many of these additional studies are not warranted. In general, greater use of medical services is not associated with better patient outcomes (11). The percentage of inappropriate MRI studies is greater when self-referring physicians order studies (12). Similarly, surgeons who own specialty hospitals are significantly more likely to operate on patients than nonowners, including procedures that have been shown to have no clinical benefit (13).

JUSTIFICATION FOR SELF-REFERRAL

One rationale for self-referral is convenience for patients. Obtaining tests at or near the physician's office reduces the time required for care and improves continuity of care. Often, however, imaging facilities are not adjacent to the physician's office. Proponents also argue that such physician investment increases access to state-of-the-art technology that would not be available otherwise (14). The evidence does not support these claims. For example, none of the physician-owned radiation therapy centers in Florida were located in rural areas or inner cities (7). Physicians who invest in ambulatory surgical centers tend to refer insured patients to them, while referring Medicaid patients to university clinics (15).

Advocates argue that if physicians take financial risks when investing in freestanding facilities, they should share in any profits. Physicians might be more willing than other investors to take such risks because they better appreciate the promise of new technologies (12, 14). Current self-referral billing, however, involves little financial risk for physicians.

PROBLEMS WITH SELF-REFERRAL

A conflict of interest occurs when physicians recommend services from which they profit financially. As noted, self-referral leads to increased costs of care and may increase inappropriate interventions. The American Medical Association (AMA) states that self-referral might "undermine the commitment of physicians to professionalism" (14). Payment to physicians for referring a patient is considered fee-splitting or a kickback, which is unethical because those physicians are not being compensated for providing or supervising medical services, but only for referring patients to another provider. Even the appearance that physicians are trying to increase profits might erode patient trust. According to the AMA, "There are some activities regarding their patients that physicians should avoid whether or not there is evidence of abuse" (14). Financial reward for physicians is traditionally regarded as a consequence of serving patients, not as a goal to be pursued for its own sake.

PROHIBITIONS ON JOINT VENTURES

It is illegal for physicians to refer Medicare or Medicaid patients for ancillary services, such as for radiology and laboratory tests, to facilities in which they have a financial interest. Exceptions are permitted for in-office ancillary services, group practices, rural areas, and services personally performed or supervised by another physician in the same group practice (16). Many states have similar prohibitions for private insurance.

Disclosure of physician ownership of outside facilities is ethically desirable, as with any conflict of interest. Disclosure, however, does not decrease referrals by physician-investors to outside facilities in which they have a financial interest (17). Patients who know that the physician has a financial incentive to increase referrals cannot judge whether recommendations for testing or treatment are sound. In addition, patients might be afraid of offending physicians if they do not go to the facility in question.

IN-OFFICE SERVICES

Ordering tests or treatments carried out by the physician or in the physician's office is distinguished from referral to outside facilities in which the physician has a financial interest (14). Procedures such as endoscopy, bronchoscopy, coronary angiography and angioplasty, and surgery are an integral part of specialist care. It would make little sense for one surgeon to evaluate the patient and then refer the patient to another surgeon for the actual procedure. Also, payment for services that physicians or their staff carry out is distinguished from kickbacks physicians receive for simply referring the patient for a service.

Although there are no legal prohibitions on physicians' referring patients to ancillary services in their office or clinic, there are ethical concerns about overutilization of services and poor quality of care. With regard to radiology studies performed in physicians' offices, deficiencies in the quality of equipment, images, and interpretations have led to certification standards for training physicians and staff, quality control, equipment, technical procedures, and interpretation of images (8). Similarly, clinical laboratories in physicians' offices must meet federal standards for certification. Moreover, physicians have an ethical obligation to set up equipment and services in their offices only if there is a demonstrated need and if they have training and experience to carry out or supervise the services.

NONFINANCIAL INCENTIVES TO PROVIDE MORE SERVICES

Social and psychological factors reinforce the financial incentives in fee-for-service medicine to provide more services. First, in the United States, both the public and physicians regard high-technology procedures, such as MRI scans, as the epitome of excellent medical care. The prestige that hospitals and physicians gain by providing these services encourages their wider use. Second, physicians commonly respond to the uncertainty inherent in clinical medicine by performing an additional test. The malpractice system encourages "defensive medicine," the ordering of interventions of small marginal benefit to patients to prevent potential lawsuits. Finally, faced with an individual patient, physicians might recommend interventions that they would not recommend as a general clinical guideline (18).

SUMMARY

1. Fee-for-service reimbursement encourages physicians to provide more services and, in some instances, to overuse services.
2. Both health care organizations and individual physicians need to ensure that clinical decisions are based on patients' best interests, not on their own self-interest.

REFERENCES

1. Jacobson M, Earle CC, Price M, et al. How medicare's payment cuts for cancer chemotherapy drugs changed patterns of treatment. *Health Aff (Millwood)*. 2010;29:1391–1399.
2. Winkelmayer WC, Chertow GM. The 2011 ESRD prospective payment system: an uncontrolled experiment. *Am J Kidney Dis*. 2011;57:542–546.
3. Palmer SC, Navaneethan SD, Craig JC, et al. Meta-analysis: erythropoiesis-stimulating agents in patients with chronic kidney disease. *Ann Intern Med*. 2010;153:23–33.
4. Wish JB. Anemia management under a bundled payment policy for dialysis: a preview for the United States from Japan. *Kidney Int*. 2011;79:265–267.
5. Hsiao WC, Dunn DL, Verrilli DK. Assessing the implementation of physician-payment reform. *N Engl J Med*. 1993;328:928–933.
6. Hillman BJ, Goldsmith J. Imaging: the self-referral boom and the ongoing search for effective policies to contain it. *Health Aff (Millwood)*. 2010;29:2231–2236.
7. Mitchell JM. The prevalence of physician self-referral arrangements after Stark II: evidence from advanced diagnostic imaging. *Health Aff (Millwood)*. 2007;26:w415–w424.

8. Hughes DR, Sunshine JH, Bhargavan M, et al. Physician self-referral for imaging and the cost of chronic care for Medicare beneficiaries. *Med Care.* 2011;49:857–864.

9. MedPAC. June 2010 Report to Congress. Available at: www.medpac.gov/chapters/Jun10_Ch08.pdf. Accessed September 11, 2012.

10. Baker LC. Acquisition of MRI equipment by doctors drives up imaging use and spending. *Health Aff (Millwood).* 2010;29:2252–2259.

11. Wennberg JE, Fisher ES, Skinner JS. Geography and the debate over Medicare reform. *Health Aff (Millwood).* 2002;(Suppl Web Exclusives):W96–W114.

12. Kouri BE, Parsons RG, Altert HR. Physician self-referral for diagnostic imaging: review of the empiric literature. *AJR.* 2002;179:843–850.

13. Mitchell JM. Effect of physician ownership of specialty hospitals and ambulatory surgery centers on frequency of use of outpatient orthopedic surgery. *Arch Surg.* 2010;145:732–738.

14. Council on Ethical and Judicial Affairs AMA. Conflicts of interest: physician ownership of medical facilities. *JAMA.* 1992;267:2366–2369.

15. Gabel JR, Fahlman C, Kang R, et al. Where do I send thee? Does physician-ownership affect referral patterns to ambulatory surgery centers? *Health Aff (Millwood).* 2008;27:w165–w174.

16. MedPAC. June 2010 Report to Congress. http://www.medpac.gov/chapters/Jun10_Ch08.pdf. Accessed November 19, 2011.

17. Office of the Inspector General. *Financial Arrangements Between Physicians and Health Care Businesses.* Washington, DC: Office of the Inspector General, U.S. Dept. of Health and Human Services; 1989.

18. Redelmeier DA, Tversky A. Discrepancy between medical decisions for individuals patients and for groups. *N Engl J Med.* 1990;322:1162–1164.

ANNOTATED BIBLIOGRAPHY

1. Hillman BJ, Goldsmith J. Imaging: the self-referral boom and the ongoing search for effective policies to contain it. *Health Aff (Millwood).* 2010;29:2231–2236.
Recent review of policy options regarding physician self-referral.

Measures to Control Health Care Costs

T he United States is expected to spend over $13,700 per capita on health care in 2020 (1). Total expenditures will be $4.6 trillion dollars, almost 20% of the gross domestic product. The cost of health care is rising faster than the gross domestic product, general inflation, and wages. The cost of employer-based health insurance hinders the country's economic competitiveness. Despite high expenditures, however, the United States continues to have worse infant mortality and life expectancy than many countries that have much lower per capita health care expenditures and also provide universal health insurance. In addition, the United States has approximately 50 million uninsured persons. Lack of health insurance is associated with serious risks, including delaying or foregoing effective treatments, worse health outcomes, and premature death (2). Gaining health insurance ameliorates many of these problems. Thus, the United States faces several challenging goals to improve health care: In addition to restraining the cost of health care, the country also needs to improve the quality of care and increase access to health care. The 2010 Patient Protection and Affordable Care Act attempted to address some of these challenges. As the United States expands health insurance coverage, total national spending on health care will increase further. Even if inefficiency and waste could be eliminated, health care costs will continue to rise because of new medical technologies and an aging population (3, 4).

Although the goal of restraining health care costs is appropriate, the means used might raise ethical concerns. The ethical guideline of justice requires physicians to be prudent in using limited health care resources and to allocate resources among patients fairly. This ethical obligation, however, might conflict with the ethical obligation to act in the individual patient's best interests. Patients might not want to forego care that potentially offers even small benefits in order to control costs (5, 6). In the 1990s, managed care provoked a public backlash because it created conflicts of interest for physicians and undermined their traditional fiduciary role (7). Physicians and policy makers need to learn from previous attempts to restrain costs.

This chapter analyzes how the self-interest of physicians and health care organizations conflicts with the patient's best interests. Chapter 30 analyzes the related issue of conflicts of interest between different patients.

CASE 32.1	Request for imaging study

Mr. H, a 43-year-old man, developed lower back pain radiating down the back of his right leg 2 days ago. This occurred after some unusually heavy gardening work. There is no history of trauma. He had a similar episode many years ago associated with a sports injury. On examination, he has decreased flexion, some paraspinous spasm, no bone tenderness, and a normal neurologic examination. His job requires him to sit for long meetings, which is uncomfortable for him. He requests a magnetic resonance imaging (MRI) scan to be sure that he does not have a bone tumor.

FINANCIAL INCENTIVES TO PHYSICIANS

TYPES OF INCENTIVES

As discussed in Chapter 31, fee-for-service reimbursement provides incentives to provide more services, thereby increasing the total cost of health care. Several alternatives to fee-for-service reimbursement have been proposed. Paying physicians predominantly by a *salary* has been adopted by several large-group organizations but is not feasible in other clinical arrangements.

Bundled payments encourage collaboration among physicians and health care institutions, which can improve patient outcomes. Examples include combining reimbursement for inpatient care with follow-up outpatient care and paying for an episode of care, such as for a heart attack, coronary bypass, or hip replacement. The bundled payment would include not just surgery but also rehabilitation, post-op care, and treatment of complications.

Global payments for management of patients with chronic conditions encourage continuity of care and coordination among providers, including specialists, nurses, pharmacists, dieticians, and physical therapists. Some proposals make physicians accountable for a population of patients, so they have incentives to provide preventive care and to coordinate care for complex, high-cost patients.

Learning from the mistakes of managed care, Medicare and Medicaid policy makers are phasing in changes from fee-for-service, at first making them voluntary and offering physicians the opportunity to earn bonuses, without putting them at risk for loss of income.

Finally, payment is partly based on *quality incentives* (so-called pay for performance). Common incentives reward adherence to evidence-based practice guidelines, such as cancer screening, inhaled corticosteroids in asthma, and statins for hypercholesterolemia, reduction of hospital-acquired infections, use of electronic health records (see Chapter 45), and patient satisfaction.

CHALLENGES REGARDING PHYSICIAN INCENTIVES

Withholding Beneficial Care

Ideally, incentives to control costs would lead physicians to eliminate only expensive services that offer little or no marginal benefit to patients. During the managed care era, strong incentives to control costs were believed to also restrict medically appropriate care. Incentives for quality of care, such as adherence to evidence-based practice guidelines, are intended to alleviate these concerns. In some cases, an exception to a clinical guidelines or utilization determination is justified (8, 9). The treating physician is in a unique position to identify and justify exceptions. Health care organizations and payers should allow legitimate exceptions and institute appeals procedures that are not unduly burdensome for physicians and patients.

Fairness to Physicians

Under bundled payment, global payment, or any prospective payment system, physicians who care for complicated, sicker patients are at a financial disadvantage. Adjustment for case mix and severity of illness is possible, but can be administratively complex, controversial, and fail to capture relevant parameters. Physicians and hospitals may avoid sicker and more complicated patients. If this occurs, more complicated patients may have difficulty accessing health care.

Undermining the Physician's Fiduciary Role

Incentives to reduce costs might lead patients to question whether physicians are acting in their best interests and reduce patient trust in physicians (10, 11). In the managed care era, the strongest objections were to "gag rules" that forbade physicians from disclosing options the insurance plan did not cover and to very steep financial incentives that put a substantial percentage of the physician's income at risk. Furthermore, an emphasis on cost containment and efficiency may lead physicians to become entrepreneurs focused on profits instead of healers focused on patient well-being (12).

Practical Concerns

There are numerous practical concerns about incentives to reduce costs. Will they be effective at achieving this goal? Because many different insurers pay physicians, even major changes in Medicare reimbursement may not change their behavior. What will be the costs of setting up new clinical care arrangements, administration, and compliance? What will be the unintended adverse effects of changes in payment? Will patient "skimming" lead to worse access for complex patients?

FINANCIAL INCENTIVES TO PATIENTS

To control costs, many insurers are offering patients incentives for cost-effective care.

PATIENT COST SHARING WHEN CHOOSING HEALTH PLANS

Increasingly, employers who provide health insurance are requiring employees to pay a portion of the monthly premiums. Typically employers contribute a fixed amount, so employees who want a more expensive plan have to pay an additional amount. The least expensive plans are health maintenance organizations (HMOs), which contract with physician groups to provide comprehensive medical care in return for capitated payments, a fixed amount per patient regardless of the actual costs of care. Patients in HMOs select a primary physician or physician group and must obtain covered services through them. Employees who want a greater choice of physicians can select other types of plans, which require them to make greater monthly contributions to premiums. In preferred provider organizations (PPOs), "preferred" physicians and hospitals accept discounted fee-for-service reimbursement rates and administrative controls in exchange for a flow of patients. PPO patients can also visit nonpreferred providers, but with higher copayments. Point of service (POS) plans allow still greater choice of physicians or hospitals for even higher premiums and copayments. When choosing a health care plan and paying health insurance premiums, patients usually want to control costs; however, when patients are sick and need medical care, they generally want interventions that might benefit them, even if they are expensive and the benefits are small.

PATIENT COST SHARING AT THE POINT OF CLINICAL SERVICES

Many insurers are increasing the copayments and deductibles, giving patients incentives to reduce use of health care services (13). With high copayments and deductibles, however, patients forego highly beneficial care as well as less effective care. Many forego highly beneficial services such as vaccination and screening tests, particularly low-income families (14). For drug benefits, tiered copayments might be $10 a month for generic drugs, $20 a month for preferred drugs on the plan's formulary, and $35 a month for nonpreferred drugs. Increased cost sharing is associated with lower adherence, more discontinuation of therapy, and greater use of emergency and inpatient services, even for drugs that improve patient outcomes (13, 15–17). It is possible to design benefits plans to eliminate copayments for evidence-based screening and prevention services, but complex plan designs may cause confusion. A randomized trial of providing heart attack patients free drugs for secondary prevention reduced subsequent vascular events, without increasing total health care costs (18).

Many patients want to discuss with physicians the value of drugs and tests relative to their out-of-pocket expenses (14, 19, 20).

INCENTIVES FOR HEALTH PROMOTION

Persons with unhealthy lifestyles, such as obesity and smoking have higher costs for health care. Many employers are offering employees financial incentives to exercise, stop smoking, and lose weight. Many people want to adopt these behaviors, but find it difficult to carry out their intentions. Several ethical issues need to be considered (21, 22).

First, it is unfair to hold people responsible for behaviors they cannot change. Heavy smokers are addicted to nicotine. People may be unable to exercise because they live in an unsafe neighborhood or may not be able to lose weight because they lack access to grocery stores that sell healthy foods. People from lower SES levels, who are already worse off, are more likely to face such challenges. Others may not be able to exercise because of arthritis, back pain, and heart disease. It may be unfair if some people have great difficulty gaining the incentive, even if they try hard. Moreover, it may be unfair to reward people for doing what others have already done on their own without rewards.

Second, some employees have concerns about privacy, undue influence by employers, and employment discrimination.

Third, the design of incentives involves tradeoffs between effectiveness, acceptability, and fairness. Should wellness programs incentivize results or attempts? The former will be more effective but may be less acceptable to employees. Should incentives be penalties or rewards? Again, the former will be more effective but less acceptable. Finally, should employers simply offer financial incentives or also take steps to facilitate the desired behavioral changes? Companies could provide walking paths, healthier food in cafeteria, and exercise classes on site, which may facilitate employees meeting targets, but may not be cost-effective.

RESPONSES BY PHYSICIANS TO INCENTIVES

When an effective test or treatment is not covered by the insurance plan, the physician must decide whether to disclose the intervention, recommend it, and help the patient obtain it (23) (*see* Table 32-1).

DISCLOSE ECONOMIC INCENTIVES TO PATIENTS

Most members of the public want to be told about physician financial incentives to reduce health care costs (24, 25). Federal Medicare and Medicaid regulations require such disclosure, as do some state laws (26). Disclosure might benefit patients in several ways. It might help patients choose a physician, physician group, or insurance plan. Moreover, it might help patients put physicians' recommendations into context, although patients are not in a good position to understand and use such information when they seek care. Disclosure might also deter insurers from setting up problematic financial arrangements that would be difficult to defend in public. Such disclosure need not reduce patient trust in physicians (27).

DISCLOSE AND RECOMMEND OPTIONS TO PATIENTS

The ethical guidelines of autonomy and beneficence require physicians to discuss alternatives that have a significantly favorable balance of benefit to risk, even if it is unlikely to be covered by the plan. The term *benefit* needs to be interpreted broadly to include psychosocial variables, such as convenience in taking medications and reassurance about not missing a serious diagnosis. Patients who are not informed of alternatives outside the insurance plan cannot be tried to be convinced about the plan to pay for care outside the system, pay out-of-pocket, or change insurance plans.

Physicians might be legally liable if, against their medical judgment, they withhold beneficial care at the insurer's behest. In a case involving premature hospital discharge, the court declared, "the physician who complies without protest with the limitations imposed by a third-party payer, when

TABLE 32-1   Responses by Physicians to Incentives to Decrease Services
Disclose financial incentives to patients.
Disclose and recommend options to patients.
Act as patient advocate.
Avoid deception.

his medical judgment dictates otherwise, cannot avoid his ultimate responsibility for his patient's care" (28).

It is ethical for physicians to take into account the cost of care when several approaches have similar outcomes for patients. When the ethical guideline of beneficence provides no strong reason to recommend one option over another, the guideline of justice might then be decisive. The prudent use of limited health care resources may be an acceptable reason to choose between options with similar risk/benefit characteristics. Physicians and patients need to acknowledge that such decisions are a form of bedside rationing that may be ethically appropriate (*see* Chapter 30). Physicians should be willing to discuss these issues openly and honestly with patients (29).

ACT AS PATIENT ADVOCATE

The guideline of beneficence urges physicians to act in the patient's best interests and serve as advocates to intercede for or speak on the patient's behalf (23). Advocacy should be based on sound clinical judgment and evidence. It is not doing whatever the patient requests. Advocating for a patient is fair only if it would also be appropriate for other physicians to advocate for their patients in similar situations, as in Case 32.1. Physicians need to make reasonable efforts to help patients obtain authorizations or make appeals to obtain care, which often requires filling out forms and making phone calls.

AVOID DECEPTION

Physicians sometimes use deception to obtain insurance coverage for a patient. In one survey, 39% of physicians reported that during the past year they had exaggerated the severity of a patient's condition, changed a patient's billing diagnosis, or reported signs and symptoms the patient did not have to help the patient get needed care (30). Such deception is more common when physicians believe that it is unfair for the plan not to cover the intervention, when they believe that the insurer's appeals process was unwieldy, and when the patient's condition is more serious (31, 32). Avoiding deception, however, is a basic ethical guideline that limits obligations to serve as patient advocates (33). Lying and deception undermine social trust because people cannot trust that other statements by physicians are truthful. Chapter 6 argues in detail that deception of insurers is not justified, except perhaps as a last resort after appeals have failed.

CASE 32.1   *Continued*

Fee-for-service reimbursement provides incentives to order imaging studies. It is very unlikely, however, in the absence of progressive neurologic signs or symptoms that Mr. H has a serious etiology for back pain. Chances are excellent that he will recover. Imaging studies have a low yield but many false positives because abnormalities are common in asymptomatic individuals. CT scans involve considerable radiation. Although an MRI scan does not involve radiation, imaging studies do not change management or improve outcomes.

Evidence-based guidelines do not recommend an MRI in this situation, even under fee-for-service reimbursement. The mere possibility that the symptoms might be caused by a serious lesion does not justify scanning or referral at this time. Anecdotal reports of patients who had a tumor discovered on an MRI for back pain should be regarded simply as anecdotes, not as persuasive evidence that the procedure is medically indicated.

Physicians who are paid for an episode of back pain rather than under fee-for-service have disincentives to order imaging studies and incentives to develop a coordinated approach to back pain. Mr. H is likely to benefit from a CD providing information about back care and a physical therapy program of active exercises as tolerated (34, 35). In addition, yoga and massage may also be beneficial (36, 37). Bundled payments can motivate physicians to establish multidisciplinary care teams with expertise in these alternative treatments, while also assuring Mr. H ready access to imaging studies and surgical specialists if his condition fails to improve. Finally, payment for an episode of care also offers incentives to address the psychosocial aspects of his illness and coping.

How can the physician respond to patient concerns that the physician is merely trying to save money (38, 39)? First, the physician should explore the patient's concerns and acknowledge the uncertainty of medical diagnosis. Is there some specific diagnosis the patient fears will be missed? Does the patient have a friend or relative whose serious illness was not diagnosed in a timely manner. Also, the doctor should explain to the patient why these interventions are not recommended at this time and also what therapies are known to promote recovery.

SUMMARY

1. Physicians should use medical resources prudently and fairly.
2. Within the constraints of health care plans, physicians need to act as patient advocates when the patient could receive significant clinical benefit from a referral, test, or therapy that the plan disallows.
3. Financial incentives that are highly likely to lead physicians to order medically inappropriate care need to be identified and restricted.

REFERENCES

1. Keehan SP, Sisko AM, Truffer CJ, et al. National health spending projections through 2020: economic recovery and reform drive faster spending growth. *Health Aff (Millwood).* 2011;30:1594–1605.
2. Committee on Health Insurance Status and Its Consequences. Institute of Medicine. *America's Uninsured Crisis: Consequences for Health and Health Care.* 2009. http://www.iom.edu/Reports/2009/Americas-Uninsured-Crisis-Consequences-for-Health-and-Health-Care.aspx. Accessed November 16, 2011.
3. Schwartz WB. The inevitable failure of current cost-containment strategies. Why they can provide only temporary relief. *JAMA.* 1987;257:220–224.
4. Eddy DM. Health system reform: will controlling costs require rationing services? *JAMA.* 1994;272:324–328.
5. Pauly MV. Medicare drug coverage and moral hazard. *Health Aff (Millwood).* 2004;23:113–22.
6. Boren SD. I had a tough day today, Hillary. *N Engl J Med.* 1994;330:500–502.
7. Hall MA. The death of managed care: a regulatory autopsy. *J Health Polit Policy Law.* 2005;30:427–452.
8. Kmetik KS, O'Toole MF, Bossley H, et al. Exceptions to outpatient quality measures for coronary artery disease in electronic health records. *Ann Intern Med.* 2011;154:227–234.
9. Ellrodt AG, Conner L, Riedinger M, et al. Measuring and improving physician compliance with clinical practice guidelines. *Ann Intern Mec.* 1995;122:277–282.
10. Blendon RJ, Brodie M, Benson JM, et al. Understanding the managed care backlash. *Health Affairs.* 1998;17:80–94.
11. Kao AC, Green DC, Zaslavsky AM, et al. The relationship between method of physician payment and patient trust. *JAMA.* 1998;280:1708–1714.
12. Kassirer JP. Managing care—should we adopt a new ethic? *N Engl J Med.* 1998;339:397–398.
13. Briesacher BA, Gurwitz JH, Soumerai SB. Patients at-risk for cost-related medication nonadherence: a review of the literature. *J Gen Intern Med.* 2007;22:864–871.
14. Kullgren JT, Galbraith AA, Hinrichsen VL, et al. Health care use and decision making among lower-income families in high-deductible health plans. *Arch Intern Med.* 2010;170:1918–1925.
15. Goldman DP, Joyce GF, Zheng Y. Prescription drug cost sharing: associations with medication and medical utilization and spending and health. *JAMA.* 2007;298:61–69.
16. Soumerai SB. Benefits and risks of increasing restrictions on access to costly drugs in medicaid. *Health Aff (Millwood).* 2004;23:135–146.
17. Huskamp HA, Deverka PA, Epstein AM, et al. The effect of incentive-based formularies on prescription-drug utilization and spending. *N Engl J Med.* 2003;349:2224–2232.
18. Choudhry NK, Avorn J, Glynn RJ, et al. Full coverage for preventive medications after myocardial infarction. °*N Engl J Med.* 2011.
19. Alexander GC, Casalino LP, Meltzer DO. Patient–physician communication about out-of-pocket costs. *JAMA.* 2003;290:953–958.

20. Shrank WH, Fox SA, Kirk A, et al. The effect of pharmacy benefit design on patient-physician communication about costs. *J Gen Intern Med.* 2006;21:334–339.
21. Volpp KG, Asch DA, Galvin R, et al. Redesigning employee health incentives—lessons from behavioral economics. *N Engl J Med.* 2011;365:388–390.
22. Madison KM, Volpp KG, Halpern SD. The law, policy, and ethics of employers' use of financial incentives to improve health. *J Law Med Ethics.* 2011;39:450–468.
23. Povar GJ, Blumen H, Daniel J, et al. Ethics in practice: managed care and the changing health care environment: medicine as a profession managed care ethics working group statement. *Ann Intern Med.* 2004;141:131–136.
24. Levinson W, Kao A, Kuby AM, et al. The effect of physician disclosure of financial incentives on trust. *Arch Intern Med.* 2005;165:625–630.
25. Licurse A, Barber E, Joffe S, et al. The impact of disclosing financial ties in research and clinical care: a systematic review. *Arch Intern Med.* 2010;170:675–682.
26. Miller TE, Sage WM. Disclosing physician financial incentives. *JAMA.* 1999;281:1424–1430.
27. Pearson SD, Kleinman K, Rusinak D, et al. A trial of disclosing physicians' financial incentives to patients. *Arch Intern Med.* 2006;166:623–628.
28. *Wickline v. State of California.* 228 Cal. Rptr. 661 (Cal. App. 1986).
29. Pearson SD. Caring and cost: the challenge for physician advocacy. *Ann Intern Med.* 2000;133:148–153.
30. Wynia MK, Cummins DS, VanGeest JB, et al. Physician manipulation of reimbursement rules for patients: between a rock and a hard place. *JAMA.* 2000;283:1858–1865.
31. Werner RM, Alexander GC, Fagerlin A, et al. The "Hassle Factor": what motivates physicians to manipulate reimbursement rules? *Arch Intern Med.* 2002;162:1134–1139.
32. Bogardus ST Jr, Geist DE, Bradley EH. Physicians' interactions with third-party payers: is deception necessary? *Arch Intern Med.* 2004;164:1841–1844.
33. Morreim EH. Gaming the system: dodging the rules, ruling the dodgers. *Arch Intern Med.* 1991;151:443–447.
34. Tilbrook HE, Cox H, Hewitt CE, et al. Yoga for chronic low back pain: a randomized trial. *Ann Intern Med.* 2011;155:569–578.
35. Deyo RA. Commentary: managing patients with back pain: putting money where our mouths are not. *Spine J.* 2011;11:633–635.
36. Hill JC, Whitehurst DG, Lewis M, et al. Comparison of stratified primary care management for low back pain with current best practice (STarT Back): a randomised controlled trial. *Lancet.* 2011;378:1560–1571.
37. Cherkin DC, Sherman KJ, Kahn J, et al. A comparison of the effects of 2 types of massage and usual care on chronic low back pain: a randomized, controlled trial. *Ann Intern Med.* 2011;155:1–9.
38. Gallagher TH, Lo B, Chesney M, et al. How do managed care physicians respond to patients' requests for costly, unindicated tests? *J Gen Intern Med.* 1997;12:663–668.
39. Levinson W, Gorawara-Bhat R, Dueck R, et al. Resolving disagreements in the patient-physician relationship: tools for improving communication in managed care. *JAMA.* 1999;282:1477–1483.

ANNOTATED BIBLIOGRAPHY

1. Kassirer JP. Managed care and the morality of the marketplace. *N Engl J Med.* 1995;333:50–52.
   Eloquent plea that professional ethics is incompatible with a profit-oriented, entrepreneurial approach to medicine.
2. Pearson SD, Daniels N, Emanuel E. Ethical guidelines for physician compensation based on capitation. *N Engl J Med.* 1998;339:689–693.
   Suggestions for a just system of incentives in managed care.
3. Hall MA, Berenson RA. Ethical practice in managed care: a dose of realism. *Ann Intern Med.* 1998;128:395–402.
   This article argues that financial incentives to physicians to limit care can be ethical and, in fact, are preferable to rules set by administrators.
4. Epstein AM. Pay for performance at the tipping point. *N Engl J Med.* 2007;356:515–517.
   Thoughtful overview of use of physician incentives to improve quality of care.
5. Povar GJ, Blumen H, Daniel J, et al. Ethics in practice: managed care and the changing health care environment: Medicine as a profession managed care ethics working group statement. *Ann Intern Med.* 2004;141:131–136.
   Consensus guidelines for ethical practice in managed care.

CHAPTER 33

Gifts from Drug Companies

ifts from drug companies to physicians formerly were ubiquitous. A study found that 97% of residents were carrying at least one item, such as reference books (90%), pens (79%), and information cards (70%) that had pharmaceutical insignia (1). In another study, 93% of medical students had been asked or required by an attending physician to attend at least one sponsored lunch (2). Eighty percent believed they were entitled to gifts. Although gifts and subsidies from drug companies might foster medical education and provide welcome perks to physicians and students, some gifts might compromise the physician's judgment or impair public trust in physicians. This chapter presents arguments for and against accepting gifts from drug companies or medical device manufacturers and suggests guidelines for such gifts (3).

TYPES OF GIFTS

In 2004, pharmaceutical manufacturers spent more than $20 billion for drug detailing to US physicians and more than $6 billion for drug samples—almost 24% of sales—more than $60,000 per physician (4). The total amount spent for promotional activities was about double the amount spent for research and development (4). Gifts and subsidies from drug companies to physicians ranged from token to lavish items. Small gifts that bear the company or product name included pens and message pads, as well as more expensive items such as umbrellas, flashlights, and clocks. Drug companies might also distribute medical books and equipment, such as reflex hammers.

MEALS AND HOSPITALITY

Drug companies provide lunch or refreshments at hospital conferences or continuing medical education (CME) courses. Conference organizers often solicit these subsidies to increase attendance. Companies also host dinners for physicians, coupled with a medical talk, commonly providing "consultants' fees" to attendees for suggesting ways to market the product.

CONTINUING MEDICAL EDUCATION AND CONFERENCES

More than 60% of funding for accredited CME now comes from commercial sources, including drug company support, advertising, and exhibitor fees (4). Drug companies commonly work with publishing and education companies to develop CME programs. Compared with CME programs sponsored by academic institutions, CME programs from these companies present fewer sessions on such topics as prevention, lifestyle changes, and doctor–patient communication (5). Drug companies might support hospital conferences by paying honoraria and travel expenses for speakers. Furthermore, physicians on speakers' bureaus for drug companies usually receive training, slides, and presentations for talks, in addition to honoraria. CME at professional society meetings receive more than 48% of their revenue for CME from commercial sponsors, in the form of grants, advertising, and exhibit fees.

DRUG DETAILING

In 2005, the drug companies hired one representative for every six licensed physicians in the United States (5). Drug representatives provide individualized information and gifts to physicians, together with free drug samples for patients. Many physicians depend on drug representatives as convenient sources of information about new drugs. Studies suggest that physician exposure to information from drug companies is associated with more prescriptions, higher drug costs, and lower quality of prescribing (6). Drug representatives have a prescribing profile for each physician, which is obtained from prescription records purchased from pharmacies. These profiles enable drug representatives to tailor their message to the individual doctor and to assess its impact (7). Drug representatives are trained to assess physicians' personality styles and to establish a personal connection with them (8).

REASONS FOR DRUG COMPANIES TO OFFER GIFTS

One commentator observed, "No drug company gives away its shareholders' money in an act of disinterested generosity" (9). There is evidence that gifts from drug companies strengthen physicians' recognition of products (10). One study found that doctors who attended a drug company–sponsored CME or who accepted funds for travel or lodging for educational symposia were more likely to prescribe the sponsor's medications. This occurred even if physicians forgot the sponsors' names or believed that they could not be influenced. Doctors who met with pharmaceutical representatives or accepted industry-paid meals were more likely to request formulary additions or to prescribe in nonrational ways. Physicians who received gifts from pharmaceutical manufacturers, even practice-related gifts, were more likely to believe that gifts did not affect prescribing behavior. Physicians who accepted free drug samples were more likely to prescribe newer (and more expensive) medications for hypertension than older medications that are recommended by practice guidelines as initial therapy (11).

REASONS FOR ACCEPTING DRUG-COMPANY GIFTS

Gifts from drug companies subsidize continuing education courses and, thereby, might enhance medical education and professional society meetings. Providing lunches and honoraria for hospital conferences might improve educational programs by increasing attendance. In an era of financial constraints, such subsidies might enable hospitals or medical schools to invite nationally prominent experts. Thus, some argue that drug-company gifts and subsidies have, overall, more benefit than harm. If physicians refused all gifts and subsidies from drug companies, then patients would pay the same amount for drugs but their physicians would receive less education. Some physicians believe that drug samples provide medications to indigent and uninsured patients; however, a lower percentage of indigent or uninsured patients report receiving drug samples than do wealthy or insured patients (12).

OBJECTIONS TO ACCEPTING DRUG-COMPANY GIFTS

Table 33-1 summarizes objections to accepting gifts from drug companies.

TABLE 33-1	Objections to Accepting Gifts from Drug Companies
Gifts create the expectation of reciprocity.	
Gifts impair objectivity.	
Gifts increase the cost of health care.	
Gifts demean the profession.	
Gifts give the appearance of conflict of interest.	

GIFTS CREATE THE EXPECTATION OF RECIPROCITY

Gifts create relationships and obligations in the recipient, such as grateful conduct, goodwill, and reciprocation (13). The problem is not that physicians immediately change prescribing practices after receiving a free lunch. Rather, as one writer has warned, "The sell is much more subtle. All the advertiser may expect is that, other things being equal, if you subsequently have to make a decision it is more likely to be in the favor of the advertiser" (14).

GIFTS IMPAIR OBJECTIVITY

Objectivity of presentations in classes, conferences, and continuing education courses might be compromised if a drug company selects speakers and topics, prepares slides for presentations, writes or edits talks, or trains the presenters (15). A speaker might selectively present or emphasize data favorable to one drug or class of drugs rather than draw from the overall body of available data (16). Even low-cost gifts, such as pens and notepads, might undermine rational prescribing by reminding physicians of specific brand-name drugs, regardless of how persuasive the evidence is that they are effective and safe (17).

GIFTS INCREASE THE COST OF HEALTH CARE

Ultimately, patients and their insurers pay for drug-company gifts to physicians. Given the sharply rising cost of drugs, it might be unseemly for physicians to receive even small gifts from drug companies. One physician criticized, "Am I supposed to believe that the members of a clinical department are so impoverished that they cannot buy their own pens or pizza and beer?" (14).

GIFTS DEMEAN THE PROFESSION

Dependence on drug-company subsidies to support CME programs demeans physicians (14). If the public realized that physicians attend conferences only if lunch is provided or the registration fee is subsidized, then they might infer that physicians place little value on keeping up-to-date with medical advances.

GIFTS UNDERMINE PATIENT AND PUBLIC TRUST

Even if gifts from pharmaceutical companies do not actually influence a physician's therapeutic decisions, they might undermine public trust. After all, physicians are not choosing medications for their own use and paying the bills themselves; they are prescribing for their patients. According to one survey, patients are more likely than physicians to believe that gifts are not appropriate and that gifts influence physician behavior (18). About 30% of patients believe that even small gifts such as a mug, pen, or lunch would influence a physician's behavior, compared with about 10% of physicians (18). Another study found that patients who believed that their physician accepted gifts were more likely to report low physician trust (19).

Outside of medicine, society has enacted strict rules regarding conflicts of interest that might undermine trust in public officials. Judges are expected to refuse gifts from persons or companies who have a financial stake in their professional decisions. Government officials may not accept gifts of more than nominal value from persons or organizations who would be affected by or gain financially from their decisions. By analogy, it might be inappropriate for physicians to accept drug-company gifts that create even the appearance of a conflict of interest.

RECOMMENDATIONS

DISCLOSE GIFTS TO THE PUBLIC

Speakers at CME programs must disclose any honoraria or consulting fees from commercial entities in the course syllabus and at the beginning of their presentations. Under the Physician Payment Sunshine Act, in 2013 drug, device, and biotechnology companies must report all payments to physicians by name that total more than US$100 a year to a publicly available database (3). Thus, members of the public will be able to determine how much money a physician received from drug companies. Physician might find it difficult to determine what gifts are acceptable and what are not. A helpful rule of thumb is, "What would your patients or the public think if they knew you had accepted these gifts?" (20). In borderline cases, it would be judicious to err on the side of declining gifts.

ALLOW CERTAIN OTHER PRACTICES

Some types of gifts or support are widely considered acceptable, with disclosure and appropriate management. At professional society meetings, drug companies often underwrite the printing of abstract books; such support is publicly acknowledged. For accredited CME courses, educational grants from commercial sponsors are permitted, provided that the sponsors may not influence the selection of speakers or the choice of topics (3). The CME course director is responsible for reviewing presentations from speakers who have financial relationships with drug or device manufacturers to ensure there is no bias. It is not known, however, how effectively these requirements are enforced.

FORBID CERTAIN PRACTICES

Certain types of gifts and support from drug companies are so likely to raise questions about bias and impropriety that they should be banned (3). For example, the American College of Physicians, the American Medical Association, the Accreditation Council for Continuing Medical Education, and the Pharmaceutical Manufacturers Association agree that it is unethical for physicians to accept direct payments to attend activities that have no educational value. The pharmaceutical industry has declared that occasional meals provided in conjunction with informational presentations must be modest (21, 22). Drug company representatives may no longer provide items for the personal benefit of health care professionals, such as tickets to a recreational event, or mugs, pens, and similar items (21, 22).

Several prominent medical schools have taken strong, comprehensive policies regarding interactions with pharmaceutical companies (3). Physicians may not accept any industry gifts, including drug samples, on campus or at clinical sites. This includes meals with conferences. Furthermore, industry representatives are not permitted in patient care areas except for in-service training on devices and are permitted in nonclinical areas only by appointment.

SUMMARY

1. Gifts from drug companies might impair objectivity, undermine public trust, and increase the cost of health care.
2. The primary concern of physicians should be their patients' best interests, not their own personal convenience or well-being.

REFERENCES

1. Sigworth SK, Nettleman MD, Cohen GM. Pharmaceutical branding of resident physicians. *JAMA.* 2001;286:1024–1025.
2. Sierles FS, Brodkey AC, Cleary LM, et al. Medical students' exposure to and attitudes about drug company interactions: a national survey. *JAMA.* 2005;294:1034–1042.
3. Lo B, Field M, eds. *Conflict of Interest in Medical Research, Education, and Practice.* 2009. http://www.iom.edu/Reports/2009/Conflict-of-Interest-in-Medical-Research-Education-and-Practice.aspx. Accessed November 16, 2011.
4. Gagnon MA, Lexchin J. The cost of pushing pills: a new estimate of pharmaceutical promotion expenditures in the United States. *PLoS Med.* 2008;5:e1.
5. Fugh-Berman A. The corporate coauthor. *J Gen Intern Med.* 2005;20:546–548.
6. Spurling GK, Mansfield PR, Montgomery BD, et al. Information from pharmaceutical companies and the quality, quantity, and cost of physicians' prescribing: a systematic review. *PLoS Med.* 2010;7:e1000352.

7. Grande D. Prescriber profiling: time to call it quits. *Ann Intern Med.* 2007;146:751–752.
8. Fugh-Berman A, Ahari S. Following the script: how drug reps make friends and influence doctors. *PLoS Med.* 2007;4:e150.
9. Rawlins MD. Doctors and the drug makers. *Lancet.* 1984;2:276–278.
10. Wazana A. Physicians and the pharmaceutical industry: is a gift ever just a gift? *JAMA.* 2000;283:373–380.
11. Ubel PA, Jepson C, Asch DA. Misperceptions about beta-blockers and diuretics: a national survey of primary care physicians. *J Gen Intern Med.* 2003;18:977–983.
12. Cutrona SL, Woolhandler S, Lasser KE, et al. Characteristics of recipients of free prescription drug samples: a nationally representative analysis. *Am J Public Health.* 2008;98:284–289.
13. Dana J. How psychological research can inform policies for dealing with conflicts of interest in medicine. In: Lo B, Field M, eds. *Conflict of Interest in Medical Research, Education, and Practice.* Washington, DC: National Academies Press; 2009:358–374.
14. Waud DR. Pharmaceutical promotions: a free lunch? *N Engl J Med.* 1992;327:351–353.
15. American College of Physicians. Physicians and the pharmaceutical industry. *Ann Int Med.* 1990;112:624–626.
16. Kessler DA. Drug promotion and scientific exchange: the role of the physician investigator. *N Engl J Med.* 1991;325:201–203.
17. Brett AS. Cheap trinkets, effective marketing: small gifts from drug companies to physicians. *Am J Bioeth.* 2003;3:52–54.
18. Gibbons RV, Landry FJ, Blouch DL, et al. A comparison of physicains' and patients' attitudes towards pharmaceutical industry gifts. *J Gen Intern Med.* 1998;13.
19. Grande D, Shea JA, Armstrong K. Pharmaceutical industry gifts to physicians: patient beliefs and trust in physicians and the health care system. *J Gen Intern Med.* 2012;27:274–279. Epub 2011 Jun 14.
20. Coyle SL. Physician-industry relations. Part 1: individual physicians. *Ann Intern Med.* 2002;136:396–402.
21. Bieri D. PhRMA's code on interactions with healthcare professionals. *Am J Bioeth.* 2010;10:18.
22. PhRMA. *Code on Interactions with Health Care Professionals.* 2008. http://www.phrma.org/about/principles-guidelines/code-interactions-healthcare-professionals. Accessed November 21, 2011.

ANNOTATED BIBLIOGRAPHY

1. Lo B, Field M. *Conflict of Interest in Medical Research, Education, and Practice.* 2009. http://www.iom.edu/Reports/2009/Conflict-of-Interest-in-Medical-Research-Education-and-Practice.aspx. Accessed November 16, 2011. Consensus report from the Institute of Medicine on conflicts of interest in medicine, including gift from drug companies. Summarizes empirical data on the topic and makes policy recommendations.
2. Fugh-Berman A, Ahari S. Following the script: how drug reps make friends and influence doctors. *PLoS Med.* 2007;4:e150. Describes the strategies drug company representatives employ when they approach physicians.
3. Steinbrook R. Financial support of continuing medical education. *JAMA.* 2008;299:1060–1062. Analyzes recent data on how CME is financed and policy alternatives for funding CME.

34

Disclosing Errors

An estimated 40,000 Americans die every year because of medical errors (1). In one survey, 42% of the public and 35% of physicians reported that an error had occurred in their own care or a family member's care (2). In only 30% of cases was the patient or family told that an error had occurred (2). Many physicians find it difficult to disclose errors to patients and colleagues because of possible recriminations from patients, setbacks to their professional reputation or livelihood, and malpractice suits. Patients want more disclosure of errors than physicians say they typically provide (3).

This chapter discusses the reasons for and against disclosing errors and suggests how physicians can respond to errors. An *error* is a failure of a plan to be completed as intended or the use of a wrong plan to achieve an aim. Errors can be either acts or omissions. Errors might—or might not—result in harm to patients; when no harm is done, the incident is called a *near miss* or a *close call*. Errors might or might not be avoidable. Adverse events are defined as undesired patient outcomes that result from medical care rather than from the underlying disease; they include situations in which the treatment plan was appropriate and carried out correctly, such as side effects of drugs.

The following case illustrates dilemmas posed by physicians' errors.

CASE 34.1   Overdose of insulin

A 54-year-old man with diabetes is hospitalized for congestive heart failure. The resident prescribes 100 units of insulin rather than the patient's usual dose of 10 units, and the patient receives the higher dose. He develops hypoglycemia, seizures, and coma. Upon recovery, the patient and his family ask physicians why the seizures occurred. The health care team is reluctant to tell them that an error occurred, fearing that they would get angry and perhaps sue them.

Traditionally, such errors were blamed on individuals who were deficient in knowledge, effort, or conscientiousness. A modern view is that most errors are due to inherent limitations in human cognition and attention and to system failures. In this view, blaming the physician is problematic (1, 4–6). First, errors like the one in Case 34.1 usually are due to a momentary loss of concentration or attention, which is beyond the doctor's voluntary control. A "slip of the pen" or a lapse in concentration could happen to the most expert and careful physician. Second, errors have multiple system causes. The pharmacist who dispensed the medication and the nurse who administered it failed to detect the incorrect dosage. The resident or attending physician might have provided closer supervision. These system problems are "accidents waiting to happen." More training for health care workers will be less effective in preventing such errors than redesigning the health care delivery system (7), including computerized ordering of medications, checklists, bar coding, and improved teamwork among physicians, pharmacists, and nurses. Focusing on improving the system of health care, rather than blaming individuals, is likely to result in higher quality of care for the population of patients as a whole.

SHOULD ERRORS BE DISCLOSED TO PATIENTS?

Since the 2001 report *To Err Is Human* from the Institute of Medicine, disclosure of errors to patients has become the standard of care (8). The Joint Commission, which accredits health care institutions, requires hospitals to tell patients when unanticipated outcomes of care occur. Finally, several states have enacted laws that require the disclosure of unanticipated outcomes of care.

REASONS NOT TO DISCLOSE ERRORS TO PATIENTS OR SURROGATES

Physician Is not Really Responsible for the Error

Physicians understandably do not want to take the blame for errors if they are not morally responsible. Only a few errors result from negligent or intentional violations of a clear standard of care or performance (4). Most are caused by systems flaws and limits in human cognition, which are beyond the physician's control.

Disclosure Would Harm Health Care Professionals

Physicians might fear that patients or families might respond to disclosure of errors by becoming angry, changing providers, or filing a lawsuit. Indeed, patients report that they would change physicians if their physician committed a life-threatening error (3). The reluctance of physicians to acknowledge errors, however, creates a vicious circle: If physicians are not forthright about errors, patients become more upset and more likely to sue. Trainees might worry that their careers will be damaged if they disclose a serious error to a supervising physician and that colleagues and supervisors might respond punitively rather than supportively (9).

REASONS TO DISCLOSE ERRORS TO PATIENTS OR SURROGATES

Disclosure Respects the Patient

Almost all patients would want even minor errors disclosed to them (10). Patients want to know what happened, why it happened, how adverse consequences will be mitigated, and how recurrences will be prevented (10–12). In addition, patients seek an apology (10). Unless the patient in Case 34.1 is told about the insulin overdose, he cannot understand this incident. He might well fear that seizures and coma will recur or that he has a grave problem, such as a brain tumor. Fearing a recurrence, he might change jobs or cut back on activities, such as driving or travel. Under the doctrine of informed consent, physicians have an affirmative duty to provide the patient or surrogate with pertinent information about his condition and the options for care. This duty to disclose goes beyond responding honestly to questions from patients. In thinking about disclosure, physicians might imagine how they would feel if a relative was harmed by an error and the health care team was not forthright about what happened.

Disclosure Benefits the Patient

Disclosure enables patients or surrogates to mitigate the harms that the error caused, for example, through additional tests, treatment, or follow-up care. Patients or families are more likely to cooperate with such measures if they understand the reasons for them. Disclosure might also allow patients to be compensated for harms resulting from errors. In Case 34.1, the patient required intensive care, a prolonged hospitalization, and a computed tomography (CT) scan following the error. It is unfair to ask the patient or an insurer to pay for this additional care. Moreover, most patients want charges for such care to be waived (13). Furthermore, it seems reasonable to compensate patients for lost income or serious disability resulting directly from errors. Patients cannot negotiate such compensation unless they or their surrogates are aware that an error occurred.

Disclosure Benefits the Physician

Disclosure might also mitigate adverse impacts on the physician's livelihood. One study found that patients are less likely to change doctors if they are told of errors and the physician accepts responsibility (13). Disclosure and apology, however, will not reduce the respondent's likelihood of seeking legal advice (13, 14). Health care institutions can institute programs that disclose adverse outcomes and offer compensation for medical errors (15). Such programs do not increase malpractice claims (16). Although disclosing an error does not shield a physician from legal liability, nondisclosure might increase the legal risk (17, 18).

WHAT TO SAY TO PATIENTS ABOUT ERRORS?

In Case 34.1, the physician clearly made an error, the patient suffered serious harm, and the error caused a poor outcome. Under these circumstances, the physician's responsibility to the patient should prevail over any self-interest in concealing the error. The physician should take the initiative in disclosing relevant information. First, physicians should explicitly acknowledge that an error occurred and offer an apology (19). When a person harms another, apologizing is the expected social response and a prerequisite to making amends and being forgiven (20). Many states do not allow expressions of sympathy made after an unanticipated outcome to be used as evidence in lawsuits. These laws, however, have major limitations: They protect institutions, not individual physicians, and do not shield explanations of the cause of errors or admissions of fault. Thus, these laws may not address physician's concerns about liability for giving patients the comprehensive disclosure and apologies that they seek (21). Second, the physician needs to explain the error and its consequences. Third, the physician should explain what can and will be done to mitigate the resulting harms to the patient and to prevent the error from recurring (11).

Some physicians might make only limited disclosure of errors—for example, telling the patient and family in Case 34.1 only that the patient's blood sugar got too low because he received more insulin than he needed, without saying that an error occurred (19). Other physicians might say, "I am sorry about what happened," but not take responsibility for the error. A partial apology, however, might be regarded by patients and families as evasive and mean-spirited. In addition, they are likely to probe for details—for example, to ask what caused his glucose to be low. Ethically, an appropriate response to concerns about a lawsuit in Case 34.1 would be for the risk manager to offer a fair out-of-court settlement. Many health care institution policies regarding errors not only mandate disclosure but also offer early settlements for medical injuries (15).

RESPONSIBILITY FOR ERRORS

The vast majority of errors are caused by systems defects or limitations in human attention and cognition, which are beyond the control of the individual physician. Few errors are caused by deficiencies in knowledge, skill, or due care. A strong argument can be made that people should not be held responsible for actions and conditions beyond their control.

The current systems approach to errors has led to calls for a "blame-free" culture because overall patients benefit more from putting in place systems to prevent errors, catch them before harm occurs, or reduce harms that do occur (7). However, it seems unfair not to hold individuals accountable for deliberate, egregious errors, for example, health care workers who commit errors habitually and willfully, despite education, counseling, and systems modifications and improvements (7).

Individual physicians are still held responsible for errors in several ways, including malpractice suits. Moreover, settlements are reported to the National Practitioner Data Bank and when applying for staff privileges, even if the error was beyond the physician's control.

SITUATIONS IN WHICH DISCLOSURE IS CONTROVERSIAL

In many cases, it might be unclear whether the physician should disclose an error to the patient or take responsibility for it.

THE ERROR CAUSED NO HARM

Errors that cause no harm to patients are called *near misses*.

CASE 34.2	Incorrect prescription

A physician prescribed a sulfonamide antibiotic to a patient with a history of allergy to those medications. A nurse discovered the error, and the prescription was changed after two doses. No adverse effects occurred.

Such near misses need to be reported to quality-improvement programs to prevent similar errors that could harm patients. Should they also be disclosed to the patient? In Case 34.2, some physicians might argue that if the prognosis or future care of the patient is not altered, there is no point in telling the patient of the error. Such physicians might hesitate to burden patients with all the uncertainties and adjustments made in the course of care. In addition, patients might lose confidence in physicians and hospitals.

Even in this case, however, there are strong reasons to disclose the error to patients. Disclosure is likely to strengthen the doctor–patient relationship because patients respect physicians for being honest. Disclosure might also promote patient well-being by allowing reconsideration of the diagnosis of drug allergy. Furthermore, patients might call attention to errors—for example, after noticing that the medication has changed. If this occurs, physicians might find it awkward to explain the change if the patient had not been told immediately. Finally, there is little risk to physicians in disclosing "near misses" because patients who suffer no harm are unlikely to get angry and cannot sue.

OUTCOME WOULD HAVE BEEN POOR EVEN WITHOUT THE ERROR

In other cases, the physician makes an error and the patient suffers a poor outcome, but the poor outcome would very likely have occurred even if there had been no error. For example, the adverse outcome might be due to the underlying disease.

CASE 34.3	Failure to administer appropriate treatment

A 52-year-old man developed vomiting and ataxia and became unconscious. In the emergency department, he had a blood pressure of 200/105, which was not treated while a CT scan was obtained. He was found to have a cerebellar hemorrhage and died in the emergency department.

In this case, standard care is to lower blood pressure before obtaining the CT scan. Once comatose, however, he would almost certainly have died even if his blood pressure had been lowered. When telling the family about the patient's death, the physicians should not say that an error was a contributing factor. Physicians must recognize, however, that determining whether an error caused an adverse outcome is difficult (7) and that their belief that the error caused no harm might be biased or self-serving. Consultation with an experienced colleague might help physicians evaluate their judgment and actions accurately.

Even if an error is not mentioned, family members might ask physicians whether everything was done to prevent an adverse outcome. This question deserves both a literal and deeper response. On the literal level, it would be deceptive to say that everything was done when the physician knows that this was not the case. On another level, the survivors might be asking whether *they* should have acted differently or whether the patient suffered needlessly.

CASE 34.3	*Continued*

The physician might say, "When someone dies in the emergency department we all ask if anything more could have been done. We will review the case to see how to improve care in the future. Once patients with this kind of bleeding into the brain lose consciousness, the bleeding is so severe that they don't recover. . . One thing is clear—he didn't suffer after he lost consciousness."

ADVERSE OUTCOME COULD NOT HAVE BEEN AVOIDED

Some procedure-related adverse events are due to a mishap, such as poor technique or a slip of the instrument. System factors, such as inadequate training or supervision, might be contributing factors. In other cases, however, the procedure was carried out skillfully.

CASE 34.4	Foreseeable complication of an invasive procedure

A 43-year-old man with interstitial lung disease undergoes a bronchoscopy and transbronchial biopsy. The procedure is performed following standard procedures. He suffers a pneumothorax that requires insertion of a chest tube for 2 days. The patient was informed of this risk prior to the procedure.

In this case, the patient suffered a known complication of an invasive procedure that was appropriately and skillfully performed. The physician needs to review the case to be certain that the standard of care was followed. The patient agreed to the procedure and accepted the risks. Although the physician must explain the unintended adverse outcome and should express regret over it, the doctor is not to blame for this complication.

DISCLOSING ERRORS BY TRAINEES TO AN ATTENDING PHYSICIAN

In teaching hospitals, errors by trainees might not be reported to attending physicians (22, 23).

DISCLOSURE OF SERIOUS ERRORS BY TRAINEES TO SUPERVISING PHYSICIANS

Students, house officers, and fellows might be reluctant to tell supervisors about errors lest they jeopardize their grades, recommendations, or future positions. Supervisors might respond judgmentally rather than supportively.

Attending physicians are ethically and legally responsible for patient care. They cannot perform this role properly if significant information about the patient is withheld. Furthermore, attending physicians might learn of such errors even if trainees do not disclose them. Most supervising physicians believe that failure to disclose errors is worse than making them in the first place (23, 24). Although trainees are expected to make some errors, covering them up raises doubts about reliability, trustworthiness, and character.

RESPONSES TO ERRORS BY TRAINEES

Supervising physicians need to respond to trainee errors on several levels.

Elicit and Acknowledge the Trainee's Emotional Distress

Appropriate emotional support needs to be provided (22, 25). The supervisor can put the trainee's feelings in context: Although it causes distress to admit an error, it is a sign of responsibility and caring. Understanding this link between emotional distress and learning might offer the resident some solace (22, 23).

Review the Medical Issues and Decisions

The supervisor can help the trainee learn from the error and make constructive changes to prevent similar errors in the future, for example, seeking advice in difficult cases, reading more about the medical problem, and confirming key clinical data personally rather than relying on someone else's report (23). Discussing errors explicitly can also help other trainees avoid similar errors (22).

Discuss How to Disclose the Error to the Patient or Surrogate

If disclosure is appropriate, then the attending physician should inform the patient together with the trainee. Such joint discussions offer trainees emotional support and role modeling.

ERRORS BY OTHER HEALTH CARE WORKERS

A physician might become aware of a definite error by another health care worker that seriously harmed a patient. For example, in Case 34.1 another clinical service or a different hospital might have made the overdose of insulin. Even if the current physician did not make the error, the patient still needs to understand what happened and try to mitigate the resulting harms. Thus, the current physician might consider whether to disclose the error to the patient.

ETHICAL ISSUES REGARDING ERRORS BY OTHER HEALTH CARE WORKERS

Patients want errors disclosed regardless of who committed them. Physicians, however, often find it more difficult to deal with errors by other health care workers. The facts of the case might be unclear, even if the physician reviews the medical record. In addition, disclosure might conflict with the current physician's self-interest. The other physician or institution might become irate or stop referring patients. Physicians in training who notice a serious error by a senior physician might fear retaliation (*see* Chapter 36). In addition, the patient or family might vent their anger on the current physician, who bears no responsibility for the error. On the other hand, if the current physicians do not discuss the earlier error, the patient and family may feel that there is a cover-up.

RESPONSES TO ERRORS BY OTHER HEALTH CARE WORKERS

Faced with a clear and serious error by another health care worker, the current physician might take several approaches.

Waiting for the patient to ask is ethically problematic because physicians have an affirmative obligation to disclose relevant information to patients.

Although asking the other physician to disclose the error might be easiest for the current physician, the previous physician might choose not to tell the patient or might provide misleading information.

If the patient is still receiving care at the institution in which the error occurred, then a joint conference might be held with the current physician, the previous physician, and the patient or family. This approach allows the other physician to take the lead in revealing the error, while ensuring that the discussion is appropriate.

If the current physician decides to tell the patient about the error, disclosure needs to be put in the context of having incomplete information about what occurred. The current physician should tell the other physician that she is going to talk to the patient and offer the other doctor the opportunity to talk to the patient first. Such consideration might maintain the relationships between the patient and the previous physician and between the two physicians.

SUMMARY

1. The decision to acknowledge an error ideally should be based on ethical guidelines, not on expedience.
2. Disclosure of errors is difficult, but failure to disclose errors undermines physicians' credibility and compromises their integrity.
3. Ultimately, the quality of medical care is enhanced if physicians are willing to admit their errors and learn from them.

REFERENCES

1. Kohn LT, Corrigan JM, Donaldson MS, eds. *To Err is Human: Building a Safer Health System.* Washington, DC: National Academy Press; 2000. http://www.iom.edu/Reports/1999/To-Err-is-Human-Building-A-Safer-Health-System.aspx. Accessed December 15, 2011.
2. Blendon RJ, DesRoches CM, Brodie M, et al. Views of practicing physicians and the public on medical errors. *N Engl J Med.* 2002;347:1933–1940.
3. Gallagher TH, Levinson W. Disclosing harmful medical errors to patients: a time for professional action. *Arch Intern Med.* 2005;165:1819–1824.
4. Runciman WB, Merry AF, Tito F. Error, blame, and the law in health care—an antipodean perspective. *Ann Intern Med.* 2003;138:974–979.
5. Reason J. Human error: models and management. *BMJ (Clinical Research Ed.).* 2000;320:768–770.
6. Reason J. Understanding adverse events: the human factor. In: Vincent C, ed. *Clinical Risk Management: Enhancing Patient Safety.* 2nd ed. London, UK: BMJ Books; 2001:9–30.
7. Wachter RM, Pronovost PJ. Balancing "no blame" with accountability in patient safety. *N Engl J Med.* 2009;361:1401–1406.
8. Gallagher TH, Studdert D, Levinson W. Disclosing harmful medical errors to patients. *N Engl J Med.* 2007;356:2713–2719.
9. Wu AW, Folkman S, McPhee SJ, et al. Do house officers learn from their mistakes? *JAMA.* 1991;265:2089–2094.
10. Gallagher TH, Waterman AD, Ebers AG, et al. Patients' and physicians' perspective regarding the disclosure of medical errors. *JAMA.* 2004;289:1001–1007.
11. Mazor KM, Greene SM, Roblin D, Lemay CA, Firneno CL, Calvi J, et al. More than words: Patients' views on apology when things go wrong in cancer care. *Patient Educ Couns.* 2011 Aug 6. [Epub ahead of print].
12. O'Connor E, Coates HM, Yardley IE, et al. Disclosure of patient safety incidents: a comprehensive review. *Int J Qual Health Care.* 2010;22:371–379.
13. Mazor KM, Simon SR, Yood RA, et al. Health plan members' views about disclosure of medical errors. *Ann Intern Med.* 2004;140:409–418.
14. Wu AW, Huang IC, Stokes S, et al. Disclosing medical errors to patients: it's not what you say, it's what they hear. *J Gen Intern Med.* 2009;24:1012–1017.
15. Mello MM, Gallagher TH. Malpractice reform—opportunities for leadership by health care institutions and liability insurers. *N Engl J Med.* 2010;362:1353–1356.
16. Kachalia A, Kaufman SR, Boothman R, et al. Liability claims and costs before and after implementation of a medical error disclosure program. *Ann Intern Med.* 2010;153:213–221.
17. Mazor KM, Reed GW, Yood RA, et al. Disclosure of medical errors: what factors influence how patients respond? *J Gen Intern Med.* 2006;21:704–710.
18. Witman AB, Park DM, Hardin SB. How do patients want physicians to handle mistakes? A survey of internal medicine patients in an academic setting. *Arch Intern Med.* 1996;156:2565–2569.
19. Gallagher TH, Garbutt JM, Waterman AD, et al. Choosing your words carefully: how physicians would disclose harmful medical errors to patients. *Arch Intern Med.* 2006;166:1585–1593.
20. Lazare A. Apology in medical practice: an emerging clinical skill. *JAMA.* 2006;296:1401–1404.
21. Mastroianni AC, Mello MM, Sommer S, et al. The flaws in state 'apology' and 'disclosure' laws dilute their intended impact on malpractice suits. *Health Aff (Millwood).* 2010;29:1611–1619.
22. Fischer MA, Mazor KM, Baril J, et al. Learning from mistakes. Factors that influence how students and residents learn from medical errors. *J Gen Intern Med.* 2006;21:419–423.
23. Wu AW, Cavanaugh TA, McPhee SJ, et al. To tell the truth: ethical and practical issues in disclosing medical mistakes to patients. *J Gen Intern Med.* 1997;17:770–775.

24. Bosk CL. *Forgive and Remember: Managing Medical Failure.* 2nd ed. Chicago, IL: University of Chicago Press; 1979.
25. Wu AW. Medical error: the second victim. The doctor who makes the mistake needs help too. *BMJ.* 2000;320:726–727.

ANNOTATED BIBLIOGRAPHY

1. Kohn L, Corrigan J, Donaldson M, eds. *To Err Is Human: Building a Safer Health System.* Washington, DC: National Academy Press; 2000.

   Argues that most errors are due to system problems and limits of human cognition and attention. Recommends a confidential system of reporting errors to prevent future errors.

2. Wu AW, Folkman S, McPhee SJ, et al. Do house officers learn from their mistakes? *JAMA.* 1991;265:2089–2094.

   House officers who accepted responsibility for serious mistakes were more likely to make constructive changes in practice, but were also more likely to experience emotional distress. Attending physicians were told of serious mistakes only 54% of the time, and patients or families were told of the mistake in only 24% of cases.

3. Gallagher TH, Waterman AD, Ebers AG, et al. Patients' and physicians' perspective regarding the disclosure of medical errors. *JAMA.* 2004;289:1001–1007.

   Explains that perspectives of physicians and patients differ markedly about disclosure of medical errors.

4. Gallagher TH, Studdert D, Levinson W. Disclosing harmful medical errors to patients. *N Engl J Med.* 2007;356:2713–2719.

   Describes growing incentives and pressures to disclose errors to patients and presents evidence suggesting that malpractice costs may decrease with greater disclosure.

CHAPTER 35

Impaired Colleagues

P hysicians who are impaired or incompetent might harm patients. Society relies on the medical profession to regulate itself, yet colleagues of impaired physicians are often reluctant to intervene, even in egregious cases. The following case illustrates common dilemmas regarding impaired colleagues.

CASE 35.1 **Drinking alcohol while on call**

Dr. New, a young internist who has recently joined a group practice, is at a party. She overhears a senior colleague, Dr. Elder, answer a page. Dr. Elder has been drinking and has slurred speech. Over the phone he prescribes 2.50 mg of digoxin, an unusually large dose. From what she hears of the conversation, Dr. New suspects that she has covered this patient, an elderly man with mild renal insufficiency, a recent hip fracture repair, and postoperative pneumonia.

Although Dr. New suspects that the patient is at risk of a drug overdose, she cannot be sure. Should she intervene to protect the patient from this suspected mistake? If so, should she confront Dr. Elder or talk to the house officer or nursing supervisor covering the service? What about other patients Dr. Elder might harm? Dr. New wants to prevent harm to patients, but she is reluctant to jeopardize a colleague's career or her own.

This chapter discusses intervening with impaired colleagues, reasons to take action, concerns about doing so, and practical suggestions. Chapter 34, which discusses errors, contains related materials. Errors by impaired or incompetent colleagues are more serious than other errors because they are more likely to be repeated. Although many medical errors are due to system problems, those discussed in this chapter are due primarily to shortcomings of an individual physician.

Common causes of impairment include alcoholism, substance abuse, and psychiatric and medical illness, such as depression and Alzheimer disease (1). Many impaired physicians can be treated effectively in programs that stress confidential rehabilitation rather than punishment (2). Physicians might also be incompetent because of inadequate knowledge and skills or careless behavior—for example, failing to round on patients.

REASONS FOR INTERVENING WITH IMPAIRED COLLEAGUES

Physicians have an ethical obligation to be competent, based on the ethical guidelines of refraining from causing harm and acting in their patients' best interests. There are also compelling ethical reasons for physicians to intervene with seriously impaired colleagues, even though the patients who might be harmed are not their own (Table 35-1).

TABLE 35-1	Reasons for Intervening With Impaired Colleagues

To prevent harm to patients
To carry out professional self-regulation
To help the impaired colleague

PREVENT HARM TO PATIENTS

People have a duty to prevent serious harm to others when it can be done at minimal risk or inconvenience to themselves (3). Modern professional codes of ethics also require physicians to protect patients from impaired colleagues (4). An impaired physician's colleagues might be in a unique position to prevent harm to patients because they have both the expertise to evaluate the quality of care rendered by colleagues and also the opportunity to do so.

In other occupations, workers whose impairment might endanger the public are aggressively identified. For example, airline pilots and train engineers are required to submit to drug testing before hiring, after accidents, and on a random basis (5). A commercial pilot who is suspected of drinking while on duty may be removed from the cockpit. Critics charge that the treatment of impaired physicians, in comparison, is too lax.

CARRY OUT PROFESSIONAL SELF-REGULATION

Society grants the medical profession considerable autonomy to regulate itself through selecting applicants for medical school and residency, defining standards of practice, certifying physicians, and disciplining members. The rationale for such professional autonomy is that laypeople do not have the expertise to determine whether physicians are impaired or incompetent. In return, society expects the profession to screen out practitioners who might endanger patients. If people believe that physicians are covering up for impaired or incompetent colleagues, they will lose trust in the medical profession and society might regulate physicians directly.

HELP THE IMPAIRED COLLEAGUE

Impaired physicians might harm themselves and their families, as well as their patients, through automobile accidents, violent episodes, or lapses in judgment. Furthermore, impaired physicians might destroy their livelihood and their families' economic security. Intervening with impaired colleagues might avert such destructive outcomes.

REASONS NOT TO INTERVENE WITH IMPAIRED COLLEAGUES

State licensing boards provide strong evidence that physicians are reluctant to intervene with impaired colleagues. Compared with the estimated prevalence of impairment, state boards receive few reports about impaired physicians (6). There might be several reasons for such reluctance.

UNCERTAINTY WHETHER PATIENTS ARE AT SERIOUS RISK

Physicians might be uncertain whether colleagues suspected of impairment are actually placing patients at risk, as in Case 35.1. Dr. New does not know the complete story. Perhaps the patient needed a high dose because he had uncontrolled atrial fibrillation or intestinal malabsorption.

RELUCTANCE TO CRITICIZE COLLEAGUES

Physicians rely on their colleagues' skills, knowledge, and judgment. Thus, doctors might hesitate to admit that a colleague is impaired because it calls such trust into question. Physicians are understandably reluctant to criticize someone who is respected. Dr. New may also feel a debt of gratitude to Dr. Elder if he has helped her establish her practice and referred patients to her. Physicians might also hesitate to probe matters that are often considered private, such as alcohol consumption. Dr. New, for example, might be reluctant to act on the basis of a personal telephone conversation that she accidentally overheard. Furthermore, doctors are understandably reluctant to undermine a colleague's reputation and livelihood. Subconsciously, physicians might identify with impaired colleagues. If they question a colleague's competence, might other physicians in turn criticize them harshly after a minor error?

RETALIATION AGAINST WHISTLE-BLOWERS

Whistle-blowers often face personal retaliation. If Dr. New confronts Dr. Elder, then he might get angry or tell her to mind her own business. If she tells other people, colleagues might label her a snitch or a tattletale. Dr. Elder might accuse her of trying to ruin his reputation or trying to build up her own practice. He might even retaliate by criticizing her work and discouraging other physicians from referring patients to her. Dr. Elder could potentially go so far as to sue her for defamation of character or lost income. Even the threat of a lawsuit might deter Dr. New from pursuing the matter. Dr. New's natural concern about her own career might conflict with her desire to prevent harm to vulnerable patients.

LEGAL ISSUES REGARDING IMPAIRED COLLEAGUES

REPORTING LAWS

Many states have adopted laws concerning reporting of impaired or incompetent colleagues (1, 7). The specific provisions of reporting laws vary from state to state. In Massachusetts, physicians must report to the state licensing board colleagues whom they suspect are practicing medicine while impaired. Other states permit such reporting but do not require it. Most states grant legal immunity from civil suits to physicians who report colleagues in good faith.

PHYSICIAN WELLNESS PROGRAMS

Most states and hospitals have set up physician health programs, which are often run by the state medical society rather than the medical licensing bureau, to treat and rehabilitate impaired physicians (1). The Joint Commission requires all hospitals to have a physician wellness committee that is coordinated with the state physician wellness program. The goal is to rehabilitate impaired physicians in a confidential manner while protecting patients. The physician may have to suspend practice or may be permitted to continue to practice in a monitored situation, depending on the circumstances. Physicians entering such programs may be granted confidentiality and immunity from disciplinary actions.

THE HEALTH CARE QUALITY IMPROVEMENT ACT

In 1986, Congress passed legislation regarding reporting of incompetent physicians. This law requires hospitals and state licensing agencies to report to the National Practitioner Data Bank most disciplinary actions related to professional incompetence or misconduct (8). In addition, insurance companies must report malpractice payments above US$10,000. To prevent incompetent or impaired physicians from simply resigning from one hospital staff, relocating, and continuing to practice elsewhere, hospitals are required to obtain information from the National Practitioner Data Bank when physicians apply for hospital privileges and periodically thereafter.

The law also confers legal immunity on persons and hospitals who report impaired colleagues in good faith. Specifically, immunity is given to persons who provide "information to a professional review body regarding the competence or professional conduct of a physician" (9). In addition, peer review bodies and persons who work with or assist them are granted legal immunity. Note, however, that in Case 35.1 these provisions would not protect Dr. New if she dealt with Dr. Elder outside the formal peer-review process.

DEALING WITH IMPAIRED COLLEAGUES

Physicians can deal with impaired colleagues in several ways (Table 35-2).

TABLE 35-2   Dealing With Impaired Colleagues
Protect patients from immediate harm
Determine whether further action is needed
Talk with the colleague directly
Report the problem to responsible officials

PROTECT PATIENTS FROM IMMEDIATE HARM

If Dr. New believes that Dr. Elder's order might seriously harm the patient, then she should take immediate action. She might consider saying, "I'm sorry to intrude, but I thought I heard you say 2.50 mg of digoxin. I'm afraid the nurses might have heard the wrong dose as well." If the matter is not resolved satisfactorily, then Dr. New could call the hospital and ask the nursing supervisor at the hospital to look into the case. Dr. New should also intervene if Dr. Elder is apparently drunk on call, even if she had no direct evidence that he had made a questionable medical decision. If Dr. Elder does not agree to have a colleague take calls for him, then it would be prudent to notify another senior physician or the chief of the department and arrange for someone else to take calls, at least until Dr. Elder regains sobriety.

DETERMINE WHETHER FURTHER ACTION IS NEEDED

After preventing immediate harm to patients, Dr. New needs to assess whether additional action is needed. Gathering more information about the impaired colleague can usually be done discreetly.

Because whistle-blowing is emotionally difficult and personally risky, physicians might take smaller steps to prevent harm to patients. Many physicians would stop referring patients to such a colleague, but would otherwise let the matter drop. Other physicians cover up for impaired colleagues rather than confront them. For example, a physician might review a colleague's work and correct that doctor's errors. Although well-intentioned, such actions are ineffective in the long run. Monitoring a colleague's clinical activities is impractical and also counterproductive because it allows the physician to deny the impairment.

TALK WITH THE COLLEAGUE DIRECTLY

A physician will often want to talk with an impaired colleague directly, particularly if the colleague is a friend. Although such conversations are uncomfortable, they can be effective. The matter can be resolved if the impaired colleague agrees to seek help—for example, by enrolling in a rehabilitation program. Alternatively, physicians impaired by physical illness might decide to retire or to restrict the scope of their practice.

REPORT THE PROBLEM TO RESPONSIBLE OFFICIALS

Dr. New does not need to solve the problem of the impaired colleague by herself. She needs only to decide whether there is sufficient suspicion of impairment to warrant further investigation. In Case 35.1, Dr. New directly observed potential harm to a patient. She can discharge her ethical obligations by reporting impaired colleagues to officials who can investigate and take appropriate action. Such officials include the chief of service, the chief of staff of the hospital, or, if a trainee is involved, the director of a training program or student clerkships. These persons are responsible for ensuring the quality of patient care and the competence of medical staff. Alternatively, Dr. New might refer her colleague to the hospital's employee assistance programs or to the state medical society's physician health program. In cases of egregious impairment or incompetence, notifying the state licensing board directly might also be advisable.

Physicians often are reluctant to confront impaired colleagues or refer them to appropriate resources. In a recent survey, about one third of physicians reported that they were not prepared to deal with incompetent colleagues (10). About 17% had direct personal knowledge of such a colleague in the past 3 years; however, only one third had reported them to the hospital, clinical, or relevant authority (10). The most common reasons were that they thought someone else would do so, that nothing would happen after the report, and fear of retribution.

In a recent survey of physicians, although 96% of physicians agreed that they should report impaired or incompetent colleagues, 45% of respondents who had encountered such physicians had not reported them (11).

The case's specific circumstances influence how physicians prefer to respond to an impaired or incompetent colleague. In one survey, most house officers said they were willing to confront a fellow house officer who was impaired by alcohol but preferred to tell the chief resident or the chief of medicine about an impaired attending physician. House officers, however, were less comfortable confronting a fellow house officer who was incompetent rather than impaired and preferred to refer such matters to a more senior physician (11).

SUMMARY

1. There are understandable practical reasons why physicians hesitate to intervene with impaired colleagues.
2. There are cogent ethical reasons for physicians to take action to prevent impaired colleagues from harming patients.
3. Physician wellness programs offer a way to rehabilitate physicians in a confidential manner, while protecting patients from harm.

REFERENCES

1. Taub S, Morin K, Goldrich MS, et al. Physician health and wellness. *Occup Med (Lond)*. 2006;56:77–82.
2. O'Connor PG, Spickard A Jr. Physician impairment by substance abuse. *Med Clin North Am*. 1997;81:1037–1052.
3. Beauchamp TL, Childress JF. *Principles of Biomedical Ethics*. 5th ed. New York, NY: Oxford University Press; 2001:113–117.
4. Snyder L, Leffler C, Ethics and Human Rights Committee, et al. Ethics manual: fifth edition. *Ann Intern Med*. 2005;142:560–582.
5. Modell JG, Mountz JM. Drinking and flying—The problem of alcohol use by pilots. *N Engl J Med*. 1990;323:455–461.
6. Feinstein RJ. The ethics of professional regulation. *N Engl J Med*. 1985;312:801–804.
7. Walzer RS. Impaired physicians. An overview and update of the legal issues. *J Legal Med*. 1990;11:131–198.
8. Yeon HB, Lovett DA, Zurakowski D, et al. Physician discipline. *J Bone Joint Surg Am*. 2006;88:2091–2096.
9. Health Care Quality Improvement Act of 1990. 42 U.S.C.A. §§11101–11151.
10. DesRoches CM, Rao SR, Fromson JA, et al. Physicians' perceptions, preparedness for reporting, and experiences related to impaired and incompetent colleagues. *JAMA*. 2010;304:187–193.
11. Reuben DB, Noble S. House officer responses to impaired physicians. *JAMA*. 1990;263:958–960.

ANNOTATED BIBLIOGRAPHY

1. Taub S, Morin K, Goldrich MS, et al. Physician health and wellness. *Occup Med (Lond)*. 2006;56:77–82.
Policy paper by the American Medical Association on the clinical, ethical, and practical issues regarding impaired physicians.

CHAPTER 36

Ethical Dilemmas Students and House Staff Face

 Every clinician in training has performed a procedure knowing that someone else could do it more skillfully.

CASE 36.1 **Performing an invasive procedure**

Obviously tired after a 9-hour wait in the emergency room, a woman with an asthma exacerbation is finally admitted to her room. "Oh no, not another needlestick!" she groans, as a medical student approaches to draw arterial blood gases. The medical student gulps, because his previous attempts have been unsuccessful or required multiple punctures.

The trainee's self-interest in learning in Case 36.1 might conflict with his patients' best interests. Learning clinical skills and taking responsibility might present inconvenience, discomfort, or even risk to patients. Ethical conflicts also arise when trainees observe unethical or substandard care by other physicians. Both trainees and patients benefit when these issues are addressed openly. Ideally, the patient's welfare should be paramount. Because of the power that senior physicians have over trainees, however, trainees who voice ethical concerns need to be protected.

LEARNING ON PATIENTS

In their training, medical students might worry that they are taking unfair advantage of patients but hesitate to discuss their concerns with supervisors (1, 2). They fear that their reputation or career might suffer or that they will be viewed as reluctant to take responsibility.

INTRODUCING TRAINEES TO PATIENTS

CASE 36.2 **Introducing students as physicians**

The attending physician introduces a medical student on a third-year clerkship to the patient as "Doctor." When the student raises concerns, the attending physician insists that students have to get over their "hang-ups" about taking responsibility, declaring, "Patients who come here know that students will be taking care of them. If they did not agree, they would go somewhere else."

Several reasons are offered for not introducing students as physicians. Patients might not trust trainees or might worry needlessly about their care. As in Case 36.2, some physicians believe that patients in a teaching hospital have given "implied consent" to trainees to care for them. There are compelling reasons, however, to introduce students truthfully. Patient trust should not be built on misrepresentation. Patients who are misled about a health care provider's role might feel betrayed if they discover the trainee's status. Informed consent requires physicians to disclose pertinent information to patients (*see* Chapter 3). State laws and accreditation requirements may also require trainees to disclose their educational status to patients (3). The argument that patients who seek care at teaching hospitals have given implied consent to be "teaching material" is untenable. The concept of "implied consent" applies only to emergency situations in which delaying treatment would seriously harm a patient who is unable to give consent.

Concerns that patients will worry inappropriately should be addressed with more information about teaching hospitals, not less. Ideally, attending physicians should introduce themselves and the other members of the team, explaining roles, how trainees are supervised, and how they enhance the quality of care. Trainees are accessible around the clock, often have more time to search the literature and answer questions, and are closely supervised. Overall, primary teaching hospitals have a lower rate of adverse patient events due to negligence than nonteaching hospitals (4). For surgical procedures, evidence is mixed. One study found increased mortality in teaching hospitals for emergency procedures but not for elective procedures (5). Another study found lower mortality with resident intraoperative involvement but higher postoperative complications (6). Most patients agree that trainees enhance the quality of their care and want to contribute to a trainee's education (7, 8).

Some trainees resort to unfamiliar titles, such as "clinical clerk," that are literally true and avoid the adverse consequences of explicitly calling oneself a student. Such titles, however, are unacceptable because they are incomprehensible to patients and are intended to mislead. "Student physician" is commonly used and emphasizes the special medical training that the student has received. Residents often introduce themselves to patients as physicians without specifying their level of training or their role (9).

CASE 36.2   *Continued*

The student should talk with the attending physician or the clerkship director about being introduced. If the attending physician has strong opinions about calling students doctors, it may be more appropriate for the clerkship director to speak with the attending physician. The student should raise explicit concerns about how his grade might be affected by a disagreement with a faculty member.

If the faculty member declines to make such an introduction, the student needs to weigh being forthright with patients against his understandable concerns about grades. Most patients will infer that students are still in training, for example, from name tags or comments by other staff. The student might explain privately to the patient, "I wanted to explain to you that I'm a medical student working closely with the other members of the team. Dr. R likes to call everyone "doctor," but I wanted to talk with you and give you a chance to ask question." Most patients appreciate such honesty.

LEARNING BASIC CLINICAL SKILLS

To learn to take a history, perform a physical examination, draw blood, and start intravenous lines, medical students need to practice on patients. Although patients are not subjected to any serious medical risks, they might be inconvenienced, lose privacy, or experience some discomfort. Out of respect for patients, the attending physician or resident should ask permission first. When asked, almost all patients agree to have students listen to a heart murmur or perform a history and physical examination. Although it is reasonable to ask patients to spend an hour with a student, it is inappropriate to ask them to spend 3 hours for an exhaustive student examination, to miss their meals, or to lose sleep.

LEARNING INTIMATE EXAMINATIONS

Although patient consent to participation by trainees in their care is always important, it is particularly important for intimate examinations, such as pelvic, rectal, breast, and testicular examinations, because of the sensitive and private nature of the procedure. Most medical schools have students learn pelvic examinations with women who are paid to do this and are trained to provide feedback to students on their performance (10). This process benefits students by decreasing their anxiety and enhancing their communication skills (11). When students carry out intimate exams with real patients, as a matter of respect for patients and their autonomy, explicit permission should be obtained (10, 12). When asked in advance without feeling pressured, the overwhelming majority of patients allow such examinations (10).

Pelvic examinations done under anesthesia offer opportunities for students to master a difficult skill. Because a woman's muscles are relaxed under anesthesia, a more thorough examination is possible. Senior physicians sometimes ask students to perform pelvic examinations on an anesthetized patient in the operating room without her consent. Consent for surgery, however, does not include consent for examination by students, so that explicit consent for student examinations is required. Under a California law, trainees may not perform a pelvic examination on an anesthetized or unconscious patient without informed consent, unless the examination is within the scope of their care for the patient (13).

LEARNING INVASIVE PROCEDURES

When trainees learn invasive procedures, such as lumbar puncture or insertion of central lines, their first patients might experience increased discomfort or even risk. The trainee's self-interest in learning and long-term goal of benefiting future patients might conflict with the short-term goal of providing the best care to current patients. Trainees frequently do not discuss their participation in invasive procedures with patients, fearing that patients will request more experienced physicians. Such requests would be understandable; physicians might consider whether they would be willing to have a trainee perform the procedure on a close relative.

In the spirit of informed consent, patients need to understand who will be performing invasive procedures and what additional risk, if any, can be attributed to trainees. For surgical procedures, almost all patients want the attending surgeon to tell them what the resident medical student will do during the operation (7, 14, 15). Patients consider such disclosure more important than medical students do (15).

Attending physicians should tell patients about the participation of students and residents in their care and introduce trainees (16, 17). Patient concerns about trainees are best resolved by providing more information. When informed and given a choice, most patients allow trainees to do procedures. Almost all patients are willing to have students perform simple procedures, such as suturing or starting an IV (18). For more invasive procedures, 27% of emergency department patients would not allow a resident to perform a lumbar puncture and 52% would not allow a resident to perform intubation (19). Most patients agree to have trainees participate in surgery (16, 17, 20). Patient requests to have a more experienced physician perform the procedure should be honored, if possible.

Trainees should carry out procedures only under adequate supervision, except in dire emergencies. Without supervision, the patient might be placed at unnecessary risk and the trainee will not be able to learn from the experience. The hospital has a responsibility to provide such supervision, and the trainee also has a responsibility to obtain it before starting the procedure. The senior physician should take over the procedure, if needed.

LEARNING ON UNCONSCIOUS OR DEAD PATIENTS

Trainees might face further dilemmas when they are asked to learn on unconscious or newly dead patients without explicit consent to do so. For example, an attending physician might tell a medical student and intern to perform pelvic examinations on a patient under general anesthesia. Pelvic examinations performed under anesthesia without explicit permission, however, violate patient privacy and autonomy (*see* Chapter 41).

Learning invasive procedures on newly dead patients without the next of kin's consent creates similar dilemmas. After a patient dies, the resident might instruct interns and students to practice intubation and inserting a central venous catheter. "The patient is dead. You can't hurt her, but you might hurt a live patient if you don't practice." Such practice increases skill and, thereby, benefits future patients (21). Some argue that dead bodies cannot be harmed. Invasive procedures, however, might be regarded as disfiguring, offensive, or a violation of the corpse's dignity (21, 22). Dead patients are not "teaching material." They deserve to be treated with respect.

Some physicians suggest that practicing invasive procedures should be permitted unless relatives specifically object. Unless family members, however, are informed of this practice, they might not know to raise objections. A better policy would be to obtain consent from survivors for practicing invasive procedures on newly dead patients (21–24). When consent is sought candidly and compassionately, most family members give permission (23, 25). In a predominantly non-White sample, however, almost one half of respondents would be angry if asked to allow trainees to learn invasive procedures on a newly deceased relative (26). Permission from survivors also helps trainees to resolve their own ambivalence over learning on patients and to appreciate that their training depends on patient altruism.

TAKING TOO MUCH CLINICAL RESPONSIBILITY

Trainees sometimes assume too much decision-making responsibility without adequate supervision (1, 2). For instance, a resident on a busy service might tell a subintern to sign his or her name on the physicians' order sheet, saying "You're a good student, and you can page me if you have a real question." It is unrealistic to expect the student to distinguish routine orders from serious management decisions. Errors in judgment or dosage can occur even with "routine" orders. Furthermore, the resident is giving the student a mixed message: "Call me for serious problems, but if you're a good student you won't bother me." Discouraging trainees' questions also reduces opportunities for learning. Students who request adequate supervision implicitly criticize the resident and might experience retaliation in grades and evaluations. They might be labeled as "not a team player," "insecure," or "reluctant to assume responsibility."

The training system might place the student in an untenable situation by exerting pressure to take too much responsibility or failing to set clear expectations or provide sufficient supervision. The institution should clarify expectations for supervising trainees and establish a procedure for residents to ask for help, which might require more involvement from the attending physician or transferring some patients to another team.

Trainees are accountable for taking too much responsibility and placing patients at increased risk. Ethically, trainees need to know their own limitations and should not exceed them.

LIMITS ON WORK HOURS

Residency accreditation bodies limit house staff work hours to prevent fatigue and burnout and to reduce medical errors. Strictly observing such limits, however, might raise ethical dilemmas.

CASE 36.3	House staff work hours

During an on-call night, an intern has admitted only two patients. After doing rounds, he has finished his tour-of-duty and is checking out when he gets paged. A 78-year-old woman that he admitted with pyelonephritis now has a temperature of 39° C, a blood pressure of 100/60, a pulse of 110, and seems confused. The cross-covering intern appears stressed; she exclaims, "Look, I've already had four admissions. How can you dump a patient like this?"

In Case 36.3, the harried cross-cover intern accuses her colleague of "dumping" a patient. This term highlights the way in which stressed physicians might focus their attention on their own well-being, rather than the patient's interests. Ironically, restrictions on house staff work hours were intended to reduce stress on physicians. The intern signing out might feel that he should help his colleague by staying longer. After all, he might be overwhelmed some day and need similar help. In this case, he does not feel tired. Moreover, the patient in early septic shock needs timely attention. It is commendable to help colleagues during unexpected emergencies. On-call systems, however, should anticipate that house officers who are on call might be overwhelmed. The interns should be able to call on the resident, the attending physician, a "float," or rapid response team for help. In the long run, asking busy interns to stay additional hours to help others only leads to more stress, fatigue, and greater risk for patients.

CASE 36.3   *Continued*

The intern ending his shift might say, "Boy, you are really getting hit. Let me try to help. I can sign her out to your resident, who can start antibiotics and stabilize her. I sure hope it lightens up later for you." In this way the outgoing intern need only spend a few extra minutes, the cross-cover physician will feel less stressed, and, most important, the patient will receive urgent care promptly.

In other cases, a resident can provide an irreplaceable benefit to a patient or family by working a little longer than the scheduled hours. For example, a resident might be in the middle of a discussion about withdrawing life-sustaining interventions or comforting a family member over a patient's death. It would be desirable for the resident to stay to finish the conversation before signing out to the covering physician. In this situation, the rapport that the physician has developed with the patient or family is not readily transferred to another doctor. Under such circumstances, strict adherence to the time clock would undermine the ideals of benefiting patients and acting with compassion. Such situations, however, should remain exceptions and should not create an expectation that trainees should routinely exceed limits of working hours.

RELATIONSHIPS WITH COLLEAGUES

CASE 36.4   **Lying or equivocating on rounds**

A 54-year-old man is admitted with severe pancreatitis. Overnight he required large volumes of fluid to maintain his blood pressure. While the intern is presenting the patient on rounds, the attending physician asks, "So what happened to his calcium?" The intern remembers that calcium is a prognostic factor that should be followed in pancreatitis. Although he checked the patient's laboratory tests, the intern cannot remember whether he specifically reviewed the calcium. He thinks he would have noticed if the calcium had not been normal.

In Case 36.4, the intern feels a tension between making a good impression on the attending physician and acting for the patient's benefit. If the intern says that the calcium was normal when it was not, then the subsequent plan of care might be inappropriate. Hence, the ethical analysis is clear: The intern should say what he did and offer to verify the value at the nearest computer terminal.

The culture of the hospital and team is important. An attending physician who tends to criticize trainees sharply deters them from telling the truth and from learning. A teaching style that stresses interns might be counterproductive. Slips in which a person forgets something are unavoidable. Usually they are due to the limits of human cognition, not neglect. Exhorting interns to be more careful or shaming them cannot remedy slips. It is more constructive for resident and attending physician to reinforce the value of truth-telling by stopping rounds to look up the value, by discussing why the calcium level is important in this case, and suggesting how to develop a routine or a checklist to ensure that essential tasks are carried out.

PROFESSIONALISM

Training programs evaluate medical students and residents for professionalism, which has been defined in terms of such core values as altruism, respect for patients and colleagues, humanism, accountability, and commitment to knowledge and high-quality care (27). These professional values are similar to what philosophers term *virtues*, characteristics and attitudes that should be inherent in a good physician. Professional values are both aspirations and expectations for behavior. They are often transmitted through a hidden curriculum, by residents rather than faculty, and through stories rather than formal teaching. Evaluations regarding professionalism are challenging because expectations may not be explicit or specific.

It is hoped that greater focus professionalism during training may reduce future misconduct. Discipline by a medical board was strongly associated with previous unprofessional behavior in the medical school (28). The strongest predictor was irresponsibility, which included unreliable attendance at clinic and not following up on patient care activities. Another factor was diminished capacity for self-improvement, including failure to accept criticism, argumentativeness, and poor attitude.

Physicians voluntarily adopt standards set by professional organizations and "profess" them to the community (27, 29, 30). Professions may be defined as occupations that seek to regulate themselves. Professional standards may be higher than legal requirements; for example, respect for patients requires physicians to do more than the legal requirements for informed consent. Critics charge that professional standards may overlook problems that concern patients, such as poor access to care and the high cost of care. Professional organizations historically have served as advocacy groups for physicians, and their efforts to obtain favorable reimbursement for physicians may conflict with patients' desires for more affordable health care. Furthermore, society may also seek standards that professional groups oppose, for example, disclosure of medical errors. The public may also want harsher sanctions for incompetent or unethical physician behavior than medical institutions are willing to enforce.

Although professionalism and clinical ethics overlap, there are several important differences. First, professional values are usually expressed in very general terms. It may not be clear how they apply in a specific case or how physicians should act when different professional values are in conflict. For example, a resident might be faced with a choice between spending time explaining a potential procedure to a patient and being late for a conference where she is presenting the case. In fact, evaluations of professionalism by faculty are inconsistent (31). Second, evaluations of professionalism sometimes reward deference to senior physicians and the academic hierarchy (32). Students allege that they sometimes are cited for unprofessional behavior when they are trying to point out unprofessional behavior by senior physicians. Third, professionalism focuses on shortcomings in personal behavior. In contrast, ethics also addresses situations where well-intentioned people disagree over the proper course of action or where important values or ethical principles are in conflict. Fourth, ethics focuses on articulating the reasons that support a certain decision in a particular situation. It is not sufficient for professionals to know the most appropriate course of action; they also must be able to justify their action to other health care workers and the patient.

UNETHICAL CARE BY OTHER PHYSICIANS

Trainees might be involved in cases in which senior physicians appear to violate ethical guidelines (32–34).

CASE 36.5   Failure to obtain informed consent for sterilization

An attending obstetrician performs a tubal ligation on a 32-year-old Latina on Medicaid who has just delivered her sixth child by cesarean section. According to the chart, the patient refused sterilization at her last prenatal visit. The resident who delivered the baby and served as the translator for the patient is outraged. The delivery room nurse confirms that no informed consent was obtained, but cautions, "Don't ruin your career over this."

Some disagreements reflect reasonable differences of clinical judgment or misunderstanding by the trainee. In Case 36.5, however, the attending physician is violating the ethical guideline of respecting patient autonomy, as well as laws on informed consent. The resident felt outraged at the event, frustrated at being powerless, guilty that she did not intervene, and ashamed that she had become an accomplice in an unethical deed. She believed that the attending physician's action was both sexist and racist.

Trainees might observe grossly substandard care by senior physicians, as when they fail to round on patients, write progress notes, or answer pages (32, 33). In cases of clearly inadequate care, the trainee has an ethical obligation to protect patients and to not mislead them. In addition, there is an ethical obligation to try to prevent harm to future patients if a pattern of impairment exists (*see* Chapter 35). There are also strong countervailing pragmatic considerations, as we discuss next.

RISKS TO WHISTLE-BLOWERS

Fear of retaliation is a legitimate practical concern for trainees (34). The obstetrics resident in Case 36.5 might receive a bad evaluation or unfavorable treatment during the rest of her training. As in all occupations, whistle-blowers might suffer harm even if their accusations prove valid. Ideally, the patient's well-being should take priority over the trainee's self-interest. Individual trainees need to decide how much personal risk as a whistle-blower they are willing to accept relative to the harm they might prevent.

SUGGESTIONS FOR TRAINEES

Involve Other Physicians

Trainees often feel that they have to resolve these troubling situations by themselves. However, they should discuss the situation with trusted colleagues and senior physicians. These discussions allow trainees to verify that they have observed unethical misconduct or markedly substandard care, rather than a reasonable difference of judgment. Such reality testing is often crucial for their peace of mind and sense of integrity. In addition, other people might provide emotional support, give advice, and intervene constructively. The chief resident, clerkship or residency director, and chief of service have an obligation to address issues of unethical or incompetent behavior (34). Furthermore, every hospital should have procedures, such as quality assurance programs or a patient ombudsperson, for investigating such cases (34).

Decide What to Tell the Patient

In addition to informing appropriate senior physicians, the trainee needs to consider what to tell patients, if anything. There are strong reasons why patients should have truthful information about events that will affect their future medical care and life plans. The sterilized woman in Case 36.5 cannot make informed decisions about reproduction if she does not know that a tubal ligation was performed.

Trainees do not need to inform the patient personally if they inform some responsible senior physician, such as the chief of service. Trainees, however, do need to answer truthfully if the patient asks the trainee directly what happened.

Protect Your Own Interests

Trainees who fulfill their obligations to patients should minimize risks to themselves (32). Some measures, such as writing an angry note in the chart or directly accusing the attending physician of being unethical, are likely to inflame the situation. Involving more senior physicians can reduce the risk of reprisals. Trainees who are unwilling to be identified as accusers can still discuss episodes with the quality assurance committee or chief of staff. In this way, if other people are willing to come forward, there will be corroborating evidence. In addition, trainees should keep records of how they raised their concerns.

SUMMARY

1. Trainees' interests in learning clinical medicine and invasive procedures might conflict with patients' interests. The ethical guideline of preventing harm to patients might conflict with trainees' career advancement.
2. The ethical ideal is for all trainees to act in patients' best interests, even at some personal risk or disadvantage.

REFERENCES

1. Christakis DA, Feudtner C. Ethics in a short white coat: the ethical dilemmas that medical students confront. *Acad Med.* 1993;68:249–254.
2. Rosenbaum JR, Bradley EH, Holmboe ES, et al. Sources of ethical conflict in medical housestaff training: a qualitative study. *Am J Med.* 2004;116:402–407.
3. Marracino RK, Orr RD. Entitling the student doctor: defining the student's role in patient care. *J Gen Intern Med.* 1998;13:266–270.
4. Brennan TA, Hebert L, Laird NM, et al. Hospital characteristics associated with adverse events and substandard care. *JAMA.* 1991;265:3265–3269.
5. Holena DN, Hadler R, Wirtalla C, et al. Teaching status: the impact on emergency and elective surgical care in the US. *Ann Surg.* 2011;253:1017–1023.
6. Raval MV, Wang X, Cohen ME, et al. The influence of resident involvement on surgical outcomes. *J Am Coll Surg.* 2011;212:889–898.
7. Kim N, Lo B, Gates EA. Disclosing the role of residents and medical students in hysterectomy: what do patients want? *Acad Med.* 1998;73:339–341.
8. Magrane D, Jannon J, Miller CT. Obstetric patients who select and those who refuse medical students' participation in their care. *Acad Med.* 1994;69:1004–1006.
9. Santen SA, Rotter TS, Hemphill RR. Patients do not know the level of training of their doctors because doctors do not tell them. *J Gen Intern Med.* 2008;23:607–610.
10. Wolfberg AJ. The patient as ally—learning the pelvic examination. *N Engl J Med.* 2007;356:889–890.
11. Jha V, Setna Z, Al-Hity A, et al. Patient involvement in teaching and assessing intimate examination skills: a systematic review. *Med Educ.* 2010;44:347–357.
12. Bibby J, Boyd N, Redman C, et al. Consent for vaginal examination by students on anaesthetised patients (letter). *Lancet.* 1988; 2:1150.
13. Cal. Bus & Prof. Code §2281 (2003).
14. Wisner DM, Quillen DA, Benderson DM, et al. Patient attitudes toward resident involvement in cataract surgery. *Arch Ophthalmol.* 2008;126:1235–1239.
15. Silver-Isenstadt A, Ubel PA. Erosion in medical students' attitudes about telling patients they are students. *J Gen Intern Med.* 1999;14:481–487.
16. Wisner DM, Quillen DA, Benderson DM, Green MJ. Patient attitudes toward resident involvement in cataract surgery. *Arch Ophthalmol* 2008;126:1235-1239.
17. Kim N, Lo B, Gates EA. Disclosing the role of residents and medical students in hysterectomy: what do patients want? *Acad Med* 1998;73:339-341.
18. Santen SA, Hemphill RR, Spanier CM, et al. 'Sorry, it's my first time!' Will patients consent to medical students learning procedures? *Med Educ.* 2005;39:365–369.
19. Santen SA, Hemphill RR, McDonald MF, et al. Patients' willingness to allow residents to learn to practice medical procedures. *Acad Med.* 2004;79:144–147.
20. Porta CR, Sebesta JA, Brown TA, et al. Training surgeons and the informed consent process: routine disclosure of trainee participation and its effect on patient willingness and consent rates. *Arch Surg.* 2012;147:57–62. doi:10.1001/archsurg.2011.235.
21. Jones JW, McCullough LB. Ethics of re-hearsing procedures on a corpse. *J Vasc Surg.* 2011;54:879–880.
22. Berger JT, Rosner F, Cassell EJ. Ethics of practicing medical procedures on newly dead and nearly dead patients. *J Gen Intern Med.* 2002;17:774–778.
23. Schmidt TA, Abbott JT, Geiderman JM, et al. Ethics seminars: the ethical debate on practicing procedures on the newly dead. *Acad Emerg Med.* 2004;11:962–966.
24. Council on Ethical and Judicial Affairs of the American Medical Association. Performing procedures on the newly deceased. *Acad Med.* 2002;77:1212–1216.
25. McNamara RM, Monti S, Kelly JJ. Requesting consent for an invasive procedure in newly deceased adults. *JAMA.* 1995;273:310–312.

26. Morag RM, DeSouza S, Steen PA, et al. Performing procedures on the newly deceased for teaching purposes: what if we were to ask? *Arch Intern Med.* 2005;165:92–96.
    intubation skills using newly deceased infants. *JAMA.* 1991;265:2360–2363.
27. ABIM Foundation, ACP-ASIM Foundation, European Federation of Internal Medicine. Medical professionalism in the new millennium: a physician charter. *Ann Intern Med.* 2002;136:243–246.
28. Papadakis MA, Teherani A, Banach MA, et al. Disciplinary action by medical boards and prior behavior in medical school. *N Engl J Med.* 2005;353:2673–2682.
29. Pellegrino ED, Thomasma DG. *For the Patient's Good: The Restoration of Beneficence in Health Care.* New York, NY: Oxford University Press; 1988.
30. Pellegrino ED. Toward a reconstruction of medical morality. *Am J Bioeth.* 2006;6:65–71.
31. Ginsburg S, Regehr G, Lingard L. Basing the evaluation of professionalism on observable behaviors: a cautionary tale. *Acad Med.* 2004;79:S1–S4.
32. Brainard AH, Brislen HC. Viewpoint: learning professionalism: a view from the trenches. *Acad Med.* 2007;82:1010–1014.
33. Caldicott CV, Faber-Langendoen K. Deception, discrimination, and fear of reprisal: lessons in ethics from third-year medical students. *Acad Med.* 2005;80:866–873.
34. Satterwhite WM, Satterwhite RC, Enarson CE. Medical students' perceptions of unethical conduct at one medical school. *Acad Med.* 1998;73:529–531.

ANNOTATED BIBLIOGRAPHY

1. Marracino RK, Orr RD. Entitling the student doctor: defining the student's role in patient care. *J Gen Intern Med.* 1998;13:266–270.
   Analyzes why medical students are often not introduced to patients as medical students.
2. Wolfberg AJ. The patient as ally—learning the pelvic examination. *N Engl J Med.* 2007;356:889–890.
   Thoughtful discussion of ethical issues in learning intimate examinations, emphasizing the need for patient consent.
3. Jones JW, McCullough LB. Ethics of re-hearsing procedures on a corpse. *J Vasc Surg.* 2011;54:879–880.
   Analysis of the ethical issues regarding learning procedures on the newly dead. Recommends that informed consent from next of kin be obtained.
4. Ginsburg S, Regehr G, Lingard L. Basing the evaluation of professionalism on observable behaviors: a cautionary tale. *Acad Med.* 2004;79:S1–S4.
   Faculty disagree over whether behaviors by medical students constitute unprofessional behavior or not. The authors caution that judgments about professionalism must pay attention to the clinical context, how the student interprets the situation, and what values he perceives to be at stake.

Ethical Issues in Clinical Specialties

VI

Ethical Issues in Clinical Specialties

CHAPTER 37

Ethical Issues in Pediatrics

Children are immature and depend on their parents or guardians emotionally and financially. They cannot make informed decisions about their care. Children must be protected from the consequences of unwise decisions that they or others make. It is tragic if a child dies or suffers serious harm because a simple, effective medical treatment was not provided.

HOW ARE ETHICAL ISSUES IN PEDIATRICS DIFFERENT?

CHILDREN ARE NOT AUTONOMOUS

Because young children cannot weigh risks and benefits, compare alternatives, or appreciate the long-term consequences of choices, they are incapable of making informed decisions. Hence, autonomy is less important in pediatrics than in adult medicine. Children's objections to beneficial medical interventions do not have the same ethical force as adults' informed refusals. Because children are immature and vulnerable, they need an adult to make decisions for them and to look after their best interests. Parents are presumed to be the appropriate decision makers for their children (1).

PHYSICIANS SHOULD BE ADVOCATES FOR CHILDREN

Doctors have a unique opportunity to identify when a child's health and well-being are jeopardized by their parents' decisions or actions. Physicians therefore have special responsibilities in these situations to prevent suffering serious, long-lasting harm.

RESPECT CHILDREN'S POTENTIAL TO BECOME AUTONOMOUS

Children's potential to become autonomous adults deserves respect. Parents mold children, and parental values deserve great deference. However, when children reach maturity they might choose different values from their parents'. Physicians need to help ensure that parental decisions do not close off a child's open future as a unique person. As children grow, they become capable of making informed decisions, and their involvement in care should increase. Physicians need to provide children with information about their conditions and opportunities to participate in decisions about their care, to the extent it is appropriate developmentally (1).

WHAT STANDARDS TO USE IN DECIDING FOR CHILDREN?

Because children cannot make informed decisions, beneficence—acting in the child's best interest—is the primary ethical guideline in pediatrics.

CHILDREN'S BEST INTERESTS

The concept of "best interests" emphasizes that children are persons separate from their parents, with their own interests and rights. Generally parents' decisions and ongoing involvement in a child's care promote the child's best interests. Assessments of a child's best interests, however, may be contested, with reasonable people disagreeing over which outcomes and risks are acceptable, and how to weigh the benefits and burdens of interventions. Moreover, promoting some of the child's interests might set back other interests of the family.

A child's best interests include both the duration and quality of life. Although quality-of-life judgments seem unavoidable, they might also be ethically problematic. It is difficult to predict a child's future quality of life. Healthy people tend to underestimate the quality of life of persons with chronic illness. Although some people believe that Down syndrome is a fate worse than death, many children with this condition experience happiness and are prized by their parents. Chapter 4 discusses best interests in detail.

CHILDREN'S PREFERENCES

To the extent that children have the capacity to make informed decisions about their medical care, their choices should be respected. Chapter 10 discusses how to determine whether a patient has the capacity to make medical decisions.

Even when children are not capable of giving informed consent, their *assent* to interventions is still ethically important if it is developmentally appropriate. It is disturbing to force interventions on a child who can understand what will be done and is actively resisting it. A child's objections, however, are not necessarily decisive. For instance, a child who objects to shots should still receive immunizations. Forced therapy, however, becomes problematic if children are older, the effectiveness of the intervention is uncertain, or the side effects are more probable, more serious, or longer lasting. The physician should listen to and respond to the child's reasons for dissenting from treatment. If interventions are carried out despite the child's objections, it is appropriate for the doctor to apologize to the child.

PARENTS' AND OTHER FAMILY MEMBERS' INTERESTS

Although the child's best interests are of primary concern, parents and other family members have interests that must also be taken into account. What is best for an individual child can be understood only in the context of what is best for the family as a whole or for other family members. Parents cannot be expected to devote all their energy and resources to one child, even though they should make some sacrifices; for example, parents might choose not to buy a house in the best school district, but instead to live closer to their jobs.

WHO SHOULD DECIDE FOR CHILDREN?

THE PRESUMPTION OF PARENTAL DECISION MAKING

Parents are presumed to be the appropriate decision makers for their children. Generally, love motivates them to do what is best for their children. In addition, parents have long-term relationships with and obligations to their children. In most cases, parents concur with physicians' recommendations—for example, agreeing to antibiotics for strep throat, bronchodilators for asthma, and surgery for appendicitis.

American culture prizes parental responsibility, family integrity, and strong parent–child relationships. Parents or guardians have considerable latitude, but not unlimited discretion, in raising children. Within limits set by society, parents have discretion to inculcate their values in children and to make choices for rearing their children. For example, children must attend school, but parents may choose the type of school.

Physicians speak of *parental permission* rather than consent to distinguish what people may decide for themselves from what they may decide for their children. Although informed adults have a right to refuse any medical intervention, parents do not have absolute power to refuse care for their children (1). As noted, parental permission should be supplemented with the child's assent when developmentally appropriate (1).

Parents commonly ask physicians what they would do if it were their child. Physicians need to clarify what the parents are asking (2). They might be asking what care would optimize their child's outcome, seeking the physician's medical judgment and reasoning. Alternatively, parents might ask whether they are making the right choice. The physician's response needs to be supportive and compassionate. If the parents want to know what the physician personally would do, it is helpful for physicians to describe the process of decision making they would use, including talking with relatives and friends, as well as what factors they would consider. If parents still want to know what the physician would do, then it is appropriate to offer a recommendation based on the parents' values and goals, which may differ from the physician's.

Emergencies

In an emergency, when a parent or guardian is not available and a delay in treatment would jeopardize the child's life or health, the physician should act in the child's best interests and immediately provide appropriate treatment without waiting for parental permission (3).

Exceptions to Parental Decision Making

Some parents are estranged from their children or unwilling to be involved in their care. Other parents lack the capacity to make informed decisions, for example, because of substance abuse or developmental disability. Strictly speaking, parents should make decisions for children unless a court has appointed someone else as guardian. Informal arrangements, however, are often made for another relative to make decisions when parents are absent or incapable of making decisions.

ADOLESCENT PATIENTS

As children mature, they develop the capacity to make informed decisions about their health care. Most states allow 18-year-olds to give informed consent or refusal to medical care without parental involvement. Younger minors may make their own decisions about health care because of their status or the condition for which treatment is sought (4, 5). State laws regarding the medical care of adolescents balance several countervailing policy goals: fostering access to treatment for important public health problems, respecting adolescents who are functionally adults, and encouraging parental involvement in their children's care. Because statutes vary according to state and medical condition, physicians need to know the laws in their jurisdiction.

Status of the Minor

Mature minors are capable of giving informed consent. Ethically, mature minors should be allowed to consent to or refuse medical treatment. Generally, adolescents above 14 or 15 years of age have such decision-making capacity, but younger children commonly have difficulty entertaining alternatives, appreciating the consequences of decisions, and appraising their future realistically. In most states, a court must declare an adolescent a matured minor.

Emancipated minors are recognized as *de facto* adults because of marriage, service in the armed forces, or living apart from parents and managing their own finances. Many states require a judicial hearing and declaration of emancipation by the courts (5).

Treatment of Specified Conditions

Most states allow minors to obtain treatment without parental permission for sensitive conditions, such as sexually transmitted infections (STIs), contraception, pregnancy, sexual assault, substance abuse, and psychiatric illness (6). The rationale is not that adolescents who seek treatment for such conditions are making informed decisions—indeed, these conditions might impair judgment or result from unwise choices. Instead, the justification is that requiring parental permission would deter many adolescents from seeking treatment for important, treatable public health problems. Even when adolescents consent to such care themselves, it is generally in their best interests to involve their parents in their subsequent care.

Parental Requests for Treatment

Parents might request that the physician test an adolescent for illicit use or pregnancy without telling the child (7). Although parents are naturally concerned, surreptitious testing is unacceptable because it violates the adolescent's emerging autonomy, creates mistrust and suspicion in the family, and undermines the physician–child relationship (7).

PHYSICIAN–CHILD–PARENT–RELATIONSHIP

Disclosing of information to children, protecting confidentiality, and truth-telling show respect for children, lead to beneficial consequences, and foster trust in the medical profession.

DISCLOSURE OF INFORMATION TO CHILDREN

Physicians should provide children pertinent information about their care in terms they can understand. Children who cannot understand medical details might still want to know what will be done to them. Doctors should also obtain the child's assent if this is developmentally appropriate.

Some parents do not want their children to know about serious diagnoses, such as cancer or HIV infection (8). Physicians should elicit the parents' concerns and fears. Parents might believe that the child will not be able to handle bad news or that peers will reject the child. Physicians can explain how children usually cope better, have fewer psychosocial problems, and adhere more closely to treatment if they understand their diagnosis and the proposed therapy. Parental requests for secrecy are particularly difficult when adolescents are capable of making health care decisions. Generally, physicians can persuade parents to allow disclosure of information to the child, provide developmentally appropriate information, and help the child cope with the news. One study of children who died of cancer found that no parent regretted talking with their child about death, but many parents who did not do so later regretted it (9).

Physicians should give forthright answers when children ask directly about their diagnosis. Deceiving the child would compromise the physician's integrity and patients' trust in the medical system.

CONFIDENTIALITY

Exceptions to Confidentiality

Physicians and other health care workers must report cases of suspected child abuse or neglect to child protective services agencies. Confidentiality is overridden to protect vulnerable children from a high likelihood of serious harm. To be justified in reporting a case, physicians do not need definitive proof of abuse and neglect, but only sufficient information to warrant a fuller investigation. In evaluating possible cases of child abuse, physicians should treat parents with respect, keeping in mind that most parents are trying their best to deal with a difficult situation. Intervention might enable parents to obtain enough assistance and support to prevent further abuse. In extreme cases, protective service agencies may remove the child from parental custody.

Disclosure to Schools

Physicians might need to disclose health information to schools. Whenever information is disclosed, physicians should disclose only information that is truly needed. For example, a school does not need to know the diagnosis, but only that the child's absence was medically indicated. Doctors might also need to arrange for the child to receive medications at school. It is useful for physicians to discuss how parents, the child, and school personnel might respond to inquiries about the child's health in ways that maintain confidentiality.

Adolescents

Adolescents commonly wish to keep certain information confidential from their parents—for instance, that they are receiving care for mental health, STDs, pregnancy, or substance abuse (10, 11). Assurances of confidentiality increase the willingness of adolescents to seek needed health care, particularly for such sensitive conditions, and to disclose information candidly to physicians. Concerns about confidentiality deter adolescents from seeking needed care. Hence, physicians should routinely discuss confidentiality with adolescents and offer them an opportunity to talk privately, apart from parents.

Many physicians provide absolute rather than conditional assurances of confidentiality (12). As Chapter 5 discussed, however, overriding confidentiality is ethically appropriate and legally mandated in several situations. Moreover, most adolescents believe that confidentiality should be overridden when a patient plans to commit suicide or has been physically or sexually abused. Thus, physicians should explain that confidentiality is not absolute and that exceptions are made in specific situations (10).

Even when adolescents are allowed to consent to treatment for sensitive conditions, parents' involvement in their subsequent care will generally be beneficial. State laws on informing parents of the adolescent's care vary both according to the condition and by state (13). For some sensitive conditions, physicians are required to notify parents or are permitted (but not required) to do so. In other conditions, physicians are prohibited from informing parents without the minor's consent. In still other conditions, doctors may use their judgment about disclosing to parents.

Generally, physicians should encourage adolescents to discuss medical decisions with their parents, who usually provide useful support and advice (11). It is often impossible to keep the parents from learning about the child's condition because of the condition's nature, the practicalities of obtaining treatment, or the need to pay for care. Doctors can offer to help adolescents disclose information to their parents. In some situations, disclosure might be counterproductive or dangerous, as when domestic violence is likely. In such situations, it would be desirable for the adolescent to confide in a trusted adult relative.

REFUSAL OF MEDICAL INTERVENTIONS

DISAGREEMENTS BETWEEN PARENTS AND PHYSICIANS

Parents sometimes refuse care that physicians believe is in the child's best interests or provide suboptimal care for the child at home. Doctors need to try to persuade parents to accept effective interventions that have few side effects (see Chapter 4). In addition, physicians, together with social workers and nurses, can mobilize emotional support and social resources to help the parents provide better care. In rare situations, physicians should ask the courts to override parental decisions—for example, when parents cannot be persuaded to accept life-saving therapy that has few side effects, such as antibiotics for bacterial meningitis in a previously healthy child. If disagreements persist, then the physician's response to parents' refusal of treatment will depend on the clinical circumstances, the benefits and burdens of treatment, and, in some cases, on the child's wishes.

INTERVENTIONS OF LIMITED EFFECTIVENESS OR GREAT BURDENS

Physicians should respect parents' informed refusals of interventions that have limited effectiveness, impose significant side effects, require chronic treatment, or are controversial. Such interventions are not clearly in the child's best interest.

EFFECTIVE INTERVENTIONS WITH FEW SIDE EFFECTS

Parents sometimes refuse treatments that are highly effective in restoring a child with life-threatening illness to health, are short term, and have few side effects (14). For example, Jehovah's Witnesses commonly refuse blood transfusions for children who undergo major trauma. Christian scientist parents often refuse antibiotics for life-threatening bacterial infections. Physicians who are unable to persuade parents to accept such interventions should seek a court order to administer the treatment (15). A court order is important because it signifies that society regards the parent's refusal as unacceptable. As one court declared, although "parents may be free to become martyrs themselves," they are not free to "make martyrs of their children" (16).

Overriding parents through the courts should be a last resort. Even if a child with asthma or diabetes is not receiving medications regularly, disrupting the parent–child bond causes emotional distress for the child. Foster placement or institutionalization might be worse for the child than care from well-meaning parents who are trying to cope with difficult circumstances.

For parental refusal of vaccinations, see Chapter 44.

EFFECTIVE BUT BURDENSOME THERAPY

Parents sometimes refuse interventions that cure a fatal disease in the vast majority of cases but highly burdensome, such as bone marrow transplantation in acute lymphocytic leukemia or combination chemotherapy in testicular carcinoma. If parents continue to refuse such therapy after repeated attempts at persuasion, some physicians seek court orders to compel treatment (17). In doing so, physicians need to take into account the need for long-term parental cooperation with the child's care. Physicians should listen to the parents' objections and show respect for their opinions and ongoing responsibility for the child. In situations where treatment is less successful, the physician's obligation to advocate for it is weaker.

ADOLESCENT'S REFUSAL OF INTERVENTIONS

In some cases, adolescents refuse effective treatments. The physician's response should depend on the seriousness of the clinical situation, the effectiveness and side effects of treatment, the reasons for refusal, the parents' preferences on treatment, and the burdens of insisting on treatment. It is difficult to force adolescents to take ongoing therapies, such as insulin shots for diabetes or inhalers for asthma. The most constructive approach is to try to understand the reasons for refusal, to address them, and to provide psychosocial support. In several cases, adolescents have run away from home rather than accept potentially curative cancer chemotherapy that has significant side effects (18). Because it is physically difficult, as well as morally troubling, to force such treatment on adolescents, these refusals have been accepted, particularly when the parents have supported the child's refusal.

INTERVENTIONS WITH NO MEDICAL INDICATIONS

Parents sometimes request medications to modify their child's behavior or enhance their school performance. Stimulant medications improve distractibility, inattention, and impulsivity in children who do not meet criteria for attention deficit/hyperactivity disorder (ADHD). If such use of stimulant medications is widespread, parents may feel pressured to use them so that their children are not at a disadvantage.

Critics contend that better alternative to such use of medications is instruction and practice to strengthen the will of a restless and unruly child (19). Proper moral education requires shaping of character. These critics contend that unlike other parental steps to help their children, such as tutoring, medications rupture the bond between effort and accomplishment and undermine the child's responsibility, self-control, and sense of right and wrong.

In rebuttal, other writers point out that these critics create a false dichotomy between medication and effort. In fact, students using stimulant medications, like drinking coffee, still must study hard to learn. It is also an oversimplification to suggest that poor school performance results primarily from a lack of will and effort. In a child with significant behavioral and learning problems who does not meet criteria for ADHD, if behavioral and counseling approaches prove ineffective, it is reasonable for informed parents to carry out a trial of medications.

HANDICAPPED INFANTS

Premature infants with low birth weight can be treated effectively in neonatal intensive care units (NICUs) and subsequently achieve normal growth and development. At extremely low birth weights, however, such as below 400 g, very few infants survive even with intensive care, and survivors commonly have severe neurologic disabilities.

The 1985 federal "Baby Doe Regulations" set limits on decisions to withhold medical treatment from disabled infants less than 1 year old. They are intended to ensure interventions such as surgery for tracheal–esophageal fistula in infants with Down syndrome. Under these regulations, treatment other than "appropriate nutrition, hydration, or medication" need not be provided if (a) the infant is irreversibly comatose, (b) treatment would merely prolong dying, (c) treatment would not be effective in ameliorating or correcting all life-threatening conditions, (d) treatment would be futile in terms of survival, or (e) treatment would be virtually futile and would be inhumane. Decisions to withhold medically indicated treatment may not be based on "subjective opinions" about the child's future quality of life. Subsequently, the Born-Alive Infants Protection Act of 2002 was intended to reject the idea that a child's care should vary according to "whether that child's mother or others want him or her" (20).

The Baby Doe Regulations have been sharply criticized, for excluding parents from decision making (20–22). A further criticism is that maximal medical interventions must be provided unless they are futile or the child is irreversibly comatose or dying. In other clinical settings, the mere possibility of survival does not require the physicians and families to employ all available medical technology (23).

SUMMARY

1. Parents are generally given great discretion to make decisions for their children, on the assumption that they will act in the child's best interests. Generally, parents and physicians should make shared decisions about the child's care.
2. A parent may not forego interventions that are almost always life-saving and have few serious adverse effects.
3. Parents may refuse interventions that have a very low likelihood of success and great adverse effects.
4. As children gain maturity, they should play an increasing role in decision making, as appropriate for their developmental stage.

REFERENCES

1. Committee on Bioethics American Academy of Pediatrics. Informed consent, parental permission, and assent in pediatric practice. *Pediatrics.* 1995;95:314–317.
2. Kon AA. Answering the question: "Doctor, if this were your child, what would you do?". *Pediatrics.* 2006;118:393–397.
3. Committee on Pediatric Emergency Medicine and Committee on Bioethics. Consent for emergency medical services for children and adolescents. *Pediatrics.* 2011;128:427–433.
4. English A, Ford CA, Santelli JS. Clinical preventive services for adolescents: position paper of the Society for Adolescent Medicine. *Am J Law Med.* 2009;35:351–364.
5. Olson KA, Middleman AB. *Consent in adolescent health care.* 2011. http://www.uptodate.com/contents/consent-in-adolescent-health-care. Accessed November 22, 2011.
6. English A. Sexual and reproductive health care for adolescents: legal rights and policy challenges. *Adolesc Med State Art Rev.* 2007;18:571–581, viii–ix.
7. Knight JR, Mears CJ. Testing for drugs of abuse in children and adolescents: addendum—testing in schools and at home. *Pediatrics.* 2007;119:627–630.
8. American Academy of Pediatrics Committee on Pediatric AIDS. Disclosure of illness status to children and adolescents. *Pediatrics.* 1999;103:164–166.
9. Kreicbergs U, Valdimarsdottir U, Onelov E, et al. Talking about death with children who have severe malignant disease. *N Engl J Med.* 2004;351:1175–1186.
10. Ford C, English A, Sigman G. Confidential health care for adolescents: position paper for the society for adolescent medicine. *J Adolesc Health.* 2004;35:160–167.
11. English A, Ford CA. More evidence supports the need to protect confidentiality in adolescent health care. *J Adolesc Health.* 2007;40:199–200.
12. Ford CA, Millstein SG. Delivery of confidentiality assurances to adolescents by primary care physicians. *Arch Pediatr Adolesc Med.* 1997;151:505–509.

13. National Center for Youth Law. *Minor Consent, Confidentiality, and Child Abuse Reporting in California*. http://www.teenhealthlaw.org/confidentiality/. Accessed November 21, 2011.

14. Asser SM, Swan R. Child fatalities from religion-motivated medical neglect. *Pediatrics*. 1998;101:625–629.

15. Wadlington W. Medical decision making for and by children: tensions between parent, state, and child. *Univ Ill Law Rev*. 1994;1994:311–336.

16. *Prince v. Massachusetts*. 321 U.S. 158 (1944).

17. Hord JD, Rehman W, Hannon P, et al. Do parents have the right to refuse standard treatment for their child with favorable-prognosis cancer? Ethical and legal concerns. *J Clin Oncol*. 2006;24:5454–5456.

18. Traugott I, Alpers A. In their own hands: adolescents' refusals of medical treatment. *Arch Pediatr Adolesc Med*. 1997;151:922–927.

19. The President's Council on Bioethics. *Beyond Therapy: Biotechnology and the Pursuit of Happiness*. 2003. http://www.bioethics.gov/reports/beyondtherapy/index.html. Accessed October 19, 2007.

20. Sayeed SA. The marginally viable newborn: legal challenges, conceptual inadequacies, and reasonableness. *J Law Med Ethics*. 2006;34:600–610.

21. Sayeed SA. Baby doe redux? The department of health and human services and the born-alive infants protection act of 2002: a cautionary note on normative neonatal practice. *Pediatrics*. 2005;116:e576–e585.

22. Bell EF. Noninitiation or withdrawal of intensive care for high-risk newborns. *Pediatrics*. 2007;119:401–403.

23. Kopelman LM. Are the 21-year-old baby Doe rules misunderstood or mistaken? *Pediatrics*. 2005;115:797–802.

ANNOTATED BIBLIOGRAPHY

1. Committee on Bioethics, American Academy of Pediatrics. Informed consent, parental permission, and assent in pediatric practice. *Pediatrics*. 1995;95:314–317.
   Lucid discussion of distinctions between assent by children, permission from parents for care, and informed consent by adults.

2. Ford C, English A, Sigman G. Confidential health care for adolescents: position paper for the society for adolescent medicine. *J Adolesc Health*. 2004;35:160–167.
   Thoughtful and current review of legal and ethical issues regarding confidentiality in caring for adolescents.

3. Traugott I, Alpers A. In their own hands: adolescents' refusal of life-sustaining treatment. *Arch Pediatr Adolesc Med*. 1997;151:922–927.
   Dilemmas occur when adolescents are old enough to run away rather than accept life-sustaining interventions.

4. Hartman RG. Coming of age: devising legislation for adolescent medical decision-making. *Am J Law Med*. 2002;28:409–453.
   Analyzes legal issues regarding the age at which adolescents may give their own consent for various treatments.

5. Truog RD, Meyer EC, Burns JP. Toward interventions to improve end-of-life care in the pediatric intensive care unit. *Crit Care Med*. 2006;34:S373–S379.
   Suggests how end-of-life decisions and care in the pediatric intensive care unit might be improved.

38

Ethical Issues in Surgery

S urgery differs from other specialties in clinically significant ways. First, surgeons intention- ally cause short-term injury to achieve long-term therapeutic goals. Patients undergo opera- tive risks, experience pain, and emerge with scars. Although all medical interventions involve risk, many surgical adverse effects are certain, rather than possible, and occur before any benefit can be realized. Second, patients turn over control of their bodies to the surgical team in the operating room. Third, operations are not standardized in the sense that drug therapies have stan- dard dosages. The surgeon's technical skill, judgment, experience, and confidence are crucial. Indi- vidual surgeons vary in their choice of incision, use of electrocautery and stapling, and selection of suture material or implanted devices. This chapter discusses how these distinctive clinical character- istics of surgery have important ethical implications.

HOW ARE ETHICAL ISSUES IN SURGERY DIFFERENT?

Several ethical guidelines are particularly salient in surgery.

1. Acting in the patient's best interests takes on added importance because patients are com- pletely dependent on the surgical team during operations. Neither patients nor their surro- gates can look out for their interests during surgery.
2. Informed consent is especially important because surgery is a major bodily invasion. Some opera- tions, such as mastectomy, colostomy, or amputation, dramatically alter patients' body image, sense of self, and daily functioning. Patients differ in what surgical risks they are willing to accept.
3. Learning procedural skills differs from learning cognitive skills. More senior physicians can supervise decision making by trainees so that the risk of mistakes is greatly reduced. With procedural skills, how- ever, the trainee has manual control of the procedure and can make a mistake before the supervising surgeon can intervene. Furthermore, there is a learning curve for surgical procedures. After surgeons complete residency or fellowship, they continue to learn new techniques, such as robotic procedures.
4. Individual surgeons are held responsible for the outcomes of surgery. Perioperative deaths raise the question of whether the surgeon erred in judgment or technique. Postoperative deaths need to be reported to the coroner. In surgical morbidity and mortality conferences, surgeons must justify why they operated and how the case was managed (1). Increasingly, hospital-specific and surgeon-specific clinical outcomes are tracked and made available to the public or insurers. More- over, surgeons usually feel personally responsible for outcomes because of their "hands-on" in- volvement in care (2).

INFORMED CONSENT IN SURGERY

Patients need information that is pertinent to their decision to have an operation. As part of the in- formed consent process, surgeons need to discuss information about the operation, the benefits and risks, the likely consequences, and the alternatives.

DISCLOSURE OF ALTERNATIVE APPROACHES

Evidence-based medicine has demonstrated that for some conditions, several options have similar outcomes. In benign prostatic hypertrophy, transurethral resection of the prostate, medical treatment, and watchful waiting are all acceptable approaches. For localized breast cancer, lumpectomy followed by radiation offers survival rates similar to more extensive surgery but less disfigurement. A number of states legally require that women with breast cancer be informed of breast-conserving treatments (3). The importance that the patient places on side effects of different approaches will be decisive. Hence, the surgeon should discuss all standard options with the patient even if the doctor believes that one is superior. However, surgeons do not need to discuss alternative or unconventional therapies whose effectiveness has not been demonstrated or that no respected subset of physicians has adopted.

DISCLOSURE OF SURGICAL INNOVATION

Surgical progress depends on innovations, which usually require stepwise refinements and generally are not evaluated in randomized clinical trials. Minor variations of established procedures, such as changing the incision, are common and low-risk (2). Some innovations, however, are major differences from accepted practice, pose more than minor risks to patients, and have not previously been described in textbooks and articles (4). Such innovations should be reviewed by peers, and patients should consent to the innovative nature of the procedure (4).

DISCLOSURE OF OUTCOMES AND EXPERIENCE

Surgical mortality and complication rates vary across institutions and surgeons. For some operations, low-volume hospitals and surgeons have markedly higher surgical mortality rates (5–7). Dissemination of hospital-specific or surgeon-specific outcomes can spur quality improvement, provided that the data are risk-adjusted and reliable (8, 9). Outcomes reporting for most operations raises a number of concerns, including inadequate risk adjustment, random variation in relatively small samples, statistically misleading comparisons, avoidance of high-risk cases, and potential patient mistrust (10). In New York and other states, public release of outcomes for coronary bypass surgery motivated quality improvement efforts in institutions with very poor outcomes (5, 11). Some insurers have also used outcomes data to direct patients to centers of excellence and to increase reimbursement for better outcomes or for participation in quality improvement programs or outcomes registries (5). However, such outcomes data have had little impact on individual patient referrals and selection of surgeons (11).

Some physicians urge that surgeons should discuss with patients their experience and outcomes when outcomes for the proposed operation vary in statistically and clinically significant ways (12, 13). Such disclosure can be based on both respecting patient autonomy and acting in the patient's best interests. In a recent survey, 63% of patients said that they could not decide whether to have an operation without being told the surgeon's experience and outcomes (14).

Disclosure of experience might also be an issue in teaching hospitals. Outcomes data are mixed. Teaching hospitals have increased mortality for emergency procedures but not for elective procedures (15). Cases with resident participation have lower morality but higher postoperative complications (16). Patients usually consider it very important to be told if a resident or a medical student is going to make the incision, hold retractors, perform rectal or pelvic examinations under anesthesia, or suture (17, 18). Thus, patients should be informed of the trainees' role during surgery and how they will be supervised (17). The faculty surgeon might say, "Dr. X is a senior resident and will be performing portions of your operation; I will be assisting and supervising Dr. X throughout" (19). Patients generally respond favorably to having trainees participate in operations (17).

Disclosure is also an issue when experienced surgeons learn new techniques, such as laparoscopic or robotic surgery. Initially, complication rates are higher with laparoscopic procedures than with open techniques and operating times are longer. When surgeons get more experience, complication rates become comparable to those of open procedures. Patients consider it extremely important to know a surgeon's experience with a new technique (14). Surgeons, however, might be concerned that patients who learn that they are inexperienced with a technique will not trust them to do the operation.

CHANGES IN THE OPERATION DUE TO UNANTICIPATED FINDINGS

A surgeon might encounter unexpected findings that require a substantially different operation than was discussed during the informed consent process. For example, suppose that during a cholecystectomy, the surgeon finds a gastric mass that is suspicious for carcinoma. Should the surgeon biopsy the mass, and, if so, should the surgeon resect the tumor if the biopsy shows carcinoma? The surgeon might believe that an opportunity to cure gastric carcinoma might be missed if biopsy and resection are not done. Furthermore, a second operation would subject the patient to additional risk. On the other hand, the patient might be upset to find that the surgeon performed a more extensive operation than discussed, even if the surgeon did so to benefit him.

How can surgeons resolve this dilemma between acting for the patient's good and respecting the patient's autonomy? Some surgeons seek blanket consent to change the operation if unexpected findings occur. An alternative is to contact the next of kin in the waiting area or by phone to discuss the proposed change in care. If the family agrees with the surgeon's recommendations, both the patient's best interests and autonomy are served. It would also be acceptable to biopsy the mass if the family cannot be immediately located and to resect the mass only if a family member's consent can be obtained.

Such cases of incidental findings need to be distinguished from cases in which the operation needs to be changed because of a complication. For instance, a surgeon might nick the spleen and a splenectomy might be required to control bleeding. In this instance, the surgeon should proceed with the splenectomy and explain to the patient after the operation that a splenectomy was done because of the intraoperative complication.

MAY A SURGEON DECLINE TO OPERATE?

In some cases, a surgeon might determine that an operation is not indicated because the risks of surgery greatly outweigh the possible benefits (20). What should the surgeon do if the patient or referring physician insists on surgery? Different reasons for not operating need to be distinguished. Some reasons are patient centered. The surgeon might believe that an operation will not benefit the patient. For instance, a patient with chronic abdominal pain might believe that the pain is caused by gallbladder disease and seek a cholecystectomy (20). If there is no objective evidence of gallstones, however, the surgeon might conclude that a cholecystectomy would be futile in a strict sense and decline to operate (*see* Chapter 9).

In other situations, the surgeon might judge that although the operation is not futile, the risks are prohibitive, as the following case illustrates.

CASE 38.1   **Decision to not operate in a very high-risk patient**

Mr. G is a 64-year-old man admitted for a myocardial infarction. He continues to have chest pain, ischemic changes on his cardiogram, and congestive heart failure. He is found to have multiple diffuse coronary lesions that cannot be revascularized. He also develops a urinary tract infection from a Foley catheter. Despite antibiotics, Mr. G subsequently develops pyelonephritis, intrarenal abscesses, and septic shock. He becomes confused and unable to participate in decisions. Percutaneous drainage guided by computed tomography is not feasible. The family appreciates that the surgery is very risky, but they believe it offers the patient the only chance of survival. The surgeon, however, believes that Mr. G's coronary disease is so unstable that he is unlikely to survive an open procedure.

Surgeons are traditionally permitted great discretion not to operate when they determine that surgery would not be in the patient's best interests. Surgeons often justify a refusal to operate by the shorthand declaration, "This patient is not a surgical candidate." Such surgical decisions are rarely challenged and discussed, but internists' unilateral decisions to withhold medical interventions are often extensively debated.

Is there an acceptable ethical basis for this distinction between surgeons and internists? Surgeons are held more responsible for the harmful consequences of operations than internists are for the harmful effects of drugs they prescribe. Making a surgical incision causes much more certain and direct harm to the patient than writing a prescription does. Furthermore, because surgery requires manual manipulations, it is undesirable to require surgeons to perform operations they consider inadvisable. An unwilling surgeon might place the patient at additional risk because of lapses of concentration or lack of confidence.

Surgeons need to appreciate that patients have different thresholds for risk. Some might accept severe short-term harms and unfavorable odds of success. Surgeons should decline to operate only if the risks are substantially greater than the likely benefits, as opposed to only slightly increased. Surgeons must guard against misrepresenting information to patients because of their own bias. For example, they should never overstate an operation's risks because they recommend against it. Furthermore, they must be careful to base decisions on medical outcomes, not their personal judgments that the patient's quality of life is unacceptably poor.

Other reasons for not operating might be surgeon centered. In some cases, surgeons question whether the risk of contracting HIV infection or hepatitis C during an operation is acceptable in view of very limited benefits to the patient (*see* Chapter 24). For example, an orthopedic surgeon might believe that a total hip replacement on a patient with AIDS presents an unacceptable risk of occupational HIV infection because bone fragments might penetrate even double gloves. In other cases, a surgeon might be reluctant to take on complex, high-risk cases that might worsen their complication rates or length of hospital stays or make it more difficult to secure contracts from managed care organizations. Yet another factor might be unreimbursed care (20). Surgeons might believe that they have accepted more than their fair share of charity cases. In these situations, the surgeon's self-interest must be acknowledged as a natural and legitimate concern. However, they must be put into perspective and addressed directly. Ultimately, the ethical ideal is for physicians to make patients' best interests paramount if they can do so without a grave setback to their own self-interest. To clarify patients' best interests, surgeons can consider what they would recommend if the patient did not have HIV infection (but another disease with a similar prognosis) or had good health insurance.

REQUESTS TO OPERATE IN WAYS THAT INCREASE RISK

Patients might consent to an operation but refuse specific interventions or techniques. Such restrictions might make their operation riskier and more complicated. These decisions need to be distinguished from patient refusals of the operation itself.

CASE 38.2   Emergency surgery on a Jehovah's Witness

Mr. D, a 54-year-old Jehovah's Witness, is admitted after a motor vehicle accident with a ruptured spleen, a hemoglobin of 6%, hypotension, chest pain, and ischemic changes on electrocardiogram. He refuses blood transfusions but agrees to surgery, understanding that he might die without transfusions. The surgeon declares, "I accept his right to refuse transfusions, but he can't make me operate with one hand tied behind my back."

In case 38.2 Mr. D has a clear indication for splenectomy. In his religion, surviving the accident is less important than avoiding the taint of transfusions, which would result in everlasting damnation (*see* Chapter 11). Operative risk increases with very severe anemia, reaching 33% when hemoglobin falls below 6 g per dl (21). Severe anemia also places this patient at greater risk for myocardial infarction and renal failure. The hospital course will be more complicated without transfusion support, and the length of stay and overall cost will probably be greater.

Some surgeons might be angry because of the need for additional time and effort and the reduced margin of error. Many surgeons intuitively make a distinction between respecting the patient's refusal of transfusions and following the patient's request to have the surgery under restrictive conditions. Philosophers distinguish negative and positive rights. Negative rights are claims to be left alone; they protect patients from unwanted interventions on their bodies. Positive rights require others to act in certain ways. Negative rights are generally considered stronger than positive rights. Thus, patients have a strong right to refuse unwanted interventions, but little power to specify how surgeons carry out their work.

Faced with requests to carry out operations with specific restrictions, surgeons generally have a legal right to decline to operate and to transfer care to another surgeon. In many cases, a more fruitful approach is to consider how to minimize additional risks due to foregoing transfusions. Use of cell salvage, hemodilution, and administering erythropoietin might reduce perioperative risk, particularly in operations with very large blood loss (22). Furthermore, traditional criteria for transfusion may be mistaken; a perioperative transfusion to maintain hemoglobin above 10 g per dl is not superior to a strategy of transfusion only if symptoms develop or to maintain hemoglobin above 8 g per dl (23). Moreover, surgeons should keep in mind the ethical ideal of putting the patient's best interests paramount. A skilled and experienced surgical team offers the patient the best chance at a favorable outcome.

In the following case, the patient objects to certain aspects of the proposed operation after the physician brings up the nature of the operation (23).

CASE 38.3	Patient refusal of emergency colostomy

Mr. N, a 74-year-old man, is admitted to the hospital with an acute abdomen. He is found to have free air under the diaphragm. The surgeon believes that the patient has perforated a peptic ulcer or a carcinoma of the colon. The surgeon explains that if the perforation is in the colon, she will perform a colostomy, which might not need to be permanent. Mr. N adamantly refuses a colostomy. "A friend got one and had one complication after another. He was so ashamed of that bag. I'd rather be dead than go through that humiliation." There is no time for the patient to talk to people who have adapted well to a colostomy. Technically, an end-to-end anastomosis is possible, but it has a much higher risk of complications.

A colleague suggests, "In an emergency I never discuss the details of the surgery. All that the patient needs to know is that he needs an operation to save his life and that the risks of surgery are small compared with the alternatives. Too much information can be dangerous because there is no time to correct misunderstandings. I would never do an end-to-end anastomosis. How would you justify it at a morbidity and mortality conference if he got a complication?"

In Case 38.3, the ethical dilemma is that the patient might be making an irreversible decision that he would greatly regret later when fully informed. The surgeon believes that the patient's refusal is based on an unrealistic appraisal of a colostomy. Most patients who are initially dismayed at the prospect of a colectomy later adjust well to living with it (24). In elective situations, most patients can be persuaded to accept a colostomy, but in an emergency there is no time for extended discussions. A surgeon dedicated to acting in the patient's best interests would want to do the less risky operation, knowing that most patients adapt to a colostomy. From this perspective, it would be terrible if the patient refused surgery because of an outcome that might not happen or might be only temporary. The colleague's concern about the morbidity and mortality conference is not just a desire to avoid personal criticism; the professional standard of care is based on what a reasonable surgeon would do under the circumstances.

In contrast, a surgeon dedicated to patient autonomy will respect the patient's refusal of colostomy even if that decision might not be fully informed. From this viewpoint, even if the operation was skillfully performed and successfully treated the perforation, it would be tragic if the patient had to live with a mutilation of his body that he did not consent to. Although the vast majority of surgical patients hold survival as their highest priority, some give higher priority to quality of life (25). Some patients might consider a colostomy so unacceptable that they would rather die than have the operation.

The surgeon in Case 38.3 has several options. One option is to refuse to operate unless the patient agrees to a colostomy if needed. This option, however, might leave the patient worse off than having an end-to-end anastomosis. Also, if the on-call surgeon declines to operate, it might be difficult to find a colleague to take over the case without delay.

CASE 38.3 | *Continued*

The surgeon try to persuade the patient to accept the colostomy, even with severe time constraints. The surgeon can ask the patient to talk over the phone with his family, primary care physician, or the chaplain, and the surgeon could explain to them why a colostomy is preferable. In addition, the surgeon might paradoxically persuade the patient by giving him control. "If you decide that you won't accept the colostomy after talking to your family and your primary care doctor, I'll do the surgery in the other, riskier way. I won't force you to have an operation you don't want. But before you decide, I'd like to understand better what about the colostomy troubles you. I'd also like you to understand why I think the colostomy is the best operation for you." The surgeon might acknowledge, "Everyone finds it hard to think about a colostomy" and might say, "I wish I had a way of doing the surgery so you didn't have a colostomy and didn't have an increased risk of complications." If persuasion fails, it is ethically appropriate for the surgeon to plan an end-to-end anastomosis, based on the patient's informed choice.

To reduce the risk of complications, some surgeons might be tempted to misrepresent what they will do in the operating room. For example, they might say they will try to do an end-to-end anastomosis if possible, even though they actually intend to do a colostomy. As Chapter 6 discusses, such misrepresentation undermines patient trust and physician integrity.

SUMMARY

1. The unique clinical circumstances of surgery impose special ethical obligations on surgeons regarding informed consent, decisions not to operate, and patient requests to carry out the operation in certain ways.

REFERENCES

1. Bosk CL. *Forgive and Remember: Managing Medical Failure*. Chicago, IL: University of Chicago Press; 1979.
2. Angelos P. The ethical challenges of surgical innovation for patient care. *Lancet*. 2010;376:1046–1047.
3. Nattinger AB, Hoffman RG, Shapiro R, et al. The effect of legislative requirements on the use of breast-conserving surgery. *N Engl J Med*. 1996;335:1035–1040.
4. Biffl WL, Spain DA, Reitsma AM, et al. Responsible development and application of surgical innovations: a position statement of the Society of University Surgeons. *J Am Coll Surg*. 2008;206:1204–1209.
5. Birkmeyer NJ, Birkmeyer JD. Strategies for improving surgical quality—should payers reward excellence or effort? *N Engl J Med*. 2006;354:864–870.

6. Birkmeyer JD, Dimick JB, Staiger DO. Operative mortality and procedure volume as predictors of subsequent hospital performance. *Ann Surg.* 2006;243:411–417.

7. Finks JF, Osborne NH, Birkmeyer JD. Trends in hospital volume and operative mortality for high-risk surgery. *N Engl J Med.* 2011;364:2128–2137.

8. Chassin MR, Loeb JM, Schmaltz SP, et al. Accountability measures—using measurement to promote quality improvement. *N Engl J Med.* 2010;363:683–688.

9. Schwarze ML. The process of informed consent: neither the time nor the place for disclosure of surgeon-specific outcomes. *Ann Surg.* 2007;245:514–515.

10. Burger I, Schill K, Goodman S. Disclosure of individual surgeon's performance rates during informed consent: ethical and epistemological considerations. *Ann Surg.* 2007;245:507–513.

11. Steinbrook R. Public report cards—cardiac surgery and beyond. *N Engl J Med.* 2006;355:1847–1849.

12. Krumholz HM. Informed consent to promote patient-centered care. *JAMA.* 2010;303:1190–1191.

13. Gates EA. New surgical procedures: can our patients benefit while we learn? *Am J Obstet Gynecol.* 1997;176:1293–1298.

14. Lee Char SJ, Hills NK, Lo B, et al. Informed consent for innovative surgery: A survey of patients and surgeons. *Surgery* In press.

15. Holena DN, Hadler R, Wirtalla C, et al. Teaching status: the impact on emergency and elective surgical care in the US. *Ann Surg.* 2011;253:1017–1023.

16. Raval MV, Wang X, Cohen ME, et al. The influence of resident involvement on surgical outcomes. *J Am Coll Surg.* 2011;212:889–898.

17. Kim N, Lo B, Gates EA. Disclosing the role of residents and medical students in hysterectomy: what do patients want? *Acad Med.* 1998;73:339–341.

18. Silver-Isenstadt A, Ubel PA. Erosion in medical students' attitudes about telling patients they are students. *J Gen Intern Med.* 1999;14:481–487.

19. McCullough LB, Jones JW, Brody BA. Informed consent: autonomous decision-making of the surgical patient. In: McCullough LB, Jones JW, Brody BA, eds. *Surgical Ethics.* New York, NY: Oxford University Press; 1998:15–37.

20. Sugarman J, Harland R. Acute yet non-emergent patients. In: McCullough LB, Jones JW, Brody BA, eds. *Surgical Ethics.* New York, NY: Oxford University Press; 1998:116–132.

21. Carson JL, Duff A, Poses RM, et al. Effect of anaemia and cardiovascular disease on surgical mortality and morbidity. *Lancet.* 1996;348:1055–1060.

22. Ferraris VA. Severe blood conservation: comment on "outcome of patients who refuse transfusion after cardiac surgery". *Arch Intern Med* 2012;172:1160-1161.

23. Carson JL, Terrin ML, Magaziner J, et al. Transfusion trigger trial for functional outcomes in cardiovascular patients undergoing surgical hip fracture repair (FOCUS). *Transfusion.* 2006;46:2192–2206.

24. Halpern J, Arnold RM. Affective forecasting: an unrecognized challenge in making serious health decisions. *J Gen Intern Med.* 2008;23:1708–1712.

25. List MA, Stracks J, Colangelo L, et al. How do head and neck cancer patients prioritize treatment outcomes before initiating treatment? *J Clin Oncol.* 2000;18:877–884.

ANNOTATED BIBLIOGRAPHY

1. McCullough LB, Jones JW, Brody BA, eds. *Surgical Ethics.* New York, NY: Oxford University Press; 1998.
Monograph on ethical issues in various surgical contexts.

2. Gates EA. New surgical procedures: can our patients benefit while we learn? *Am J Obstet Gynecol.* 1997;176:1293–1298.
Argues that surgeons should disclose their own experience and outcomes during the informed consent process.

3. Burger I, Schill K, Goodman S. Disclosure of individual surgeon's performance rates during informed consent: ethical and epistemological considerations. *Ann Surg.* 2007;245:507–513.
Schwarze ML. The process of informed consent: neither the time nor the place for disclosure of surgeon-specific outcomes. *Ann Surg.* 2007;245:514–515.
Analyses of whether to disclose to patients surgeon-specific outcomes.

4. Birkmeyer NJ, Birkmeyer JD. Strategies for improving surgical quality—Should payers reward excellence or effort? *N Engl J Med.* 2006;354:864–870.
Ethical and policy analysis of different approaches for using surgeon-specific or institution-specific outcomes data to improve quality of care.

5. Biffl WL, Spain DA, Reitsma AM, et al. Responsible development and application of surgical innovations: a position statement of the Society of University Surgeons. *J Am Coll Surg.* 2008;206:1204–1209.
Suggests criteria for when surgical innovation should be peer reviewed and require informed consent from the patient.

39

Ethical Issues in Obstetrics and Gynecology

E thical dilemmas in obstetrics and gynecology are particularly difficult because care for a pregnant woman and care for her fetus are inextricably linked. Furthermore, decisions about reproduction and sexuality involve intimate and private topics, such as sexuality, reproduction, and childrearing, which are often socially contested.

HOW ARE ETHICAL ISSUES IN OB-GYN DIFFERENT?

THIRD PARTIES SEEK TO INFLUENCE HIGHLY PERSONAL ISSUES

Many women want control of their reproductive decisions and have strong preferences in family planning and childbirth. At the same time, some public leaders and religious groups hold strong views regarding children, family, and the appropriate role of women and seek to shape women's decisions about reproductive health (1). Debates over reproductive health in the United States may be passionate and highly politicized. On the one hand, some seek to reaffirm traditional attitudes toward women, reproduction, and sexuality. On the other hand, feminist critics assert that society and physicians exercise inappropriate control over women through policies regarding reproductive health care. Some women also believe that pregnancy and childbirth have become overly technologic and medicalized.

PHILOSOPHIC QUANDARIES THAT SCIENCE CANNOT RESOLVE

Decisions about reproduction inevitably raise philosophic or religious questions that science cannot resolve.

- Is the fetus a person with moral and legal rights?
- When does personhood begin: at conception, viability, birth, or some other time?
- Do women have an ethical right of reproductive liberty that encompasses a right to abortion?

Theologians, philosophers, public officials, and the public have debated these conundrums without reaching agreement or common ground. Consensus is unlikely to emerge, and public policies need to be developed despite deep disagreements.

UNPRECEDENTED DILEMMAS IN ASSISTED REPRODUCTION

Assisted reproductive technologies (ARTs) allow pregnancy to occur in unprecedented ways. With ARTs and gamete donation, different persons can fill the roles of genetic, gestational, and childrearing parents. Dramatic dilemmas have arisen over the disposition of frozen embryos after a couple has separated, ART for postmenopausal women, and "surrogate motherhood," in which the gestational mother has no genetic link with the fetus and will not raise the child after birth. Such dilemmas force people to reconsider fundamental, often unspoken beliefs about parental responsibility and roles.

INTERTWINED INTERESTS OF THE PREGNANT WOMAN AND FETUS

Everyone hopes that children will be born healthy. It is tragic when a child is born with a serious preventable illness or congenital anomaly. The pregnant woman has a moral responsibility to take reasonable steps to reduce harm and provide benefit to the child who will be born (2). Physicians have a responsibility to represent the interests of such future children, who cannot represent themselves. These moral responsibilities are based on the desire to prevent harm to children who will be born; they do not require a belief that the fetus is a person with rights (2).

Fetal movements and fetal heartbeat can be visualized with ultrasound and other imaging techniques. Doctors can diagnose many conditions in utero, such as congenital abnormalities or fetal distress. Furthermore, physicians can treat the fetus through interventions on the mother, such as prenatal vitamins, tocolytic agents in premature labor, corticosteroids in prematurity, and fetal blood transfusion for Rh isoimmunization. In light of this ability to diagnose and treat fetal disorders, it seems reasonable to consider the fetus a patient, along with the pregnant woman, provided that she intends to carry the fetus to term and presents for prenatal care (2). Thinking of the fetus as a patient helps prevent inadvertent injury to the fetus by reminding physicians and pregnant women to consider how care for the woman might affect the fetus.

The idea that the fetus is a patient acknowledges that interventions directed to the fetus are also interventions on the pregnant woman that might cause her unacceptable side effects or disrupt other important aspects of her life (3). For example, in premature labor, terbutaline causes tremor and anxiety in the pregnant woman. Long-term bed rest for premature labor might prevent the pregnant woman from caring for her other children or working at a job that supports her family. Most pregnant women accept side effects, inconvenience, and disruption of their life for the sake of the child who will be born. Pregnant woman need not accept every intervention that might benefit the fetus, however, regardless of the degree of benefit, risks, or impact on her life. Responsibilities to a fetus who will become a child have limits; logically they should not exceed responsibilities that parents have to living children (1). Parents are not obligated to provide all potentially beneficial interventions to children after birth or to minimize all harms to them.

Some concepts of the fetus as patient are conceptually flawed because they mistakenly regard the fetus as an independent entity that can be treated apart from the pregnant woman (2, 3). Furthermore, these views fail to recognize that the pregnant woman herself is a patient with needs, interests, and rights (3). The requirement of informed consent cannot be waived because a woman is pregnant.

INFORMED CONSENT IN OBSTETRICS AND GYNECOLOGY

Several situations in obstetrics and gynecology raise particular ethical issues regarding consent. With increasing attention to patient autonomy in modern medicine, the informed preferences of the pregnant woman are today given greater weight. Chapter 36 discusses the importance of informed consent when students learn how to conduct pelvic examinations.

INFORMATION ABOUT FAMILY PLANNING AND ABORTION

Some physicians have strong moral and religious objections to these interventions (3). They believe it would violate their conscience to write a prescription for birth control or perform an abortion. Institutions should make reasonable accommodations to conscientious objections, and patients should be referred to facilities that provide care (*see* Chapter 24).

REPRODUCTIVE HEALTH FOR ADOLESCENTS

Girls below 18 years of age, who are often sexually active, might seek care for contraception, sexually transmitted diseases, or pregnancy. Many people believe that allowing minors to obtain such care without parental consent undermines family values and encourages promiscuity and irresponsibility. Many adolescents, however, present for reproductive care after they have already been sexually active or become pregnant. In most states, adolescents may seek reproductive health care without parental consent. The rationale is that it is preferable for adolescents to have access to such care rather than to forego it because they are reluctant or unable to obtain parental approval. Usually, it is in the adolescent's best interest to involve their parents in their care, and physicians generally should encourage them to do so. In some cases, however, adolescents might have compelling reasons for not involving parents—for example, in cases of domestic violence or incest. Chapter 37 discussed ethical issues in adolescent medicine in detail.

ELECTIVE CESAREAN SECTION AT TERM

Operative and anesthetic advances have decreased the risks of elective cesarean section deliveries. With reductions in operative adverse effects, the risk/benefit balance may no longer be unfavorable (4, 5). Attitudes toward elective cesarean section at term have shifted dramatically (6), and many obstetricians report that they would choose it for themselves or their partner (7). When pregnant women inquire about elective C-section at term, physicians should discuss options and present relevant information. Women whose requests are based on fear of childbirth need to be identified, as counseling and support usually lead them to change their minds and accept vaginal delivery (8). Several experts recommend that physicians should try to dissuade patients but ultimately respect their informed decisions (4, 5).

OBSTETRIC EMERGENCIES

Some obstetric decisions need to be made in crisis situations. An uncomplicated pregnancy at term might unexpectedly and rapidly become an emergency if severe fetal distress develops or if the umbilical cord is wrapped around the fetus's neck. A cesarean section might need to be carried out immediately to prevent severe, irreversible harm to a child. As with any emergency situation, the informed consent process may be truncated if delaying care to obtain consent would cause serious harm and most patients would agree to the intervention if fully informed. In an emergency, a cesarean section may be performed on the basis of the pregnant woman's assent rather than informed consent. That is, the patient agrees to the doctor's recommendations without being informed of all the procedure's risks and benefits. Almost all pregnant women agree to recommended emergency cesarean sections (9).

FORCED CESAREAN SECTION DELIVERIES

If a pregnant woman cannot be persuaded to accept a cesarean section that the physician believes is required, some doctors ask the courts to authorize the operation. The trend in recent appellate rulings is that a competent pregnant woman may refuse a cesarean section even if a viable fetus's welfare is at stake (3). Courts note that competent adults may refuse treatment, that cesarean sections are a significant bodily invasion, and that the medical need for the procedure is often inaccurate or overstated. In many cases in which court orders were sought for cesarean section, the woman delivered a healthy child vaginally without complications at stake (3). In addition, forced cesarean sections undermine women's trust in physicians and are disproportionately sought on women who do not speak English and women of color. Nonetheless, trial courts sometimes still order cesarean sections, and, in one case, criminal charges were brought against a woman at stake (3).

STERILIZATION

Sterilization without a woman's consent is a grave violation of her autonomy. In the early 1900s, nonvoluntary eugenic sterilization was carried out in the United States on women who had mental retardation, resided in psychiatric institutions, and were prisoners (10). African American women were disproportionately subjected to nonvoluntary sterilization. In response to these abuses, many states have enacted procedural requirements, such as waiting periods, to ensure that sterilization decisions are voluntary and informed (10).

Sterilization is commonly considered for severely mentally disabled persons. It might be in the best interests of a person who will never have the capacity to make informed reproductive decisions or to provide basic care for a child (11). Generally, a court hearing is required to sterilize a woman who is not capable of giving informed consent (10).

ABORTION

Debates over abortion in the United States are contentious. Prolife advocates contend that the fetus is a person with a right to live and that abortion is murder. Prochoice advocates claim that women have a right to control their bodies and their reproductive choices and often contend that a fetus becomes a person only after birth. Disagreements over abortion are associated with different views on women's roles and the meaning of their lives (12). Debates have become increasingly polarized.

The Supreme Court has made several important rulings on abortion. In *Planned Parenthood v. Casey* (1992), the Supreme Court affirmed the landmark 1973 *Roe v. Wade* decision, which protected a woman's right to choose to abort her fetus. In *Casey*, the court held that states may ban abortion after fetal viability, as long as exceptions were made to protect the woman's health or life and as long as the restriction's "purpose or effect [was not] to place substantial obstacles in the path of a woman seeking an abortion before the fetus attains viability" (13). Many states require parental notification if a minor seeks an abortion; these states must have a procedure for adolescents to seek judicial authorization for the procedure instead of parental notification. Physicians need to understand the laws in their state.

Some requests for abortion are particularly problematic (14). For example, a pregnant woman might seek an abortion because of the sex of her fetus even though there is no increased risk of sex-linked genetic disease. The parents might desire a son or daughter to balance their family. Some cultures or religions prize male children more than females, and some doctors may want to respect those norms. There are strong ethical objections, however, to selecting the sex of a fetus (15). The practice reflects and contributes to discrimination against women. Furthermore, some critics argue that sex selection violates the proper parental role and expectations. In this view, children should be unconditionally accepted, not regarded as products made to the parents' specifications. Although parents commonly have a preference about the child's sex, a physician is not morally justified to abort a healthy fetus solely because of its sex (16). If the obstetrician cannot persuade the woman to withdraw her request, then the doctor is justified in withdrawing from the case.

MATERNAL–FETAL MEDICINE

Most pregnant women agree with their physician's recommendations for interventions that benefit the fetus. In some cases, however, women might reject such recommendations despite the doctor's continued attempts at persuasion.

PRENATAL TESTING

During pregnancy, women commonly have screening tests for rubella, syphilis, gonorrhea, Rh type, and diabetes. The Centers for Disease Control and Prevention (CDC) now recommend routine prenatal HIV testing (17). In many prenatal blood tests, the patient usually assents rather than gives full informed consent. The physician does not discuss the risks, benefits, and alternatives of each test, and testing is carried out unless the patient objects. Another way to describe routine testing is that women may opt out of testing but do not need to give affirmative consent. Going beyond routine testing, most states require mandatory prenatal testing for syphilis (18). The ethical justifications for routine and mandatory prenatal screening tests are prevention of harm to children who will be born, the poor uptake of voluntary testing, and the judgment that the infringement of the woman's autonomy is acceptable.

SCREENING FOR CHROMOSOMAL ABNORMALITIES

Pregnant women might request interventions whose balance of benefits to risks physicians consider unfavorable. For example, young pregnant women at low risk for genetic abnormalities might request screening for chromosomal abnormalities such as Down syndrome. A decade ago, many providers declined to carry out amniocentesis or chorionic villus sampling if the risk of miscarriage was greater than the probability of a serious chromosomal abnormality; however, the options for screening have proliferated, with different approaches having different risks, benefits, and uncertainties. Recently, the noninvasive technique of serum biochemical markers plus fetal ultrasound have been shown to be effective and safe. It is now recommended that the various options for screening for chromosomal abnormalities be offered to all pregnant women receiving prenatal care, regardless of age (19).

Women vary in their desire for information regarding the risk of such birth defects. Some women might place a high value on information about the fetus and reassurance that the pregnancy is progressing normally, even though there is little likelihood of a serious abnormality (20). Moreover, women might want to know of congenital abnormalities even if they would still carry the fetus to term. Furthermore, their values may differ from those of physicians. In accordance with the principle of respect for patient autonomy, the indications for screening for chromosomal abnormalities have broadened to include the pregnant woman's informed preferences. The physician should check that the mother understands the benefits and risks of the various options and help the woman deliberate about the decision. Ultimately, however, the woman's informed choice should be decisive.

PRENATAL SCREENING USING FETAL DNA IN MATERNAL SERUM

Cell-free fetal DNA can now be detected in maternal blood, allowing noninvasive prenatal screening for birth defects early in pregnancy (21). Because it is noninvasive, there is no risk of miscarriage. As free fetal DNA replaces invasive procedures like CVS or amniocentesis for definitive diagnosis, prenatal testing may become acceptable to more pregnant women. Already Rh incompatibility and sex can be determined as early as 7-week fetal gestation. It is expected that tests for chromosomal abnormalities such as Down syndrome will become clinically available. Furthermore, genomic sequencing of fetal DNA fragments will soon become available, allowing multiple tests for genetic abnormalities to be run on a single maternal blood sample. Such multiplex testing raises concerns about informed consent and what limits, if any, should be placed on the technology (21).

CARE OF PREGNANT WOMEN WITH OTHER MEDICAL PROBLEMS

When pregnant women have serious medical problems, such as cancer, depression, or seizures, physicians face dilemmas. On the one hand, suboptimal treatment of the mother's condition may harm the fetus as well as the mother. In some cases, physicians may feel frustrated if a pregnant woman does not adhere to her recommended medical regimen. Physicians need to help the woman understand the benefits of taking medications regularly, identify barriers to compliance, and work with her to address them, as with any patient. Some physicians consider asking the courts to compel treatment for the pregnant woman in order to protect the fetus (22). It is neither ethically acceptable nor feasible, however, to force an informed woman to take medications against her objections.

On the other hand, physicians are also concerned about the risks interventions pose to the fetus. However, such concern for the fetus must not lead physicians to inappropriately withhold effective therapies from the woman (1). Physicians often overestimate the risks and do not consider the risks of not intervening. In conditions such as depression or epilepsy, aggressive treatment for the pregnant woman promotes the physical health of the child who will be born as well as the health of the woman. Furthermore, it will be in the child's best interests for the mother to be healthy. For example, the teratogenic risks of antidepressants may be outweighed by the benefits to the fetus from better control of maternal major depression (23). The pregnant woman should make informed decisions about the care of her medical problems and about what risks to the fetus are acceptable in view of the intervention's overall benefits. It is inappropriate for physicians to withhold effective interventions from the mother or to insist that the pregnant woman obtain an abortion as a condition of treating her medical conditions.

SUBSTANCE AND ALCOHOL ABUSE DURING PREGNANCY

Many states have enacted laws to try to prevent harm to the fetus caused by prenatal substance abuse. About one-half of the states permit involuntary civil commitment of pregnant women who use certain illegal drugs (24). In a few states, drug abuse during pregnancy triggers child abuse laws (24, 25). No state mandates drug screening during pregnancy. Use of criminal sanctions against pregnant substance abusers is problematic. Physicians and hospitals may not conduct drug testing of pregnant women for criminal prosecution without a warrant or explicit consent (25). Except in South Carolina, courts have refused to apply existing criminal laws on child endangerment or delivery of drugs to a minor to drug-using pregnant women. Criminal charges are not applied evenly across racial and socioeconomic categories (26). There is some evidence that punitive approaches to drug and alcohol abuse during pregnancy are counterproductive, deterring women from seeking prenatal care or being candid with physicians (26). Focusing on substance abuse treatment is more likely than criminal punishment to benefit the health of the fetus and the mother (3, 27).

HOME BIRTHS

Some pregnant women desire a more natural, less technologic childbirth and want to deliver at home. They and the midwife may ask a physician to serve as backup in case complications occur. It is appropriate for physicians to respect women's informed choices regarding site of delivery, even if contrary to their recommendation, and to use their expertise to minimize risks that might otherwise occur with home births (28).

ASSISTED REPRODUCTIVE TECHNOLOGIES

Because physicians take an active and essential role in ARTs, they feel a responsibility for the well-being of the child who might be born (29). Many physicians would hesitate to provide infertility treatments to women with drug addiction, serious developmental delay, or severe psychiatric illness because they believe the woman would not be a good parent. Other physicians might be reluctant to assist single, unmarried, or lesbian women because they believe that only married women should be parents.

Concern for the well-being of children who will be born is laudable. Physicians should help women and couples who seek ARTs appreciate the difficulties of infertility treatments and childrearing. The physician might also make recommendations on the basis of the patient's situation, needs, and goals. Furthermore, it would be irresponsible for physicians to provide ARTs to women who are incapable of giving informed consent or to women who have abused their children. However, physicians should distinguish concerns that are based on clinical evidence from their personal views of parenthood and family. Some characteristics, such as marital status, poorly predict good parenting (29). Many married couples fail as parents, but many persons who are single or in nontraditional relationships are successful parents.

Some women over 40 seek infertility treatments (29). Many are committed to raising a child, have strong social support, and have carefully considered their decision. However, some writers believe that the natural span of childbearing years should be respected (30). Because having a child is such a private decision, it is problematic for third parties to impose their personal views of who is worthy of being a parent.

SUMMARY

1. Obstetrics and gynecology raise ethical issues that may be particularly controversial.
2. Doctors need to appreciate that the patient's values might differ from their own, try to understand how the woman's decision might make sense from her perspective, and negotiate a mutually acceptable plan for care.

REFERENCES

1. Lyerly AD, Mitchell LM, Armstrong EM, et al. Risk and the pregnant body. *Hastings Cent Rep.* 2009;39:34–42.
2. Chervenak FA, McCullough LB, Brent RL. The professional responsibility model of obstetrical ethics: avoiding the perils of clashing rights. *Am J Obstet Gynecol.* 2011;205:315.e1–5.

3. ACOG Committee Opinion #321: maternal decision making, ethics, and the law. *Obstet Gynecol.* 2005;106:1127–1137.

4. Minkoff H. The ethics of cesarean section by choice. *Semin Perinatol.* 2006;30:309–312.

5. Kalish RB, McCullough LB, Chervenak FA. Patient choice cesarean delivery: ethical issues. *Curr Opin Obstet Gynecol.* 2008;20:116–119.

6. Ecker JL, Frigoletto FD Jr. Cesarean delivery and the risk-benefit calculus. *N Engl J Med.* 2007;356:885–888.

7. Al-Mufti R, McCarthy A, Fisk NM. Survey of obstetricians' personal preference and discretionary practice. *Eur J Obstet Gynecol Reprod Biol.* 1997;73:1–4.

8. Rouhe H. Should women be able to request a caesarean section? No. *BMJ.* 2011;343:d7565. doi:10.1136/bmj.d7565.

9. Lescale KB, Inglis SR, Eddleman KA, et al. Conflicts between physicians and patients in non-elective cesarean delivery: incidence and adequacy of informed consent. *Am J Perinat.* 1996;13:171–176.

10. ACOG Committee Opinion. Number 371. July 2007. Sterilization of women, including those with mental disabilities. *Obstet Gynecol.* 2007;110:217–220.

11. Caralis D, Kodner IJ, Brown DE. Permanent sterilization of mentally disabled individuals: a case study. *Surgery.* 2009;146:959–963.

12. Murray TH. Moral obligations to the not-yet-born child. *The Worth of a Child.* Berkeley, CA: University of California Press; 1996:96–114.

13. *Planned Parenthood of Southeastern Pennsylvania v. Casey.* 112 US 674 (1992).

14. Harris LH, Cooper A, Rasinski KA, et al. Obstetrician-gynecologists' objections to and willingness to help patients obtain an abortion. *Obstet Gynecol.* 2011;118:905–912.

15. The President's Council on Bioethics. *Beyond Therapy: Biotechnology and the Pursuit of Happiness.* 2003. http://bioethics.georgetown.edu/pcbe/reports/beyondtherapy/. Accessed September 12, 2012.

16. The New York State Task Force on Life and the Law. *Assisted Reproductive Technologies: Analysis and Recommendations for Public Policy.* New York, NY: The New York State Task Force on Life and the Law; 1998:165–169.

17. Wolf LE, Lo B, Gostin LO. Legal barriers to implementing recommendations for universal, routine prenatal HIV testing. *J Law Med Ethics.* 2004;32:137–147.

18. Acuff KI. Prenatal and newborn screening: state legislative approaches and current practice standards. In: Faden RR, Geller G, Powers M, eds. *AIDS, Women and the Next Generation.* New York, NY: Oxford University Press; 1991:121–165.

19. Sharma G, McCullough LB, Chervenak FA. Ethical considerations of early (first vs. second trimester) risk assessment disclosure for trisomy 21 and patient choice in screening versus diagnostic testing. *Am J Med Genet C Semin Med Genet.* 2007;145:99–104.

20. Kuppermann M, Learman LA, Gates E, et al. Beyond race or ethnicity and socioeconomic status: predictors of prenatal testing for Down syndrome. *Obstet Gynecol.* 2006;107:1087–1097.

21. Greely HT. Get ready for the flood of fetal gene screening. *Nature.* 2011;469:289–291.

22. Brown SD, Truog RD, Johnson JA, et al. Do differences in the American Academy of Pediatrics and the American College of Obstetricians and Gynecologists positions on the ethics of maternal–fetal interventions reflect subtly divergent professional sensitivities to pregnant women and fetuses? *Pediatrics.* 2006;117:1382–1387.

23. Stewart DE. Clinical practice. Depression during Pregnancy. *N Engl J Med.* 2011;365:1605–1611.

24. Jos PH, Perlmutter M, Marshall MF. Substance abuse during pregnancy: clinical and public health approaches. *J Law Med Ethics.* 2003;31:340–350.

25. Harris LJ, Paltrow L. The statuf of pregnant women and fetuses in U.S. criminal law. *JAMA.* 2003;289:1697–1699.

26. ACOG Committee Opinion No. 422: at-risk drinking and illicit drug use: ethical issues in obstetric and gynecologic practice. *Obstet Gynecol.* 2008;112:1449–1460.

27. Armstrong EM. Drug and alcohol use during pregnancy: we need to protect, not punish, women. *Womens Health Issues.* 2005;15:45–47.

28. Ecker J, Minkoff H. Home birth: what are physicians' ethical obligations when patient choices may carry increased risk? *Obstet Gynecol.* 2011;117:1179–1182.

29. The New York State Task Force on Life and the Law. *Assisted Reproductive Technologies.* New York, NY: The New York State Task Force on Life and the Law; 1998:177–213.

30. The President's Council on Bioethics. *Reproduction and Responsibility: The Regulation of New Biotechnologies.* http://bioethics.georgetown.edu/pcbe/reports/reproductionandresponsibility/. Accessed September 12, 2012.

ANNOTATED BIBLIOGRAPHY

1. The New York State Task Force on Life and the Law. *Assisted Reproductive Technologies.* New York, NY: The New York State Task Force on Life and the Law; 1998:177–213.
   The President's Council on Bioethics. *Reproduction and Responsibility: The Regulation of New Biotechnologies.* http://bioethics.georgetown.edu/pcbe/reports/reproductionandresponsibility/. Accessed September 12, 2012.
   Two works that present ethical and public policy analyses regarding assisted reproductive technologies.
2. ACOG Committee Opinion #321: maternal decision making, ethics, and the law. *Obstet Gynecol.* 2005; 106:1127–1137.
   Argues against punitive and coercive approaches to protecting the fetus, which violate the woman's right to informed consent, are often based on unsound clinical judgments and are selectively applied to the most vulnerable women.
3. Minkoff H, Chervenak FA. Elective primary cesarean delivery. *N Engl J Med.* 2003;348:298–302.
   Argues that elective cesarean delivery at term is a medically and ethically acceptable option.
4. Jos PH, Perlmutter M, Marshall MF. Substance abuse during pregnancy: clinical and public health approaches. *J Law Med Ethics.* 2003;31:340–350.
   Analysis of ethical and legal issues regarding substance abuse during pregnancy.

40

Ethical Issues in Psychiatry

S ome patients have such severe psychiatric illness that they might seriously harm themselves and others. Treating their psychiatric illness might restore their decision-making capacity and their control over their actions. To protect them from the grave consequences of nonautonomous decisions and actions, physicians might need to restrict their freedom temporarily. Involuntary court-ordered interventions raise ethical concerns because they deprive patients of liberty. In the past, many psychiatric patients were subjected to extreme measures, such as lengthy confinement in inhumane institutions and psychosurgery.

HOW ARE ETHICAL ISSUES IN PSYCHIATRY DIFFERENT?

SEVERE PSYCHIATRIC ILLNESS MIGHT IMPAIR AUTONOMY

Severe psychiatric illness might hinder patients from making informed decisions; distinguish right from wrong; appreciate the consequences of their actions; control their thoughts, impulses, and actions; or care for themselves. When such patients are severely symptomatic, they might have different values, preferences, and judgments than when their illness is in remission.

TREATMENT MIGHT RESTORE THE PATIENT'S AUTONOMY

Treating the underlying psychiatric illness can restore the patient's decision-making capacity and ameliorate psychiatric symptoms. Thus, a short-term infringement on the patient's freedom, such as court-ordered treatment, might restore the patient's autonomy in the long term.

PHYSICIANS CAN PREVENT SERIOUS HARM

Physicians are in a unique position to identify patients who are rendered nonautonomous by psychiatric illness and to prevent serious harm. Society, therefore, has authorized physicians to restrict such patients' liberty in certain circumstances.

PSYCHIATRIC THERAPIES CHANGE THOUGHTS AND FEELINGS

Psychiatric medications can alter how people think and feel. Many patients believe that effective psychiatric therapies restore their true self by removing delusions, disturbed thinking, and mood disorders. However, some patients object that medication transforms them into a different person or alters their thought processes, mental state, and essential characteristics in unacceptable ways.

CONFIDENTIALITY ENCOURAGES CARE FOR MENTAL ILLNESS

During therapy, patients reveal their innermost emotions, fears, and fantasies. Maintaining confidentiality respects the personal and sensitive nature of such information, encourages patients to seek mental health care and to be candid with physicians, and protects patients from stigma and discrimination. Recent federal privacy regulations, as well as some state laws, give special protection to psychotherapy notes by requiring specific patient authorization to disclose them. Dilemmas arise because protecting severely impaired psychiatric patients or third parties may require confidentiality to be overridden.

ACCESS TO PSYCHIATRIC CARE

Despite efforts to achieve insurance parity for medical and psychiatric conditions, many patients have limited access to mental health care. Health insurers often restrict the frequency or duration of mental health care. Many patients with severe psychiatric illness are uninsured, and public mental health services are underfunded. Many patients have additional problems, such as homelessness, alcoholism, or substance abuse, that further complicate access to care.

INVOLUNTARY PSYCHIATRIC COMMITMENT

Involuntary commitment is a dramatic exception to the ethical guideline of respecting people's liberty. Because it infringes on freedom so profoundly, it must be carefully justified.

RATIONALE FOR INVOLUNTARY COMMITMENT

Intervention is warranted to prevent patients who lack the capacity to make informed decisions from causing serious harm to themselves or to others. Depriving them of liberty for a short time might allow treatment to restore their autonomy (1). After depression, bipolar disorder, or schizophrenia is treated, most patients no longer choose to kill themselves or harm others. In contrast, persons who are likely to harm others but are not mentally ill may not be detained against their will unless they have committed a crime (1).

STANDARDS FOR INVOLUNTARY COMMITMENT

States have different criteria for involuntary commitment, but typically require that because of mental illness patients are (1):

- dangerous to themselves, for example suicidal, or
- unable to care for themselves, for example unable to provide food, clothing, and shelter, or
- dangerous to others, for example through threatening, attempting, or committing violence, or
- (in some states) at high risk of deteriorating to the point where they will require involuntary commitment.

PROCEDURES FOR INVOLUNTARY COMMITMENT

Physicians need to be familiar with the law in their state. On an emergency basis, patients typically may be held against their will for brief periods (usually a few days). During an emergency, patients can also be treated against their will to prevent serious physical injury to themselves or others or, in some states, to prevent an irreversible deterioration of their condition. A court hearing must be held to determine whether the patient may be confined for a longer period.

Legal hearings are time-consuming, and many physicians believe that they are an unwarranted intrusion of the legal system into medical practice. However, the public demands rigorous safeguards because involuntary psychiatric hospitalization is a serious deprivation of liberty and has been abused in the past.

OUTPATIENT COMMITMENT AND INVOLUNTARY TREATMENT

Outpatient commitment may be considered in several situations (2). First, outpatient commitment may be instituted on the basis of the patient's advance directives. While in remission, a patient may indicate that he would want outpatient commitment if his condition deteriorated so that inpatient commitment was highly likely. The patient may, therefore, direct physicians and surrogates to override his refusal of treatment to avoid more severe impairment and involuntary hospitalization.

Second, outpatient commitment may be a less restrictive alternative to inpatient commitment. Almost all states allow involuntary outpatient commitment, but most set identical thresholds for inpatient and outpatient commitment. New York and several other states allow preventive involuntary outpatient commitment to prevent a relapse or deterioration that would lead to involuntary inpatient commitment (3). Patients must have a history of "noncompliance with treatment for mental illness that led to hospitalization or have a history of serious violent behavior toward self or others" (3). Such assisted outpatient treatment must be the least restrictive alternative for the patient. Procedures to issue such orders may be started by relatives or roommates of the patient, as well as by mental health, medical, or social service providers or probation or parole officers (3). New York also provides enhanced services and care coordination to patients who are committed. Such outpatient commitment reduces hospitalization and the risk of being arrested and does not deter patients from voluntarily seeking mental health services after the court order is lifted (4).

These two justifications for outpatient commitment have a sound ethical basis as more humane and less restrictive than repeated involuntary hospitalizations. A third situation is controversial. Some patients accept outpatient commitment as a condition of receiving social services, such as disability payments or housing, or to avoid prison for minor crimes. Although they technically need not accept outpatient treatment, the alternatives are distinctly unattractive. Critics charge that social services should be viewed as rights and should not be used as leverage on patients (5). Opponents also object that such programs divert attention and resources from the underlying problem of inadequate outpatient services (5).

MITIGATING ADVERSE CONSEQUENCES

After psychiatric patients are involuntarily hospitalized, they might view the physicians as adversaries who can no longer be trusted. Such feelings might make psychiatric therapy difficult. Physicians should try to stress shared therapeutic goals. An experienced psychiatrist has suggested saying, "It would be a shame if you killed yourself while your depression clouded your judgment. Let's get you undepressed; then, if you still want to kill yourself, I can't stop you" (1). Such a statement demonstrates concern, suggests that therapy might ameliorate the mental illness, and reassures patients that ultimately they are in control.

Patients who are hospitalized involuntarily have certain legal rights (1), including a right to treatment and a right to the least restrictive alternative, as well as rights of visitation, communication, privacy, and freedom of movement, subject to legitimate restrictions.

SUICIDAL PATIENTS

When patients attempt or threaten suicide, physicians have an ethical obligation to intervene.

RATIONALE FOR SUICIDE INTERVENTION

The ethical justification for suicide intervention is to prevent serious, irreversible harm to persons who lack decision-making capacity. Suicidal patients are almost always impaired by severe depression or other severe mental illness (4). Their actions do not result from autonomous choices, but rather from mental illness. Interventions to prevent suicide provide time to treat the underlying mental illness or let it enter a remission. Empirical studies demonstrate the effectiveness of suicide prevention. If persons are prevented from committing suicide, then only about 10% to 20% subsequently kill themselves (6).

Even strong proponents of patient autonomy recognize the need to intervene to prevent nonautonomous persons from killing themselves (7). Some suicidal threats, although representing a "cry for help," might not warrant involuntary commitment and might be treated through less restrictive measures, such as arranging for voluntary psychiatric treatment, mobilizing assistance from family and friends, removing the means of suicide, and getting patients to promise to call for help. Imposing involuntary commitment is a last resort and should be continued only as long as necessary to protect the nonautonomous patient. In contrast, it is ethically problematic to restrict the liberty of autonomous persons to protect them. Some patients with terminal illnesses with decision-making capacity might make a deliberate decision to end their lives. The ethics of physician-assisted suicide is hotly debated (*see* Chapter 19).

WHEN IS A PATIENT SUICIDAL?

When patients are severely depressed or mention suicide, physicians should ask specific questions to determine the likelihood of a serious suicide attempt. Fears that raising the topic of suicide will suggest or even encourage it are unfounded and deter physicians from gathering crucial information and initiating effective treatment. Many depressed patients feel relieved to discuss suicide with a caring and nonjudgmental physician.

PATIENTS WHO ARE DANGEROUS TO OTHERS

Widely publicized cases have focused attention on the physician's obligation to prevent psychiatric patients from killing third parties. Patients with serious psychiatric illnesses might disclose to physicians plans to kill or injure third parties, actual attempts, or overt acts of harm. Thus, the physician might be in a unique position to prevent serious harm to potential victims. Social norms and criminal sanctions might not deter psychiatric patients who cannot control their violent impulses. In this situation, the landmark Tarasoff case established that confidentiality should be overridden to prevent serious harm to third parties (6).

CASE 40.1   The Tarasoff case and the duty to prevent harm

A university student, Prosenjit Poddar, confided to his psychologist that he was planning to kill a woman, readily identifiable as Tatiana Tarasoff, who had rejected him romantically. The therapist and his superiors at the student health service decided that Poddar should be committed involuntarily and asked the campus police to detain him. The police did so but released him because he appeared rational. The director of psychiatry ordered no action to place Poddar under involuntary detention. Subsequently Poddar went to Tarasoff's home and stabbed her to death.

Although therapists feared that the decision would deter patients from seeking mental health services and disclosing their violent thoughts, this has not occurred. Most states now require therapists to protect identifiable persons threatened with serious violence by psychiatric patients (8). Generally, the duty is limited to identifiable patients and actual threats.

STEPS TO PREVENT HARM

The duty to prevent harm to potential victims of psychiatric patients requires several steps (9). First, the physician needs to evaluate the threat of violence. Asking about violence does not give patients the idea of harming others or encourage them to do so. It is useful to ask whether the patient has ever seriously injured another person or thought about doing so (9).

Predictions of violence by physicians are not very accurate. In one study, 53% of psychiatric patients whom physicians predicted would be violent in fact committed violent acts over the subsequent 6 months; in comparison, 36% of psychiatric patients whose psychiatrists had no concerns about violence committed violent acts (10). Doctors need to do the best they can within the limits of clinical judgment. The standard of care is what a reasonable physician would do under the circumstances.

After determining that the threat of violence is severe and probable, the physician must decide how to respond. A number of actions might protect the victim, such as changing the patient's medications, increasing the frequency of therapy sessions, having the patient give up weapons, hospitalizing the patient voluntarily, committing the patient involuntarily, and notifying the police (9).

The law in many states specifically requires warning the threatened victim. Such warning does not replace steps to reduce the risk of violence. Physicians should notify patients before they override confidentiality and explain why they are required to do so (9). Patients might agree with warning the threatened person (1). Many patients are ambivalent about violence and welcome help with expressing their emotions or dealing with interpersonal conflicts. When beginning therapy with patients who have a history of violence, physicians should discuss the situations in which confidentiality may be overridden (1).

REFUSAL OF PSYCHIATRIC TREATMENT

Patients who are involuntarily committed may have a right to refuse psychiatric treatment. The rationale is that confinement without treatment can sometimes accomplish the goal of care—preventing harm to self or others (1). The ethical guideline of preventing harm has more moral force than the guideline of doing good (*see* Chapter 4). Thus, the obligation to prevent harms to nonautonomous psychiatric patients or to third parties is stronger than the duty to help them recover their well-being. Moreover, forced administration of medications to unwilling patients is intrusive, inhumane, and impractical in the long run. Even if psychiatric medications were forcibly administered to inpatients, patients can (and often do) discontinue them after discharge.

Because competency is determined with regard to specific tasks, a patient who is not competent to refuse commitment may still be competent to refuse psychiatric medications. Administering medications to competent patients against their will violates their liberty and bodily integrity. Patients often view the risks and benefits of psychiatric therapies differently from physicians. Many psychiatric patients refuse drugs because of unacceptable side effects or because medications alter their brain and personality. Finally, past abuses have led the public to question physicians' judgments that treatment is beneficial and necessary.

On the other hand, confining patients, but not treating them with effective medications has been criticized as letting people "rot with their rights on" (11). To critics, it is cruel and pointless to withhold from severely impaired patients the very treatments that are likely to restore their autonomy and well-being. In this view, short-term involuntary treatment for the underlying psychiatric illness is a lesser infringement on the patient's freedom than prolonged involuntary hospitalization without treatment.

Several states require a court hearing if a psychiatric patient who has been involuntarily committed refuses treatment (1). The court determines whether the patient is competent to make an informed decision to refuse treatment. If so, the refusal must be honored. If the patient is not competent, the court may order treatment.

The patient's capacity to make informed decisions, therefore, is crucial to whether the patient's refusal of psychiatric therapy will be respected (*see* Chapter 10). Assessing the decision-making capacity of psychiatric patients can be particularly difficult. People with major depression might underestimate the benefits of treatment and overestimate the risks (12). They might be convinced that the treatment will fail or that they will experience a serious side effect of therapy. Similarly, manic patients might believe that nothing is wrong with them and, therefore, they do not need treatment.

Most refusals of inpatient treatment are resolved in a few days. In one study, only 7% of inpatients refused antipsychotic medication for longer than 24 hours (13). Common reasons for refusal were psychotic or idiosyncratic thought processes, side effects of medications, denial of mental illness, and alleged ineffectiveness of medications. Cases were resolved in several ways. In 50% of cases, patients eventually took medication voluntarily, after nursing staff, psychiatrists, or family reassured, coaxed, or persuaded them (1). In 23% of cases, either the psychiatrist discontinued antipsychotic drugs or the patient was discharged without them—that is, the physician ultimately did not consider these medications essential. Finally, in 18% of cases the psychiatrists obtained a court order for involuntary administration of the medication. In all the cases that went to court, the judge authorized involuntary treatment.

REFUSAL OF MEDICAL TREATMENT

Patients with serious psychiatric illness might refuse recommended therapy for concurrent medical problems. As with any patient refusal, the first step is to ask whether the patient lacks decision-making capacity (*see* Chapter 11). A psychiatric diagnosis *per se* does not imply that a patient lacks the capacity to make an informed decision about medical treatment. A competent patient's refusal should be respected if attempts at persuasion are unsuccessful. If the patient lacks decision-making capacity, decisions should be based on advance directives or made by surrogates (*see* Chapters 12 and 13).

Dilemmas arise when psychiatric patients who lack decision-making capacity actively resist medical treatment that is clearly in their best interests. Resorting to physical force or deception is ethically troubling and may seem inhumane. Forced treatment might also undermine the doctor–patient relationship and make it more difficult for patients to take responsibility for other aspects of their lives. Finally, involuntary medical treatment is impossible in the long term. In a structured inpatient setting, cajoling, and negotiation might enable the staff to get the patient to take the medicine. However, the patient can discontinue medicines after discharge.

PSYCHOTROPIC DRUGS IN LESS SEVERE CONDITIONS

Selective serotonin reuptake inhibitors (SSRIs) are effective not only in major depression, but also in other conditions, such as dysthymia or social anxiety. Some patients with these conditions report that SSRIs make them feel better than they normally do. Their mood brightens, and anxiety, social inhibition, obsession, compulsion, and fear diminish. Some patients report that such medications allow them to become themselves again, gain their true identity for the first time, or function in social situations where they previously felt extreme anxiety or inhibitions.

Critics object to the use of psychoactive medications in persons with "merely melancholy or inhibited temperaments" (14). In their view, using medications in this context is not a proper goal of medicine (14). From their perspective, people should achieve a more flourishing life through self-examination and arduous effort, not through brain-altering medications. Furthermore, from their viewpoint, some negative feelings should not be blunted; it is part of the human condition to experience sadness or outrage. These critics fear that people taking medications will lose "what sorrow teaches, discontent provokes" (14).

Such broad philosophical objections overlook severe symptoms and functional impairment that people might experience. Generalized social anxiety disorder is much more severe than shyness or performance anxiety; people with it avoid or fear most social and work situations and experience distress and functional impairment. Clinical trials show that both cognitive-behavioral therapy and pharmacologic therapy with SSRIs are effective for this condition (15).

Furthermore, these critics present a problematic view of the physician's role and responsibilities. Discounting the patient's experience and distress is disrespectful. Also, critics need to examine empirical evidence. Is exhorting patients to greater efforts at self-improvement effective when patients are impaired by intrusive feelings and thoughts that they cannot control? Omitting the option of medications that have been shown to be effective is inconsistent with the ethical ideal that physicians should act in the best interests of the patient, as defined by the patient's values. Finally, it is questionable whether physicians should try to impose their view of the good life on their patients who have not selected them for that view.

SUMMARY

1. When psychiatric patients are suicidal, unable to care for themselves, or are dangerous to others, physicians have ethical and legal obligations to prevent harm.
2. These obligations may override respecting patient autonomy and maintaining confidentiality.
3. In fulfilling this duty, physicians also need to use their clinical skills and judgment to encourage effective treatment for the underlying psychiatric disorders.

REFERENCES

1. Appelbaum PS, Gutheil TG. *Clinical Handbook of Psychiatry and the Law.* 4th ed. Philadelphia, PA: Lippincott Williams & Wilkins; 2007.
2. Saks ER. Involuntary outpatient commitment. *Psychol Public Policy Law.* 2003;9:94–106.
3. Office of Mental Health NYS. An explanation of Kendra's law. http://www.omh.ny.gov/omhweb/Kendra_web/Ksummary.htm. Accessed November 28, 2011.
4. Swartz MS. Introduction to the special section on assisted outpatient treatment in New York State. *Psychiatr Serv.* 2010;61:967–969.
5. Monahan J, Bonnie RJ, Appelbaum PS, et al. Mandated community treatment: beyond outpatient commitment. *Psychiatr Serv.* 2001;52:1198–1205.
6. Miller RD. Need-for-treatment criteria for involuntary civil commitment: impact in practice. *Am J Psychiatry.* 1992;149:1380–1384.
7. Beauchamp TL, Childress JF. *Principles of Biomedical Ethics.* 5th ed. New York, NY: Oxford University Press; 2001:176–194.
8. Appelbaum PS. *Almost a Revolution: Mental Health Law and the Limits of Change.* New York, NY: Oxford University Press; 1994.
9. Anfang SA, Appelbaum PS. Twenty years after Tarasoff: reviewing the duty to protect. *Harv Rev Psychiatry.* 1996;4:67–76.
10. Lidz C, Mulvey EP, Gardner W. The accuracy of predictions of violence to others. *JAMA.* 1993;269:1007–1011.
11. Appelbaum PS, Gutheil TG. "Rotting with their rights on": constitutional theory and clinical reality in drug refusal by psychiatric patients. *Bull Am Acad Psychiatry Law.* 1979;7:306–315.
12. Grisso T, Appelbaum P. *Assessing Competence to Consent to Treatment: A Guide for Physicians and Other Health Professionals..* New York, NY: Oxford University Press; 1998.
13. Hoge SK, Appelbaum PS, Lawlor T. A prospective, multicenter study of patients' refusal of antipsychotic medication. *Arch Gen Psychiatry.* 1990;47:949–956.
14. The President's Council on Bioethics. *Beyond Therapy: Biotechnology and the Pursuit of Happiness.* 2003. http://bioethics.georgetown.edu/pcbe/reports/beyondtherapy/. Accessed September 12, 2012.
15. Schneier FR. Clinical practice. Social anxiety disorder. *N Engl J Med.* 2006;355:1029–1036.

ANNOTATED BIBLIOGRAPHY

1. Appelbaum PS, Gutheil TG. *Clinical Handbook of Psychiatry and the Law.* 4th ed. Philadelphia, PA: Lippincott Williams & Wilkins; 2007.
   Excellent book on ethical and legal issues regarding psychiatric patients. Contains practical clinical advice on managing patients with severe psychiatric disorders.
2. The President's Council on Bioethics. *Beyond Therapy: Biotechnology and the Pursuit of Happiness.* . http://bioethics.georgetown.edu/pcbe/reports/beyondtherapy/. Accessed September 12, 2012.
   Critique of the widespread use of psychiatric medications for enhancement, rather than for major psychiatric illness.
3. Swartz MS. Introduction to the special section on assisted outpatient treatment in New York State. *Psychiatr Serv.* 2010;61:967–969.
   Lucid overview of involuntary outpatient commitment and its rationale and outcomes. Other articles in this issue present outcomes research regarding the New York policy.

Current Controversies

41

Ethical Issues in Organ Transplantation

After receiving a kidney, liver, heart, or lung transplant, many patients with end-stage disease can return to active lives. Organ donors undergo interventions to benefit the recipient. The ethical concern is that the donor's well-being might be compromised to benefit someone else. Thus, consent for donation and minimizing harm to donors are essential to maintain public trust.

The need for organ transplantation far exceeds the supply of donated organs. At the end of 2011, more than 92,000 people were on active waiting lists for transplants, whereas the number of organ transplants in 2011 was about 35,000. Thus, difficult decisions about allocating donated organs cannot be avoided. Patients on the waiting list and potential donors need to believe that allocation procedures are fair and trustworthy. This chapter discusses the donation of organs and the selection of recipients.

DONATION OF CADAVERIC ORGANS

ETHICAL CONCERNS ABOUT CADAVERIC DONATION

Harm to Donors

When transplantation was initiated, concerns were raised that cadaveric organ transplantation hastened or caused the donor's death. Criteria were developed for determining death in patients whose brains had ceased to function, but whose hearts were still beating (*see* Chapter 21).

Conflicts of Interest

Because of concerns that potential organ donors might have their deaths hastened, decisions about the potential donor's care must be separate from and take priority over decisions about procurement and transplantation (1). The physician for the potential donor may not be part of the transplantation team. Also, in the United States, payments for donation are prohibited to prevent abuse and exploitation of potential donors.

Respect for Organ Donors

Cadaveric donation raises concerns about respect for human remains, for the decedent's wishes regarding disposition of the body, and for the wishes of survivors (2). If people do not want to be organ donors, their wishes must be respected.

THE CURRENT SYSTEM FOR CADAVERIC DONATION

The United States has a voluntary system for organ donation. The Uniform Anatomical Gift Act allows people to use an organ donor card to grant permission to use their organs for transplantation after their death. This card is usually part of a person's driver's license. However, many Americans have not signed such cards, ever if they support organ transplantation. Some fear that if they agree to organ donation, they will receive suboptimal care (2). Hospitals must report all inpatient deaths to local organ procurement organizations, which contact eligible families to request donation.

Only about 50% of relatives of patients with brain death give permission for organ donation (2). Many families do not understand the concept of brain death, and some perceive the organ procurement process as insensitive (2). Some cultural beliefs pose barriers to organ donation (3). For instance, many Asian or Latino families believe that bodies must be buried whole or else spirits will suffer after death.

DONATION AFTER CICRULATORY DETERMINATION OF DEATH (DCDD)

Most cadaver donors are declared dead by brain criteria and have effective circulation until the organs are harvested. Some donors, however, are declared dead by circulatory and respiratory criteria rather than neurologic criteria for "brain death" (2, 4). Chapter 32 discusses DCDD in detail, particularly the ethical concerns.

This approach raises several ethical concerns (5, 6). First, is the donor really dead? The time from the development of asystole to declaration of death is typically about 2 to 5 minutes, beyond the period when circulation can spontaneously return. Some protocols, however, harvest organs after a shorter period of asystole to reduce warm ischemia time and improve recipient outcomes. Second, does the process of donating organs cause or hasten death? Some steps to preserve organs, such as an infusion of heparin and inserting large-bore catheters to facilitate infusion of organ-preservation solution after death, are clearly not for the benefit of the donor and should be done only with explicit consent.

PROPOSALS TO INCREASE THE DONATION OF CADAVERIC ORGANS

Many proposals have been made to increase cadaveric organ donation, and some have been adopted in other countries (2, 7). However, some of these proposals might undermine public trust in transplantation and, in the long term, make people less willing to donate.

Mandated Choice

Persons would be required to state their preferences about organ donation when renewing drivers' licenses or filing income taxes. This requirement would relieve relatives of the stress of making decisions about donation. In surveys, most Americans support this policy.

Following Donor Cards

Under existing statutes, organs may be retrieved from people who had signed donor cards even if the next of kin does not agree. Ethically, it is consistent with respecting patient advance directives. As a practical matter, however, objections from family members are honored because of concerns about adverse publicity that might undermine public trust.

Presumed Consent

Currently, organs are harvested only if the patient or family has given explicit consent. Under this proposal, organs would be harvested unless the patient or family specifically objects. Although this approach has been adopted in some countries (8, 9), many people in the United States object (2).

ORGANS FROM LIVING DONORS

Transplantation of kidneys and portions of liver and lung from living donors is increasing (10). Most live donors are persons who have a preexisting emotional relationship with the recipient, such as relatives, friends, and coworkers. A few donors are "Good Samaritans" who have no previous relationship with the recipient. Donation from persons who are not genetically related is feasible because human leukocyte antigens (HLA) compatibility does not enhance survival of liver and lung transplants and is less important in living kidney transplants than cadaveric transplants. The quality of organs from live donors is higher because of more thorough medical screening and shorter ischemia time compared with cadaveric donors. Transplants from live donors do not delay transplants to other patients on the waiting list because the total number of donors is increased.

ETHICAL ISSUES REGARDING LIVE DONATION

Harm to Donors

Surgeons might violate the guideline of "do no harm" when they operate on a healthy person to benefit another person. A highly publicized death of a living liver donor in 2002 led to a decline in live donations. Other risks include postoperative bile leak, pain, and lost income.

To limit risks, persons may not serve as living donors if they have medical conditions that significantly increase operative risk or if they have abnormal organ function. To further reduce risk of living liver donation, some have advocated that it be carried out only at experienced centers .

Motives of Donors

Donation to relatives and friends is understandable because people want to help and care for persons they have close relationships with. Donating to a stranger, however, raises ethical concerns (11). On the one hand, forming a close emotional bond to a stranger in need can be an extraordinary form of altruism and humanitarianism. On the other hand, it can also be driven by a desire for publicity, financial gain, or internal psychological conflicts. Thus, offers by strangers to donate need to be carefully reviewed to rule out problematic motives (12).

Consent From Donors

Because a live donor undergoes serious risks to benefit another person, it is essential that the decision to donate be free and informed. Many live donors choose to donate immediately, however, before they learn of the risks of donation. People commonly base important decisions on emotion rather than reason. Altruism does not fit a model of rational utilitarian deliberation about personal risks and benefits. However, donors should be able to explain their decision to donate in a coherent manner, even though they might give less weight than most people to the possibility of a serious risk. The donor's decision should remain stable after the donor receives more information and has time to reflect.

Consent should be voluntary as well as informed (13). A patient's relative might feel family pressure to donate and may need help to carry out an intention to refuse. Doctors may offer a general excuse that someone is not a suitable donor, without specifying why. However, it would be ethically problematic for a physician to provide a false medical reason as an excuse (14), as with any deception by a physician (see Chapter 6).

The "gift of life" through live donation entails obligations and burdens (13, 15). Generally, gifts impose reciprocal obligations and expectations on the recipient. The gift of an organ is so extraordinary that it might become a "tyranny" (15). A live donor might take a "proprietary interest" in the recipient's life (15). A sense of indebtedness might make it difficult for the recipient to remain independent of the donor. Many transplantation programs generally do not reveal the identities of donors and recipients to each other if they are not already acquainted.

Use of children as live donors raises particular ethical concerns because they cannot give consent for themselves and depend on others to protect their interests. Although adults may make extraordinary sacrifices for others, they may not require children to do so. Hence, children should be live donors only as a last resort if no suitable adult donor can be identified, if the recipient is a close family member, and the child assents (16). To assure that a child donor's interests are protected, approval from a donor advocacy team should be obtained.

Payment to Donors

In some impoverished countries, paying live donors is common (17). In India, paid kidney donors reported that they were financially worse off after surgery despite receiving payments (18).

Furthermore, paid donors from developing countries might pose risks to recipients because of a significantly higher rate of HIV and hepatitis B and C. Although some writers have advocated a regulated market to decrease the gap between the need for transplantation and the supply of organs (19), documented exploitation, coercion, and abuse are a compelling reason to reject such proposals (17, 20). Because of a flourishing black market in countries where payment for organs is illegal, is seems unlikely that a regulated market can be enforced (21). In the United States as well as other countries, buying and selling of organs is illegal.

Reimbursement for Donors

Proposals have been made to give living donors incentives, such as reimbursement of out-of-pocket expenses such as loss of income due to disability resulting from surgery, free medical care for complications of donation, and high priority for transplantation should they need it (22, 23). These financial incentives can be distinguished from payments because they do not result in a net financial gain for donors; instead, they make donors return to the position they would have been in had they not donated their organs.

Confidentiality of Recipient

The recipient might have a medical condition that might affect the potential donor's willingness to donate. For example, the recipient might have cancer that might recur in the transplanted organ and reduce the likelihood of long-term success. Moreover, some donors may not want to help patients whose liver failure was caused by alcoholic liver disease or HIV infection brought about by their own actions and choices. According to the principle of informed consent, prospective living donors should receive information that is pertinent to their decision to donate. Because patient confidentiality is also important, potential recipients must give permission to disclose such information to potential donors (24).

CURRENT SYSTEM FOR LIVE DONATION

Live donors undergo extensive education and medical and psychosocial evaluation (10, 12). This process ensures that decisions to donate are informed, free, and altruistic and that the donor is not at increased medical risk from donation.

PAIRED DONATION

Paired kidney donations overcome incompatibilities between donors and their intended recipients. A living donor directs the donated organ to a compatible recipient, while another donor donates to the first donor's recipient (25). Three-way or chain exchanges extend this approach by including additional pairs of donors and recipients. Although such donations increase the number of people who receive transplants, they also raise ethical concerns (25). First, pressure on potential donors may increase, since incompatibility is no longer a contraindication to donation. Second, because a donor might withdraw from donation once his intended recipient has received an organ, harvesting of organs is performed simultaneously for each donor–recipient pair.

SELECTION OF RECIPIENTS

Because the number of people needing transplants far exceeds the number of donated organs, difficult allocation decisions must be made.

HISTORICAL BACKGROUND

When dialysis was developed in the 1960s, only a limited number of dialysis machines were available, and committees ranked candidates according to their perceived social worth (26). Responding to concerns that selection was based on prejudice and unwarranted value judgments, Congress funded dialysis for all patients with end-stage renal disease. In transplantation, however, allocation decisions cannot be avoided because of a shortage of organs.

Because people donate cadaveric organs without knowing who will receive them, a fair allocation procedure is essential to maintain public willingness to donate organs (27). Moreover, it is unfair to ask people to donate if there is no opportunity to receive a transplant.

The following section discusses general ethical principles for allocating organs. Specific selection criteria are too detailed to be discussed here but can be found at www.unos.org. Different considerations receive priority for different organs (27).

BENEFICENCE

From a utilitarian perspective, scarce organs should go to those patients who will receive the greatest net medical benefit (27). Relevant outcomes include the likelihood and duration of recipient survival and quality of life, compared to not receiving a transplant. Although this criterion appears objective, it involves complex value judgments.

Many physicians consider it pointless to transplant a scarce organ that is very likely to be rejected because of recipient nonadherence. Active injection drug use or alcoholism and a history of nonadherence are commonly regarded as contraindications to transplantation (28, 29). Critics, however, contend that psychosocial factors might "cloak biases about race, class, social status, and other factors that, if stated openly, would not be tolerated" (30). Furthermore, such obstacles might be overcome with rehabilitation and psychosocial support.

JUSTICE

The guideline that scarce resources should be distributed fairly or equitably is indisputable in the abstract but difficult to specify. Several approaches to operationalize equity have been considered (27, 31).

Time on the Waiting List

The precept of "first-come, first-served" seems intuitively fair if there are no other compelling reasons to distinguish among candidates; however, time on the waiting list can be manipulated by placing patients on the waiting list earlier in the course of illness or at several regional transplantation networks. Better-educated and wealthier patients are more likely to take advantage of these possibilities. To make time on the waiting list fairer, only patients meeting minimum clinical criteria may be placed on the list (27).

Medical Need

To assist those in greatest need, in liver and heart transplantation, patients who would die soon without transplantation are given priority over more stable patients. Cadaveric livers are assigned according to the Model for End-Stage Liver Disease (MELD) system, a severity of illness score based on laboratory tests, which predicts the risk of death while on the waiting list. Significant geographical disparities remain, however, with sicker patients in larger organ-procurement areas waiting longer for transplants than patients in smaller organ-procurement areas (32–34).

Geographic Location

Waiting times for liver transplantation vary up to fivefold among various geographical regions, even among sickest candidates who are most likely to die without transplantation (33). To reduce these disparities in waiting times, we might allocate organs on a regional or national basis to those with the greatest medical need, with less emphasis on keeping organs in the geographic area in which they are donated (32, 33). This policy is justified by the idea that organs belong to the nation as a whole and that where a person resides or is on the waiting list is not a morally relevant allocation criterion (27). This proposed change would provide more organs to large referral centers, which transplant sicker patients and have better outcomes. Opponents object that such redistribution penalizes states that make efforts to increase donations and might worsen outcomes by increasing cold ischemia time (33).

Anticipated Benefit of Transplantation

An increasing number of elderly patients are placed on transplant waiting lists. If they receive an organ from a younger cadaveric donor, they might die years before the graft is projected to stop functioning. Younger transplant candidates would have more years of use from such an organ. Thus, it has been proposed to better match cadaveric kidneys with longer projected graft survival to recipients with long estimated survival. The specifics of these proposals, however, are controversial and unproven (35).

Ability to Pay

Transplantation is generally performed only on patients who can pay for it. Medicare covers kidney transplantation for all Americans. Most private insurers and most state Medicaid programs cover liver and heart transplantation. Americans who lack health insurance must raise money for transplantation of these organs, for example, through public appeals.

Allocating organs by ability to pay, although routinely practiced, has been strongly criticized (27). It seems unfair to ask all people, rich and poor alike, to be organ donors if the poor or uninsured would not be eligible recipients.

Previous Transplantation

The success rate in transplanting a second organ after one transplanted organ fails is substantially lower than in first-time transplants (36). The guideline of promise keeping or loyalty is often used to justify retransplantation; having made a commitment to the patient, the surgeons cannot now abandon him or her. Critics contend, however, that retransplantation might be a denial of the inevitable limits of human life and an unwillingness to say "enough is enough" (37).

Citizenship

Should people who are not long-term US residents receive organs harvested in the United States? Particular objections have been directed at foreigners who come to the United States specifically to obtain a transplant. It seems unfair, however, to exclude foreign nationals who contribute to the US economy and who would be asked to serve as organ donors.

Ethnic Background

Even though African Americans are more likely than Caucasians to develop chronic renal failure, they are less likely to receive a kidney transplant: they are less likely to be evaluated for transplantation, to be placed on waiting lists, and to find a donor (38). Also, they have longer waiting times on transplantation lists. The point system for prioritizing cadaveric kidneys gives priority to HLA matching, which improves graft and patient survival. Because the prevalence of ABO and HLA antigens differs among ethnic groups, African Americans are less likely to find a highly matched Caucasian donor. Most donors are Caucasian. Thus, allocation rules that optimize graft survival disadvantage African Americans. Changing the point system to decrease the importance of HLA matching improved access of African Americans to renal transplants, while decreasing average graft survival only slightly (38).

UNOS policy forbids explicit consideration of gender, race, or social factors, such as wealth or celebrity status in allocating cadaveric organs.

DIFFERENCES IN ALLOCATING VARIOUS ORGANS

The ethical guidelines of beneficence and justice are balanced differently for different organs (27). For renal failure, dialysis is an effective alternative to transplantation and the level of HLA matching is a predictor of cadaveric graft survival. Hence, urgency is not considered, and HLA matching is given weight. In contrast, in liver failure, because there is no alternative to transplantation, the highest priority is given to patients in the most critical condition. HLA matching is not considered because it has little impact on outcomes. Different ethical considerations might conflict. For example, liver recipients with the most urgent need have worse outcomes and greater costs than more stable patients.

PATIENT BEHAVIORS THAT CAUSE DISEASE

If patients who received a liver transplant for alcoholic liver disease begin to abuse alcohol again, they have an increased risk of transplant failure due to recurrent liver disease or failure to adhere to posttransplant care (39). The issue of transplantation in alcoholic liver disease has been heatedly debated on. On the one hand, some argue that patients should be held responsible for repeatedly and knowingly putting in jeopardy a scarce, lifesaving resource (40). In this view, patients who develop end-stage liver disease "through no fault of their own" should have higher priority than persons with alcoholism (41). Moreover, the public might be less willing to donate organs if they are given to alcoholics. On the other hand, restrictions on liver transplantation for alcoholics may be considered unfair (28, 42) because alcoholism has genetic and environmental components that are beyond the person's control. Moreover, criteria for disqualification are inconsistent and arbitrary, and treatment for alcohol dependence may not be offered (28). Furthermore, judgments of moral responsibility are not made for other illnesses.

Selected patients with alcoholic liver disease have liver transplant survival rates comparable to those of patients with other liver diseases (29). Most transplant centers require a period of abstinence from alcohol and adherence to medical care for patients with alcoholic liver disease as a surrogate for their posttransplant behavior. Such abstinence may also permit the liver to recover, so that transplantation may no longer be needed (29). Similarly, substance abusers must undergo drug testing to document abstinence. Patients should receive referrals for counseling and rehabilitation.

DIRECTED DONATION TO STRANGERS

CASE 41.1	Advertising for an organ donor

In 2004, Mr. K, a 32-year-old newlywed man with advanced liver cancer, placed an ad on billboards: "I need a liver. Please help save my life." The next month he received a cadaveric liver that was donated specifically to him. Seven months later he died. It was not known whether his death was due to recurrent liver cancer, complications of transplantation, or other causes.

Cadaveric organs, as well as organs from living donors, may be donated to a specific individual. Most directed cadaveric organs are from relatives or friends who die unexpectedly. Some organs, however, are directed to people who are the subject of news stories, solicitations on the Internet, or advertisements. The directed donation in Case 41.1 was severely criticized as unfair (43). Some patients with localized liver cancer are given higher priority to increase their chances of transplant before widespread metastases develop. In Case 41.1, Mr. K already had advanced disease and, therefore, was low on the waiting list. Advertisements portray a transplantation candidate as deserving an exception to usual allocation criteria. Everyone on the waiting list, however, has powerful stories of why he needs a transplant. Advertisements allow the wealthy and well-educated to jump ahead of people who are higher on the list because they are more likely to die without a liver transplant. Organ donation depends on a public perception of fairness, that no candidate is favored because of social standing, fame, or wealth. Claims that public appeals to donate to a specific individual increase the total number of available organs are not based on strong empirical data (44). To address these concerns about fairness, it has been proposed that publicly solicited organs must go to the first person on the waiting list, unless the recipient and the donor had a preexisting emotional relationship (44).

SUMMARY

1. Although transplantation can return patients with end-stage illness to active lives, it raises difficult issues of informed choice, acceptable risk in donation, and fair allocation.

2. Living donation presents particular ethical challenges because healthy donors undergo risks to benefit others and because consent needs to be both informed and free.
3. Transparency and accountability in the transplantation process are essential to maintain public willingness to donate organs.

REFERENCES

1. DeVita MA, Caplan AL. Caring for organs or for patients? Ethical concerns about the Uniform Anatomical Gift Act (2006). *Ann Intern Med.* 2007;147:876–879.
2. Committee on Increasing Rates of Organ Donation. *Organ Donation: Opportunities for Action.* Washington, DC: National Academies Press; 2006.
3. Hippen BE. A modest approach to a new frontier: commentary on Danovitch. *Transplantation.* 2007;84:464–466.
4. Bernat JL, Capron AM, Bleck TP, et al. The circulatory-respiratory determination of death in organ donation. *Crit Care Med.* 2010;38:963–970.
5. Steinbrook R. Organ donation after cardiac death. *N Engl J Med.* 2007;357:209–213.
6. Miller FG, Truog RD. *Death, Dying, and Organ Transplantation.* New York, NY: Oxford University Press; 2012.
7. Childress JF. How can we ethically increase the supply of transplantable organs? *Ann Intern Med.* 2006;145:224–225.
8. Rithalia A, McDaid C, Suekarran S, et al. A systematic review of presumed consent systems for deceased organ donation. *Health Technol Assess.* 2009;13:iii, ix–xi, 1–95.
9. Rithalia A, McDaid C, Suekarran S, et al. Impact of presumed consent for organ donation on donation rates: a systematic review. *BMJ.* 2009;338:a3162.
10. Pavlakis M. Live kidney donation: a 36-year-old woman hoping to donate a kidney to her mother. *JAMA.* 2011;305:592–599
11. Neuberger J. Making an offer you can't refuse? A challenge of altruistic donation. *Transpl Int.* 2011;24:1159–1161.
12. Dew MA, Jacobs CL, Jowsey SG, et al. Guidelines for the psychosocial evaluation of living unrelated kidney donors in the United States. *Am J Transplant.* 2007;7:1047–1054.
13. Biller-Andorno N. Voluntariness in living-related organ donation. *Transplantation* 2011;92:617-9.
14. Ross LF. What the medical excuse teaches us about the potential living donor as patient. *Am J Transplant.* 2010;10:731–736.
15. Fox RC, Swazey JP. *Spare Parts.* New York, NY: Oxford University Press; 1992:31–42.
16. Ross LF, Thistlethwaite JR Jr. Minors as living solid-organ donors. *Pediatrics.* 2008;122:454–461.
17. Scheper-Hughes N. Keeping an eye on the global traffic in human organs. *Lancet.* 2003;361:1645–1648.
18. Sehgal A, Galbraith A, Chesney M, et al. How strictly do dialysis patients want their advance directives followed. *JAMA.* 1992;267:59–63.
19. Bakdash T, Scheper-Hughes N. Is it ethical for patients with renal disease to purchase kidneys from the world's poor? *PLoS Med.* 2006;3:e349.
20. The declaration of Istanbul on organ trafficking and transplant tourism. *Transplantation.* 2008;86:1013–1018.
21. Biller-Andorno N, Capron AM. "Gratuities" for donated organs: ethically indefensible. *Lancet.* 2011;377:1390–1391.
22. Arnold R, Bartlett S, Bernat J, et al. Financial incentives for cadaver organ donation: an ethical reappraisal. *Transplantation.* 2002;73:1361–1367.
23. Delmonico FL, Arnold R, Scheper-Hughes N, et al. Ethical incentives—not payment—for organ donation. *N Engl J Med.* 2002;346:2002–2005.
24. Roland ME, Lo B, Braff J, et al. Key clinical, ethical, and policy issues in the evaluation of the safety and effectiveness of solid organ transplantation in HIV-infected patients. *Arch Intern Med.* 2003;163:1773–1778.
25. Wallis CB, Samy KP, Roth AE, et al. Kidney paired donation. *Nephrol Dial Transplant.* 2011;26:2091–2099.
26. Fox RC, Swazey JP. *The Courage to Fail: A Social View of Organ Transplants and Dialysis.* 2nd ed. Chicago, IL: University of Chicago Press; 1978.
27. Childress JF. Putting patients first in organ allocation: an ethical analysis of the U.S. debate. *Camb Q Healthc Ethics.* 2001;10:365–376.
28. Webb K, Shepherd L, Day E, et al. Transplantation for alcoholic liver disease: report of a consensus meeting. *Liver Transpl.* 2006;12:301–305.
29. Bathgate AJ. Recommendations for alcohol-related liver disease. *Lancet.* 2006;367:2045–2046.
30. Robertson JA. Patient selection for organ transplantation: age, incarceration, family support, and other social factors. *Transplant Proc.* 1989;21:3431–3436.
31. Stegall MD. The development of kidney allocation policy. *Am J Kidney Dis.* 2005;46:974–975.
32. Washburn K, Pomfret E, Roberts J. Liver allocation and distribution: possible next steps. *Liver Transpl.* 2011;17:1005–1012.
33. Committee on Organ Procurement and Transplantation Policy. *Organ Procurement and Transplantation: Assessing Current Policies and the Potential Impact of the HHS Final Rule.* Washington, DC: National Academy Press; 1999.

34. Trotter JF, Osgood MJ. MELD scores of liver transplant recipients according to size of waiting list: impact of organ allocation and patient outcomes. *JAMA.* 2004;291:1871–1874.
35. Hippen BE, Thistlethwaite JR Jr, Ross LF. Risk, prognosis, and unintended consequences in kidney allocation. *N Engl J Med.* 2011;364:1285–1287.
36. Ubel PA, Arnold RM, Caplan AL. Rationing failure: the ethical lessons of the retransplantation of scarce organs. *JAMA.* 1993;270:2469–2474.
37. Fox RC, Swazey JP. *Spare Parts.* New York, NY: Oxford University Press; 1992:204–205.
38. Danovitch GM, Cecka JM. Allocation of deceased donor kidneys: past, present, and future. *Am J Kidney Dis.* 2003;42:882–890.
39. Beresford TP, Everson GT. Liver transplantation for alcoholic liver disease: bias, beliefs, 6-month rule, and relapse—but where are the data? *Liver Transpl.* 2000;6:777–778.
40. Brudney D. Are alcoholics less deserving of liver transplants? *Hastings Cent Rep.* 2007;37:41–47.
41. Moss AH, Siegler M. Should alcoholics compete equally for liver transplantation? *JAMA.* 1991;265:1295–1298.
42. Cohen C, Benjamin M. Alcoholics and liver transplantation. The Ethics and Social Impact Committee of the Transplant and Health Policy Center. *JAMA.* 1991;265:1299–1301.
43. Steinbrook R. Public solicitation of organ donors. *N Engl J Med.* 2005;353:441–444.
44. Hanto DW. Ethical challenges posed by the solicitation of deceased and living organ donors. *N Engl J Med.* 2007;356:1062–1066.

ANNOTATED BIBLIOGRAPHY

1. Committee on Increasing Rates of Organ Donation. *Organ Donation: Opportunities for Action.* Washington, DC: National Academies Press; 2006.
   Consensus report recommending greater use of donation after circulatory determination of death in order to decrease the gap between the need for transplants and the supply of organs..
2. Childress JF. Putting patients first in organ allocation: an ethical analysis of the U.S. debate. *Camb Q Healthc Ethics.* 2001;10:365–376.
   Washburn K, Pomfret E, Roberts J. Liver allocation and distribution: possible next steps. *Liver Transpl.* 2011;17:1005–1012.
   Ethical analysis of organ allocation options and application to liver transplantation.
3. Delmonico FL, Arnold R, Scheper-Hughes N, et al. Ethical incentives—not payment—for organ donation. *N Engl J Med.* 2002;346:2002–2005.
   Argues that modest financial incentives to reward organ donation are ethically defensible, whereas payment for organs is not.
4. Bakdash T, Scheper-Hughes N. Is it ethical for patients with renal disease to purchase kidneys from the world's poor? *PLoS Med.* 2006;3:e349.
   Pro and con debate over paying renal donors.

42

Ethical Issues in Genomic Medicine

Since the sequencing of the entire human genome in 2002, DNA-based tests have become increasingly available for such conditions as cystic fibrosis (CF), familial colon and breast cancer, hemochromatosis, and polycystic kidney disease. Current high-throughput genotyping allows researchers to assay 500,000 single nucleotide polymorphisms (SNPs) and carry out genomewide association studies for common polygenic conditions, such as diabetes, obesity, hypertension, and coronary artery disease (1). Typically, the reported odds ratios are low, around 1.2 to 1.3. DNA tests can also predict response to therapy, identifying patients who are more likely to respond or to develop adverse effects. Such testing may allow personalized or precision medicine (2).

Several types of DNA testing need to be distinguished (3).

DNA testing for predisposition to adult-onset genetic diseases might lead to preventive and therapeutic interventions for the person who is tested, through improved presymptomatic screening, diagnosis, and prognostication.

Carrier screening for recessive conditions affects only future reproductive decisions. *Prenatal genetic testing* raises additional ethical controversies regarding procreation and abortion.

DNA profiling of a patient's cancer tissue may allow physicians to target therapies to specific mutations in cancer cells (2).

With rapid advances in genomics, physicians in all specialties will increasingly be asked to advise patients about genetic testing. This chapter discusses the clinical limitations of DNA-based screening tests, genetic discrimination, informed consent for genetic testing, confidentiality of test results, and genetic enhancement. We use the term *genomics* to refer to the DNA sequence of chromosomes; genetics refers simply to the science of inheritance.

WHAT IS DIFFERENT ABOUT GENOMICS?

Genetic or genomic information is commonly viewed as qualitatively different from other clinical information. On closer analysis, however, this claim is untenable in some respects.

PEOPLE OVERESTIMATE THE IMPACT OF GENES

The media have characterized the human genome as a "blueprint" for life or as a "future diary," implying that a person's DNA sequence determines his or her future and that genomic information has greater predictive power than other medical information. To be sure, some severe diseases are caused by single-gene mutations that have complete penetrance, such as Huntington disease. However, most genes have incomplete penetrance or variable expressivity, so that their presence does not reliably predict the occurrence of disease or its severity. Furthermore, most common conditions are polygenic. For example, a person's risk of hypertension and diabetes depends on several genes, including genes that might be protective or modify the expression of other genes. Many laypeople mistakenly regard genetic influences as all-or-none, rather than as probabilities. Furthermore, health and illness are determined by education and environmental factors, such as diet, exercise, and exposure to viral illness, as well as by heredity.

GENETICS PROVIDES INFORMATION ABOUT RELATIVES

All genetic information, whether a family history or a DNA test, provides information about relatives, as well as the proband (4). Ethical dilemmas arise regarding the confidentiality of genomic information if the proband refuses to share information that is shared by all relatives and would enable them to take steps to prevent or treat a serious disease.

GENOMIC TESTING HAS SIGNIFICANT RISKS

The risks of genomic tests are psychosocial rather than medical. Persons found to be at risk for adult-onset illness might be labeled as abnormal even if they are asymptomatic. Patients might experience psychological distress, which generally is mild, after learning either positive or negative test results (5). Breaches of confidentiality might cause stigma and discrimination.

Genetic and genomic information might be considered especially personal and sensitive. People might regard information about their heredity and future health as highly private and not to be widely disclosed. They might believe that genetic information reveals something essential about themselves, which would not otherwise be apparent. Furthermore, genetic information might reveal information about relatives or family secrets, for example, about adoptions and nonpaternity. Genomic testing might also contradict a person's beliefs about parentage or ancestry.

GENETIC INFORMATION MIGHT BE STIGMATIZING

Scientifically flawed ideas about inheritance were used in the late 19th and early 20th centuries to support ideas of racial superiority and discriminatory social policies (6). Eugenic laws were passed forbidding marriage or mandating sterilization of people categorized as feebleminded, insane, and criminals. In addition, miscegenation laws and restrictive immigration policies were enacted. Given this history, some people fear that genetic research today might be used to support discriminatory social policies (7).

GENOMIC KNOWLEDGE MIGHT UNDERMINE TRADITIONAL BELIEFS

Critics fear that advances in genetic science might contradict moral and religious teachings about human nature or undermine human dignity (8). For example, some people oppose preimplantation genetic diagnosis as fostering a desire for the "perfect" baby, disrespecting persons with disabilities, violating the natural order, and undermining the awe of procreation (8). Advances in genetics might also change beliefs about individual responsibility. Identification of genes that predispose to alcoholism or drug addiction might allow persons with these conditions to escape responsibility for their behaviors, because people generally are not considered responsible for inherited conditions.

WHEN IS DNA-BASED GENETIC TESTING APPROPRIATE?

Every clinical test should meet several criteria before being accepted into clinical practice (9, 10). *Analytic validity* means that the test is reliable and accurate: If the test is repeated, the same results will be reported. *Clinical validity* means that the test predicts the presence or absence of a clinical disease or condition. In the past, reports of genes associated with depression, schizophrenia, and Parkinson disease were not confirmed in subsequent studies (11). In technical terms, the test must have high positive and negative predictive values. *Clinical utility* means that testing must lead to better outcomes for the patient. The potential benefits of testing must outweigh the risks, and the balance of benefits to risks must be acceptable to the patient. For most conditions, a screening test is justified only if there is an intervention that will prevent the disease or if treatment is more effective when started early in the disease (12). Earlier diagnosis *per se* is not usually considered a justification for a policy of screening for risk factors. A test, however, might have *personal utility* without clinical utility. Some patients might desire screening for predisposition for a serious adult-onset illness even if there is no prevention or treatment known to be effective. Similarly, patients may want genomic tests that predict prognosis, even if there is no treatment available. If they were found to be at risk, they might change plans regarding education, career, or marriage. Other individuals simply want to know information about their future, even if it is imperfect.

Thus, genomic tests for susceptibility to adult-onset diseases are most justified if the disease is serious, the test has high positive predictive value, and prevention or treatment is effective. However, many DNA tests are ordered in situations that do not meet these criteria (13). The following examples illustrate diseases for which DNA-based genetic tests are in appropriate or not warranted.

BRCA1 AND BRCA2

These autosomal dominant genes for susceptibility to breast cancer account for about 2% to 3% of cases of breast cancer. In families with a high incidence of breast and ovarian cancer, mutations in BRCA1 are associated with up to an 85% lifetime risk of developing breast cancer and a 40% risk of ovarian cancer (14). Women who test positive for BRCA mutations should undergo more intensive mammography screening, starting at an earlier age than recommended for the general population. Moreover, they can consider preventive measures, which include chemoprevention with tamoxifen or raloxifene and prophylactic mastectomy and oophorectomy, which have medical and psychosocial ramifications (15, 16). BRCA testing has important limitations. As with other genomic tests, false-negative tests might occur if no specific mutation has been identified in the family, if the test kit used did not detect the mutation in the family, or if inheritance in the family is due to a different gene than BRCA.

HEREDITARY NONPOLYPOSIS COLORECTAL CANCER (HNPCC)

This autosomal dominant syndrome is caused by mutations in mismatch-repair genes. The most common mutations, MLH1 and MSH2, occur in up to 3% of cases of newly diagnosed colorectal cancer (17–20). In persons with these mutations, the lifetime risk of colorectal cancer is about 80%, and such cancers are more likely to be earlier onset and synchronous. Screening colonoscopy starting around age 20 to 25 cuts the risk of colorectal cancer in half and decreases overall mortality by 65%. Thus, genomic screening is useful because it identifies persons who should have earlier colonoscopy. Negative tests, however, have low predictive value. Because many other mutations can cause this syndrome, testing for only these two mutations has a sensitivity of only 60%.

HEMOCHROMATOSIS

Hemochromatosis is a syndrome of cirrhosis, diabetes, and gonadal failure due to iron overload. About 1 in 200 persons of Northern European descent are homozygous for the mutation C282YP. The clinical validity of population-based DNA screening is unproven because of low penetrance and variable expressivity (21, 22).

FACTOR V LEIDEN

This abnormal clotting factor, which occurs in 5% of Northern Europeans, increases the risk of venous thromboembolism. In women taking oral contraceptives, there is a 30-fold increase in relative risk. DNA testing is useful in persons with unexplained thromboembolic disease, but population screening is not recommended because the absolute risk is very low (23).

RESULTS OF WHOLE-GENOME SEQUENCING

As the price of whole-genome sequencing drops, it will become less expensive than an analysis of one or two genes. Currently, many genomic sequences are "variants of unknown significance." As genomic knowledge increases, however, their significance will be clarified. If clinical significance is established and results change recommendations for care, would physicians have an ethical obligation to recontact patients to update the interpretation of previous sequencing results (24)?

While such recontact would benefit patients, it may be burdensome or impractical for the physician who ordered the tests, who may have no ongoing relationship with the patient or may not monitor new genomic discoveries (24).

DIRECT-TO-CONSUMER GENOMIC TESTING OVER THE INTERNET

Genomic tests for susceptibility are available over the Internet (11, 25, 26). Patients might ask physicians about such testing, or bring in results of DNA tests obtained over the Internet. Tests might concern physical characteristics such as eye color or height, as well as susceptibility to adult-onset medical conditions. Sometimes, testing is combined with recommendations for skin care, antiaging, or nutritional products. These Internet tests currently are not regulated by the FDA. Patients send a buccal swab or blood spot. If a state requires a physician to order the test, a physician employed by the company, who has not met the patient, does so. Consumers pay out-of-pocket for the test and receive the results directly, whereas in clinical practice patients receive results through their physician. Testing can be anonymous, and the consumer's physician or insurer need not know the results.

For many common polygenic conditions, the validity and clinical utility of DNA-based tests has not been established. In coronary artery disease, the risk attributable to reported polymorphisms is much less than the attributable risk due to established clinical risk factors, such as smoking, hypertension, and hypercholesterolemia. Furthermore, it is not well understood how additional genes might modify or protect against these risks. Moreover, the specific genes responsible for the association and their mechanism of action have not been elucidated. Despite concerns that these tests might lead to "unnecessary medical interventions or false reassurance or missed diagnoses" (11), experience to date indicates that such results have little impact on either emotions or health-related behaviors (25). Although anecdotal reports suggest that genomewide sequencing might motivate patients to adopt healthier behaviors and accept preventive interventions, current evidence does not support this hypothesis (27).

Other ethical concerns regarding direct-to-consumer genomic testing include the quality of the testing and counseling provided by telephone or over the Internet (25). Furthermore, the company has a vested interest in encouraging testing, even if clinical utility is low. Finally, there are confidentiality concerns because the Internet company may not be subject to HIPAA privacy regulations.

ANCESTRY TESTING

On the Internet, several companies offer genomic testing to help people learn their genealogy or continent of origin. People have many reasons for obtaining such tests, including to satisfy curiosity about their heritage or the geographical origins of their ancestors, to connect to their homeland, to identify genetic relatives, and to obtain benefits such as race-based scholarships or Native American casino profits. These tests have a number of limitations (28). Mitochondrial DNA (inherited through the maternal lineage) or Y-chromosome DNA (inherited through the paternal lineage) tests trace inheritance only through a single genetic lineage, so that contributions from many other distant ancestors is not taken into account. Moreover, these tests sample only a limited amount of the subject's DNA, classifications are derived from small, selected population samples, and there are no quality control requirements. Given these limitations, it is not surprising that a person who sends a sample to different companies for genetic ancestry testing often receives inconsistent results. Genetic ancestry testing might have adverse psychological consequences. Test results might contradict clients' beliefs about their ethnic heritage (28), but Internet companies seldom warn clients of this risk.

GENETIC DISCRIMINATION

Screening for genetic disorders might lead to stigmatization and discrimination. Asymptomatic persons at increased risk for adult-onset genetic conditions might regard themselves, or be regarded by others, as impaired. Although there is no evidence of widespread discrimination on the basis of genetic testing, fears about it are widespread and might prevent persons from accepting genetic testing in clinical care or participating in research (29).

INSURERS

In the United States, health and life insurance companies have incentives to use genetic testing to avoid adverse selection, which occurs when patients increase coverage after they learn they are at risk for diseases but insurers do not have that information (30). Insurers who are unaware of such risk would sell coverage at relatively low rates to individuals who are at increased risk for claims. Insurers, therefore, want to know any pertinent medical information that the applicant knows and seek to limit coverage for preexisting diseases, exclude the diseases from coverage, or set prohibitive premiums. To prevent such practices, most states have prohibited genetic discrimination in health insurance (31).

Widespread genetic testing might be incompatible with the current US system of individual risk rating and exclusion of high-risk persons from coverage (32). With increases in genomic screening, more and more individuals will be found to be at risk for some genetic disease. If many such persons were in effect excluded from coverage, then the very purpose of health insurance, to cover the costs of health care when illness strikes, would be negated (33).

EMPLOYERS

Employers also have incentives to use genetic screening. Excluding employees who are likely to become sick might increase future productivity and cut health insurance premiums. Employers might also want to identify workers at genetic risk for occupational diseases because it might be cheaper to exclude them from the workplace than to reduce occupational exposure. Genetic testing, however, might be a tragedy for employees identified as at risk for adult-onset conditions. They might be unable to find employment, even if they are asymptomatic and able to work productively.

ANTIDISCRIMINATION LAW

In 2008, the federal Genetic Information Nondiscrimination Act (GINA) was passed. It prohibits health insurers from using a person's genetic information to set eligibility or premiums. Employers may not use a person's genetic information to make employment decisions, such as hiring, job assignments, promotions, and firing (34). Neither health insurers nor employers may request or require a person or family to provide genetic information. The law does not apply to disability, long-term care, and life insurance. The 2010 Patient Protection and Affordable Care Act extends GINA by banning insurers from determining eligibility based on health status, medical condition, or receipt of health care and from setting premiums based on health status (31).

INFORMED CONSENT FOR GENOMIC TESTING

Careful attention to informed consent can maximize the benefits of genomic testing and minimize its risks.

IMPORTANCE OF INFORMED CONSENT

Informed consent is particularly important for genomic testing because individuals differ on whether the benefits of testing outweigh the risks. Some persons at risk will want more prognostic information, even if its significance is uncertain and no proven preventive or therapeutic intervention is available. Others might decline testing because they do not perceive themselves to be vulnerable or are concerned about losing insurance (29, 34).

CHALLENGES TO INFORMED CONSENT

Genetic concepts and probabilities are difficult to comprehend. Misunderstandings about genomic testing and the interpretation of results are widespread among health professionals and laypeople alike. The availability of testing for multiple conditions over the Internet without a physician's order further complicates consent.

NONDIRECTIVE GENETIC COUNSELING

Nondirectiveness has been a core tenet in genetic counseling. People interpret this term in different ways (35). Commonly it means that the counselor presents all sides of an issue in an unbiased manner, that the counselor's personal views should not influence the client's decision, and that the client's or couple's decision is respected (36). Historically, the ideology of nondirectiveness developed as a reaction to eugenicist policies and from the desire to distance prenatal genetic diagnosis from controversies over abortion (35).

In prenatal genetic testing, genetic counselors are often directive (37). In one study, 28% of genetic counselors said they would recommend testing or screening to a client (36). Another study found that genetic counselors gave advice an average of almost six times per session and that clients did not object (38). Some concerns about nondirectiveness might be resolved if counselors respond to clients' questions about what to do by suggesting issues to consider in making the decision, rather than by giving a direct recommendation (39).

The stance of nondirectiveness is ethically problematical for several reasons. First, patients commonly request advice or help determining which option is most consistent with their values. Second, nondirectiveness might violate ethical guidelines of beneficence. Physicians should recommend highly predictive screening tests for adult-onset conditions. Finally, the physicians have some obligation to be directive if patients are making a decision that is ethically troubling (36). As we discuss later, physicians should encourage patients to share genetic test results with relatives who might be at high risk for a preventable serious disease.

RECOMMENDATIONS

Provide Pretest Education

Education about the risks and limitations of testing is desirable before testing is carried out. When multiple genomic tests are run on one specimen, pretest counseling is not feasible.

Make a Recommendation Regarding Testing

In some situations, genomic tests are highly predictive of future disease, and effective prevention or early treatment is available. Doctors should recommend such tests. At the other extreme, some tests have no established analytical validity. Physicians should recommend against such testing and explain why. Some patients might still want to be tested because the results will have personal utility; their informed choices should be respected.

GENOMIC TESTING IN CHILDREN

Testing children for susceptibility to adult-onset diseases raises special ethical concerns because testing during childhood deprives children of the opportunity to make informed decisions whether or not to be tested (40). Since many adults choose not to be tested, it cannot be assumed that children would agree with testing when they reach maturity. Thus, genomic testing is best deferred until the child reaches maturity, unless there are effective preventive measures to be instituted during childhood if the test is abnormal.

CONFIDENTIALITY OF GENOMIC RESULTS

Genetic testing provides information about relatives as well as the individual being tested. Persons identified as having a predisposition to a serious adult-onset genetic illness have a moral duty to inform relatives who might also be at risk. An ethical dilemma can arise for physicians when the patient objects to such disclosure.

> **CASE 42.1** **Disclosure of abnormal results to relatives**
>
> *A 48-year-old man with colon cancer with a strong family history of colon cancer is found to have an MLH1 mutation for HNPCC. Relatives with this allele have an 80% lifetime risk of colon cancer, often at an early age. He refuses to inform his sister, with whom he had a falling out several years ago regarding his marriage. "After what she did to me and my wife, I wouldn't help her in any way."*
>
> *The physician should offer to send a letter to the sister or to the sister's physician advising her that she is at risk for HNPCC and advising her to be tested, so that the patient need not have any direct contact with his sister. About one quarter of patients with HNPCC who would not contact a relative would agree to have their physician do so (41).*

WHEN IS OVERRIDING CONFIDENTIALITY JUSTIFIED?

The guidelines in Chapter 5 on exceptions to confidentiality can be applied to genetic testing. The potential harm to identifiable third parties is serious and likely if a high risk of cancer is missed. Moreover, the test might lead to an effective intervention to avert the risk—annual screening colonoscopy beginning at a much earlier age than usually recommended. There is no less invasive means for warning relatives at risk, because the presence of an MLH1 mutation has much greater predictive power than a family history of cancer. Since genetic information is shared among relatives, the presumption of confidentiality of genetic test results on one individual might be reversed. Genetic results might be considered part of a familial "joint account" to be shared with relatives unless there are good reasons not to do so (4). There are good reasons both to override confidentiality in this situation (42, 43) and also to maintain it (44, 45). The proband might feel wronged if confidentiality is breached. Practically speaking, a proband who does not want a relative contacted can refuse to cooperate with identifying and contacting the relative. In addition, overriding confidentiality might undermine the willingness of other persons to be tested for genetic conditions. Some distinguish overriding confidentiality to prevent infectious disease from this case because the person with a genetic condition does not cause the risk to others (45). The rationale behind overriding confidentiality, however, is the prevention of serious and likely harm to unknowing third parties, regardless of the cause of the risk.

Legal issues are uncertain (46). Appellate rulings involving overriding confidentiality of genetic information are inconsistent, but one court ruled that a physician must take reasonable steps to warn immediate family members (46). This duty to warn may require more than informing the patient that the disease is inherited. However, disclosure of test results to relatives over the patient's objections might violate federal or state laws on privacy and confidentiality. Thus, physicians cannot simply follow the law, but must rely on their ethical judgment.

In most tests for adult-onset conditions, the predictive power is low or there are no effective preventive or therapeutic measures (43) so that overriding confidentiality is unjustified. In screening for autosomal recessive conditions, such as cystic fibrosis, there are no compelling reasons to override confidentiality. Relatives who might be carriers are at no risk for illness, and their offspring will be at risk only if their partners are also carriers.

RECOMMENDATIONS
Discuss Disclosure During Pretest Counseling

Discussing the importance of disclosure during informed consent for testing can prevent most dilemmas about disclosure to relatives.

Urge Disclosure of Positive Results to Relatives

Physicians should urge patients to disclose positive results to relatives when the information would lead to a change in their medical care (47). Physicians can elicit patients' concerns about informing relatives and help them resolve the problem.

Disclosure Against the Wishes of the Patient Should Be a Last Resort

In exceptional situations, there may be compelling ethical reasons to disclose results of genetic testing to relatives over the objections of the patient. Such disclosure should be a last resort after failing to persuade the patient to allow notification. The physician should tell the patient that notification will occur and give him the option to notify relatives directly. Relatives at risk should be offered the information; if they do not want to know it, their refusal should be respected.

GENETIC ENHANCEMENT

In the future, gene transfer might offer the possibility of enhancing athletic or cognitive performance. This dilemma is sometimes framed as enhancement or "beyond therapy": A medical intervention is being used to augment and improve a person's native capacity, not to treat a serious disease. In this view, success from other means is less worthy of admiration and praise (8). Even if genetic enhancements were shown to be safe and effective, critics object that they would exacerbate existing health and social disparities and create pressure for competitors or other students to use them. Others object that such enhancements disrupt the connection between effort and success. From this perspective, success is praiseworthy only if it results from the fulfillment of one's natural capacities, developed through effort and discipline. In this view, success from other means is less worthy of admiration and praise (8).

In rebuttal, others argue that biotechnologic enhancements do not differ in kind from better equipment, diet, and training, which are also more accessible to the wealthy and still require vigorous training. To achieve short-term advantage and glory, some people might accept long-term serious adverse effects. From this viewpoint, the sole justification for banning such interventions in athletic competition is an agreement on the rules of the game, which are based on socially constructed conventions, not on deep moral principles.

SUMMARY

1. In advising patients about genomic testing, physicians need to be aware of the clinical limitations of testing, the risk of discrimination, the importance of informed consent, the importance of confidentiality, and the implications for relatives.

REFERENCES

1. Pearson TA, Manolio TA. How to interpret a genome-wide association study. *JAMA*. 2008;299:1335–1344.
2. Committee on a Framework for Development a New Taxonomy of Disease; National Research Council. *Toward Precision Medicine: Building a Knowledge Network for Biomedical Research and a New Taxonomy of Disease*. Washington, DC: National Academies Press; 2011. http://www.nap.edu/catalog.php?record_id=13284. Accessed December 16, 2011.
3. Offit K. Personalized medicine: new genomics, old lessons. *Hum Genet*. 2011;130:3–14.
4. Lucassen A, Parker M. Confidentiality and sharing genetic information with relatives. *Lancet*. 2010;375:1507–1509.
5. Marteau TM, Croyle RT. Psychological responses to genetic testing. *BMJ*. 1998;316:693–696.
6. Kevles DJ. *In the name of eugenics: genetics and the uses of human herdity*. New York, NY: Alfred A. Knopf; 1985.
7. Nuffield Council on Bioethics. *Genetics and Human Behavior: The Ethical Concerns*. London, UK: Nuffield Council on Bioethics; 2002.
8. The President's Council on Bioethics. *Beyond Therapy: Biotechnology and the Pursuit of Happiness*. 2003. http://bioethics.georgetown.edu/pcbe/reports/beyondtherapy. Accessed September 14, 2012.
9. Secretary's Advisory Committee. *Enhancing the oversight of genetic tests: recommendations of the SACGT*. 2000. http://www.od.nih.gov/oba/sacgt/gtdocuments.html. Accessed November 16, 2007.
10. Hudson K, Javitt G, Burke W, et al. ASHG Statement on direct-to-consumer genetic testing in the United States. *Obstet Gynecol*. 2007;110:1392–1395.
11. Offit K. Genomic profiles for disease risk: predictive or premature? *JAMA*. 2008;299:1353–1355.
12. Newman TB, Kohn MA. *Evidence-Based Diagnosis*. New York, NY: Cambridge University Press; 2009.

13. Giardiello FM, Brensinger JD, Petersen GM, et al. The use and interpretation of commercial APC gene testing for familial adenomatous polyposis. *N Engl J Med.* 1997;336:823–827.
14. Nelson HD, Huffman LH, Fu R, et al. Genetic risk assessment and BRCA mutation testing for breast and ovarian cancer susceptibility: systematic evidence review for the U.S. Preventive Services Task Force. *Ann Intern Med.* 2005;143:362–379.
15. Hartge P. Genes, cancer risks, and clinical outcomes. *N Engl J Med.* 2007;357:175–176.
16. Robson M, Offit K. Clinical practice. Management of an inherited predisposition to breast cancer. *N Engl J Med.* 2007;357:154–162.
17. Gala M, Chung DC. Hereditary colon cancer syndromes. *Semin Oncol.* 2011;38:490–499.
18. Lynch HT, Boland CR, Rodriguez-Bigas MA, et al. Who should be sent for genetic testing in hereditary colorectal cancer syndromes? *J Clin Oncol.* 2007;25:3534–3542.
19. Lindor NM, Petersen GM, Hadley DW, et al. Recommendations for the care of individuals with an inherited predisposition to Lynch syndrome: a systematic review. *JAMA.* 2006;296:1507–1517.
20. Kaz AM, Brentnall TA. Genetic testing for colon cancer. *Nat Clin Pract Gastroenterol Hepatol.* 2006;3:670–679.
21. Bryant J, Cooper K, Picot J, et al. A systematic review of the clinical validity and clinical utility of DNA testing for hereditary haemochromatosis in at-risk populations. *J Med Genet.* 2008;45:513–518.
22. Whitlock EP, Garlitz BA, Harris EL, et al. Screening for hereditary hemochromatosis: a systematic review for the U.S. Preventive Services Task Force. *Ann Intern Med.* 2006;145:209–223.
23. Evaluation of Genomic Applications in Practice and Prevention (EGAPP) Working Group. Recommendations from the EGAPP Working Group: routine testing for Factor V Leiden (R506Q) and prothrombin (20210G>A) mutations in adults with a history of idiopathic venous thromboembolism and their adult family members. *Genet Med.* 2011;13:67–76.
24. Pyeritz RE. The coming explosion in genetic testing—is there a duty to recontact? *N Engl J Med.* 2011;365:1367–1369.
25. Caulfield T, McGuire AL. Direct-to-consumer genetic testing: perceptions, problems and policy responses. *Annu Rev Med.* 2012;63:23–33.
26. Wolfberg AJ. Genes on the Web—direct-to-consumer marketing of genetic testing. *N Engl J Med.* 2006;355:543–545.
27. Bloss CS, Schork NJ, Topol EJ. Effect of direct-to-consumer genomewide profiling to assess disease risk. *N Engl J Med.* 2011;364:524–534.
28. Royal CD, Novembre J, Fullerton SM, et al. Inferring genetic ancestry: opportunities, challenges, and implications. *Am J Hum Genet.* 2010;86:661–673.
29. Greely HT. Banning genetic discrimination. *N Engl J Med.* 2005;353:865–867.
30. Dodge JH. Predictive medical information and underwriting. *J Law Med Ethics.* 2007;35:36–39.
31. Hudson KL. Genomics, health care, and society. *N Engl J Med.* 2011;365:1033–1041.
32. Rothstein MA. Genetic exceptionalism and legislative pragmatism. *J Law Med Ethics.* 2007;35:59–65.
33. Ashcroft R. Should genetic information be disclosed to insurers? No. *BMJ.* 2007;334:1197.
34. Hudson KL. Prohibiting genetic discrimination. *N Engl J Med.* 2007;356:2021–2023.
35. Hodgson J, Spriggs M. A practical account of autonomy: why genetic counseling is especially well suited to the facilitation of informed autonomous decision making. *J Genet Couns.* 2005;14:89–97.
36. Bartels DM, LeRoy BS, McCarthy P, et al. Nondirectiveness in genetic counseling: a survey of practitioners. *Am J Med Genet.* 1997;72:172–179.
37. Williams C, Alderson P, Farsides B. Is nondirectiveness possible within the context of antenatal screening and testing? *Soc Sci Med.* 2002;54:339–347.
38. Michie S, Bron F, Bobrow M, et al. Nondirectiveness in genetic counseling: an empirical study. *Am J Hum Genet.* 1997;60:40–47.
39. Kessler S. Psychological aspects of genetic counseling: nondirectiveness revisited. *Am J Med Genet.* 1997;72:164–171.
40. Borry P, Evers-Kiebooms G, Cornel MC, et al. Genetic testing in asymptomatic minors: background considerations towards ESHG Recommendations. *Eur J Hum Genet.* 2009;17:711–719.
41. Kohut K, Manno M, Gallinger S, et al. Should healthcare providers have a duty to warn family members of individuals with an HNPCC-causing mutation? A survey of patients from the Ontario Familial Colon Cancer Registry. *J Med Genet.* 2007;44:404–407.
42. Andrews LB, Fullarton JE, Holtzman NA, et al., eds. *Assessing Genetic Risks: Implications for Health and Social Policy.* Washington, DC: National Academy Press; 1994.
43. The American Society of Human Genetics Social Issues Subcommittee on Familial Disclosure. Professional dislcosure of familial genetic information. *Am J Hum Genet.* 1998;62:474–483.
44. Wickle JTR. Late onset genetic disease: where ignorance is bliss, is it folly to inform relatives? *BMJ.* 1998;317:744–747.
45. Sulmasy DP. On warning families about genetic risk: the ghost of Tarasoff. *Am J Med.* 2000;109:738–739.
46. Offit K, Groeger E, Turner S, et al. The "duty to warn" a patient's family members about hereditary disease risks. *JAMA.* 2004;292:1469–1473.
47. Forrest LE, Delatycki MB, Skene L, et al. Communicating genetic information in families—a review of guidelines and position papers. *Eur J Hum Genet.* 2007;15:612–618.

ANNOTATED BIBLIOGRAPHY

1. Hudson KL. Prohibiting genetic discrimination. *N Engl J Med.* 2007;356:2021–2023.
   Hudson KL. Genomics, health care, and society. *N Engl J Med.* 2011;365:1033–1041.
   Analysis of the antidiscrimination protections in the Genetic Information Nondiscrimination Act and the Affordable Health Care and Patient Protection Act.
2. Caulfield T, McGuire AL. Direct-to-consumer genetic testing: perceptions, problems and policy responses. *Annu Rev Med.* 2012;63:23–33.
   Analyses of direct-to-consumer genomic testing.
3. Royal CD, Novembre J, Fullerton SM, et al. Inferring genetic ancestry: opportunities, challenges, and implications. *Am J Hum Genet.* 2010;86:661–673.
4. Offit K, Groeger E, Turner S, et al. The "duty to warn" a patient's family members about hereditary disease risks. *JAMA.* 2004;292:1469–1473.
   Lucassen A, Parker M. Confidentiality and sharing genetic information with relatives. *Lancet.* 2010;375:1507–1509.
   Analyses of clinical, ethical, and legal issues regarding disclosure of genetic information to relatives.

Ethical Issues in Public Health Emergencies

I n recent years, public health emergencies have required physicians, the public, and public health officials to consider how the doctor–patient relationship may change during a public health emergency. In 2001, the bombing of the World Trade Center and outbreaks of inhalation anthrax raised concerns about bioterrorism. In 2003, severe acute respiratory distress syndrome (SARS) rapidly spread to many countries through international travel. More recently, concerns about an avian influenza pandemic have led to guidelines for addressing a shortage of influenza vaccine. These incidents dramatize how grave threats to public health may require mandatory public-health interventions, such as quarantine and isolation, and raise dilemmas about how to protect the public health, while still respecting individual freedom and treating different groups equitably (1–3). Some patients will not accept restrictions on their freedom of movement, while others will want preventive measures that public health policies do not recommend.

This chapter analyzes the dilemmas that physicians will confront because some patients will disagree with public health measures, both in emergencies and in ordinary practice.

RECENT PUBLIC HEALTH EMERGENCIES

INHALATIONAL ANTHRAX FROM BIOTERRORISM

In October 2001, Congressional staff who were exposed to anthrax contained in a letter were offered prophylactic antibiotics within hours. In contrast, prophylactic antibiotics for postal workers were delayed, even after several workers were hospitalized with what was found to be anthrax pneumonia. Concerns were raised that predominantly African American postal workers received less timely attention than predominantly Caucasian Congressional staff. As seasonal upper respiratory infections peaked, prescriptions for ciprofloxacin, the recommended drug for inhalational anthrax, increased so much that a shortage was feared. These anthrax outbreaks illustrate how knowledge about an outbreak is incomplete and evolving, that public health measures may be perceived as unfair, and how people may request measures that are not recommended by public health officials.

SEVERE ACUTE RESPIRATORY DISTRESS SYNDROME

In 2002–2003, the SARS epidemic illustrated how emerging infections may spread rapidly through international airplane travel. Public health responses varied markedly in different nations, but mandatory measures, such as quarantine and isolation, were widely instituted (4). In China, officials locked patients and health care workers in hospitals that experienced many cases of SARS. In Canada, in contrast, exposed persons were quarantined in their homes.

EXTREMELY DRUG-RESISTANT TUBERCULOSIS

In March 2007, a US citizen with extremely drug-resistant tuberculosis (XDR-TB) flew from the United States to travel to Europe for his wedding and honeymoon, although public health officials recommended that he not travel (5). At the end of his return flight, a federal isolation order was issued. Public health officials in several countries had to contact hundreds of airline passengers who might have been exposed to XDR-TB. Furthermore, the case illustrates how procedures for mandatory public health measures need to be in place before an emergency occurs.

HOW DO ETHICAL ISSUES IN PUBLIC HEALTH DIFFER?

Public health differs from clinical practice in several important ethical ways. In clinical practice, physicians are guided by the well-being of individual patients and their informed consent. During a public health emergency, the government may institute mandatory interventions, such as surveillance, testing, quarantine, isolation, and directly observed treatment, which infringe on the liberty and autonomy of individuals.

FOCUS ON POPULATION OUTCOMES

Public health focuses on the benefits and risks to a population, rather than to individual patients. The goal is to improve aggregate measures of community health, such as reducing the incidence of SARS, XDR-TB, or pandemic influenza or reducing their mortality. Achieving public health goals may require measures that are not in the best interests of individual persons.

INDIVIDUAL LIBERTY AND AUTONOMY MAY BE OVERRIDDEN

The government has the authority to impose mandatory public health measures in response to a serious, probable threat to the public that the governor declares to be a public health emergency. *Quarantine* restricts the movement of persons who have been exposed or might have been exposed to a communicable disease. The goal is to prevent transmission of infection during the incubation period. *Isolation* separates a person known to have a communicable disease from other people, during the period when he can communicate the disease to others. These measures place heavy burdens on those who are detained, restricting freedom, violating privacy, and putting them at risk for economic losses and stigmatization (6). Other mandatory medical interventions may also be imposed, such as testing, vaccination, and treatment.

In ordinary clinical practice, the patient decides whether to accept or decline an intervention. The ethical tension between the interests of the individual and the well-being of the public should be acknowledged and addressed in public health programs.

Public officials should follow several requirements when imposing mandatory interventions (1–3):

- The threat to public health must be serious and likely.
- The intervention should be effective in addressing the threat.
- The intervention should be the *least restrictive alternative* that addresses the threat.
- *Procedural due process* should be available to persons deprived of their liberty autonomy. Persons who are subjected to compulsory measures should have the right to an open, impartial, and timely appeal of their case.
- Policies should be *implemented equitably*. The benefits and burdens of the intervention should be equitably distributed across society, consistent with the epidemiologic features of the threat. In the past, public health measures were sometimes applied in a discriminatory manner, and persons and groups affected by epidemics often were stigmatized (1). Any perception that some groups are being treated unfairly will undermine public support for compulsory measures.

These requirements assure that the balance of benefits to harms in overriding individual autonomy is acceptable and that violations on individual liberty are minimized.

Public health officials may enforce public health mandates through the state's police powers. Public health measures, however, usually require the cooperation of affected persons. The use of force may undermine cooperation. Isolation and quarantine raise social, financial, and logistical challenges (7). Hence, public health officials generally invoke compulsory measures only as a last resort, after less restrictive measures have failed. It is not necessary to have complete enforcement of isolation or quarantine to stem an outbreak (7).

CHANGE IN THE PHYSICIAN'S ROLE

The physician has less decision-making power in a public health emergency. Public health policies during an emergency are set by public health officials, not by individual clinicians, and may be enforced by the state's police powers. Physicians should presume that public measures are reasonable and fair if they are developed through appropriate decision-making procedures. If doctors have questions or disagreements, then they should raise them with officials, rather than try to override guidelines (8).

WEAKER EVIDENCE BASE

The evidence base for interventions in public health emergencies often is weaker than the evidence base for clinical practice. Knowledge about new conditions is incomplete and increases over the course of an emergency. Public health officials, however, may need to act quickly despite uncertain and incomplete information.

REQUESTS FOR NONRECOMMENDED INTERVENTIONS

In public health emergencies, physicians in clinical practice will encounter patients who reject restrictions on their autonomy as unwarranted or unfair. In this section, we discuss how physicians should respond when patients request interventions that are not recommended in public health guidelines. In a later section, we discuss how physicians should respond when patients refuse to comply with public health restrictions.

CASE 43.1	Patient who requests antibiotics

During the anthrax outbreaks in the fall of 2001, a 48-year-old man requests a prescription for ciprofloxacin. He is a Federal Express driver who has had no exposure to anthrax, but is concerned that he is at high risk for exposure because anthrax has been transmitted through the mail. "Look at what happened to those postal workers in Washington. Two of them died, and there were delays in getting them antibiotics. If I see white powder, I want to take the antibiotics right away." After the physician explains that there are concerns about a national shortage of the antibiotic of choice if a massive outbreak occurs, the patient retorts, "That's ridiculous. Look at those office workers in Congress who weren't even exposed. They got medicine in a few hours. They weren't told there was shortage."

In usual clinical practice, when patients request interventions that are not indicated, physicians attempt to persuade the patient that they are unnecessary (*see* Chapter 32) but generally accede to such requests, as long as the intervention does not present undue risk to the patient. In contrast, during a public health emergency, interventions may be in short supply and not available for persons outside of public health criteria (8).

PROTECT THE PUBLIC HEALTH

During public health emergencies, physicians, like all citizens, have a new primary obligation—to act for the common good. Physicians need to consider how a decision for one patient may impact on the spread of an epidemic, on public trust, and on perceptions of fairness.

FOLLOW PUBLIC HEALTH GUIDELINES FOR ALLOCATION

If effective interventions will be in short supply during severe public health emergencies, allocation and triage will be unavoidable. During an influenza pandemic, the need for triage should be expected, as the following case illustrates (6).

| **CASE 43.2** | **Vaccination during an influenza pandemic** |

An influenza pandemic is expected to occur, most likely due to an H5N1 strain of avian influenza. Vaccine against a pandemic strain will be in short supply because the vaccine can be manufactured only after an outbreak begins so it can be directed at the specific viral antigens causing the pandemic. Moreover, the influenza vaccine manufacturing process is complex, and only a few companies are capable of producing it.

During an outbreak of pandemic influenza, a healthy 68-year-old lawyer asks his primary care physician for vaccination. "We've just bought a new home and had first grandchild. I can't afford to get sick, and my family can't afford to lose me." Public health guidelines for vaccination during a pandemic give low priority to healthy people of this age. During vaccine shortages early in a pandemic, they are unlikely to be vaccinated.

Guidelines for the allocation of influenza vaccine during a pandemic have been proposed. Currently, US guidelines give first priority to persons needed to respond to the pandemic (such as workers in vaccine manufacturing plants and essential medical personnel) and then to those at highest risk for influenza-associated hospitalization and death (9). For example, people 6 months to 64 years of age with two or more high-risk conditions are in the second highest priority group. In a lower priority level are healthy people 65 years and older, who have lower mortality. These priorities have the utilitarian rationale of saving the greatest number of lives by giving priority to those at highest risk of dying. Scarce resources are allocated to those in greatest need. All human lives are valued equally in this context. In addition, groups who have a poor response to influenza vaccine receive lower priority, such as nursing home residents and patients with severe immunodeficiency.

Other ethical principles, however, may be more appropriate for allocating scarce resources during a public health emergency (10). Some propose a life-cycle allocation procedure (11): Every person should have an opportunity to live through all the stages of life. Under this principle, children would have priority over elderly persons. This principle is consistent with the common belief that the death of a child or young adult is more tragic than the death of an elderly person who has already had the opportunity to have a family and career and grow old.

PERCEPTIONS OF FAIRNESS

Public acceptance of priorities for allocating scarce resources during a public health emergency will be greater if the policies are implemented fairly. If many patients receive interventions even though they are not in high-priority groups, people may conclude that the guidelines are unfair or are being unfairly implemented or that the threat is greater than officials acknowledge. Any perception that public health measures are worsening existing health disparities will undermine willingness to accept restrictions.

ACT IN THE BEST INTERESTS OF THE PATIENT

In so far as it is possible, physicians should maintain their usual role of acting in the best interests of the patient, while respecting public health guidelines.

Advocate for Appropriate Exceptions to Restrictions

A particular case may be a justified exception to public health policies. An exception should be fair in the sense that it would also apply to all patients in a similar clinical situation, not just the particular patient.

Elicit and Address Patient Concerns and Emotions

Physicians should acknowledge that fear and a sense of loss of control are natural human reactions to public health emergencies. Trying to reassure people by telling them not to worry is unlikely to be effective. Patients may be more willing to pay attention to public health after their own needs are acknowledged. It also might be possible to address the patient's concerns and needs without violating public health guidelines.

CASE 43.1   *Continued*

It may be acceptable to write a prescription for ciprofloxacin that can be filled if exposure occurs for someone in a high-risk occupation. The guidelines for antibiotics during an anthrax episode were voluntary rather than mandatory. If access to ciprofloxacin were strictly limited, the physician could prescribe other antibiotics that might also be effective and were not in short supply. When patients have a prescription and access to follow-up care, they may decide not to fill the prescription.

During the SARS epidemic, patients often could be reassured if they believed they could see the physician promptly if their condition worsened or failed to improve. Also, patients may be reassured by knowing what warning signs to watch for.

CASE 43.2   *Continued*

The physician should try to respond to the patient's understandable concerns through empathic listening and by reminding him of measures that he can take to reduce his risk of being infected, such as social distance. To avoid this scenario, public health officials might limit the number of doses available to physicians' offices, instead distributing most doses through vaccination clinics. This would reduce the need for treating physicians to deny vaccinations to patients with whom they have an ongoing relationship.

REFUSAL OF PUBLIC HEALTH INTERVENTIONS

During a public health emergency, physicians can expect to encounter patients requesting to be exempted from public health restrictions.

CASE 43.3   **Patient who rejects quarantine**

During the SARS epidemic in 2002, a 48-year-old businessman presents with fever, cough, and malaise. Five days before he returned from a trip to a country where SARS cases have been reported, but he was not near the area where SARS cases have been reported. He says his symptoms are no different from what he commonly experiences after such long travel. Because SARS cases have been reported in his city, public health officials are requiring physicians to report such cases for consideration of home quarantine. He objects strongly. "If I had known that, I wouldn't have come in. I have a lot of meetings that I can't do over the phone. My business would go down the tubes if I were put in quarantine."

In clinical practice, when patients refuse recommended interventions, their informed wishes are respected. In public health emergencies, however, individual autonomy is not paramount. Compulsory measures may be imposed to prevent transmission to others and to control an outbreak of a serious infection.

FOLLOW PUBLIC HEALTH GUIDELINES

Physicians need to be clear about the limits of their discretion in public health emergencies. In some situations, doctors may have little control over public health measures. Reporting of emerging infections or infections related to bioterrorism may be mandatory and done directly by hospitals or clinical laboratories, rather than individual physicians. In other situations, isolation and quarantine may be voluntary rather than mandatory; if this is the situation in Case 43.2, the physician may exercise discretion.

ACT IN THE BEST INTERESTS OF THE PATIENT (8)
Advocate for Changes in Guidelines or Exceptions

Doctors should communicate any disagreements with public health guidelines to responsible officials. For example, a policy of quarantine for all persons who have traveled to a particular country may not be warranted if cases of the disease have been reported only from a well-defined area of a large country. Justifications for exceptions need to have a sound public health basis. It would be ethically inappropriate to argue that patients who would suffer economic losses should be exempted from home quarantine.

Establish Common Ground With the Patients

When patients refuse public health measures, physicians can try to find areas of agreement. For example, most patients do not want to infect their family. Also business people may suffer greater harm to reputation and business relationships if they flout public health measures and others are infected as a result. Furthermore, cooperating with public health officials may enable patients to have access to special tests that are not otherwise available.

Mitigate the Risks of Mandatory Public Health Interventions

Physicians can assuage the adverse psychosocial consequences of quarantine or isolation by keeping in telephone contact with patients and by addressing their feelings of isolation. In addition, physicians can help address practical concerns, for example, by referring patients for social services and for legal assistance as needed.

REFRAIN FROM DECEPTION

Patients might ask doctors to intentionally misrepresent their condition to exempt them from public health policies. For instance, patients may ask physicians to certify that they do not have a reportable condition. Such deception is ethically problematic for physicians (*see* Chapter 6). Moreover, the harms of such deception outweigh the benefits when adverse consequences to other patients and the public health are taken into account.

CRISIS STANDARDS OF CARE

In disasters, such as natural disasters, pandemics, or bioterrorism, the need for medical care might overwhelm the supply of health care workers, hospital beds, medicines, and equipment. Scarce life-saving resources might need to be allocated according to emergency public health directives. Ethical norms would not change; health care workers would need to provide the best care they reasonably can under the circumstances. However, legal standards of care may change (12). Emergency care might be triaged, some services might be relocated from emergency departments and hospitals to alternate facilities, and licensing, certification, and credentialing might be altered.

If an influenza pandemic occurs, then allocation decisions will also need to be made for antiviral therapy and for mechanical ventilation for persons who develop respiratory failure. Triage of patients with respiratory failure will be particularly difficult because some persons will die because life-sustaining treatment is withheld (10). Chapter 30 discusses the related topic of allocation of resources in ordinary clinical care.

REFUSAL TO CARE FOR CONTAGIOUS PATIENTS

During epidemics, physicians and other health care workers may be at increased risk for contracting the disease. During the SARS epidemic of 2002–2003, a disproportionate percentage of cases and deaths occurred among physicians and nurses caring for hospitalized patients with SARS. During an influenza pandemic, despite receiving vaccine, health care workers are likely to also be at increased risk. Some health care workers might refuse to care for patients because of fears of contracting a fatal illness. Chapter 24 discusses such refusal to care for patients.

CONTROVERIES OVER VACCINATIONS

Day-to-day public health practice also present ethical dilemmas. Although vaccines are credited with sharply reducing the mortality and morbidly of childhood contagious diseases such as polio, pertussis, diphtheria, measles, mumps, and rubella, they still raise controversies.

CHILDHOOD IMMUNIZATIONS

Some parents object to childhood immunizations because of religious beliefs, concerns about side effects, or opposition to modern medicine. Concerns about adverse effects persist even though scientific studies show no association with vaccines. The original study that alleged a link between vaccination and autism was falsified and recently retracted (13). Immunizations are required for entrance into school, although many states allow parents to refuse on the basis of religious or other objections or do not enforce requirements. If the number of unimmunized children is small and herd immunity exists, physicians should try to understand the parents' concerns, acknowledge that vaccines have risks, and try to persuade them that the benefits outweigh the risks (14, 15). Unvaccinated children, however, can transmit infection to children who cannot be vaccinated (e.g., because of very young age or medical contraindications) or have failed to develop an immune response. If an epidemic does break out, public health officials enforce requirements for immunization.

HUMAN PAPILLOMA VIRUS VACCINE

Human papilloma virus (HPV) vaccine dramatizes controversies over the role of adolescents and parents in decisions regarding medical care related to risky behaviors (16–18).

CASE 37.1　HPV vaccine

The HPV vaccine is more than 90% effective in preventing new infections and precancerous cervical lesions caused by the HPV types that it covers. The vaccine is expected to prevent cancer through preventing sexual transmission of HPV types that cause cervical cancer. Because the vaccine must be given before HPV infection is acquired, the Centers for Disease Control and Prevention recommends routine vaccination for 11- and 12-year-old girls. "Routine" means that the vaccine is administered without extensive discussion or expressed consent unless the parent or child objects.

Proposals for mandatory HPV vaccination as a condition of entry into middle school were driven by a vaccine manufacturer and by advocacy groups funded by it (19). Strong objections were raised to requiring mandatory vaccination for infections that could not be communicated by casual contact in the classroom, undermining parental choice, discussing adolescent sexuality before parents thought it was appropriate, and allegedly promoting sexual promiscuity (16, 17, 19). Some opponents also mistrusted government and rejected other childhood vaccinations. Although HPV vaccine raises some similar issues as abortion, it need not be as contentious. Unlike abortion, HPV vaccine cannot be considered morally wrong *per se*: its long-term goal is cancer prevention, an undisputable benefit.

Mandatory public health policies can be ethically justified if voluntary measures have failed, no less coercive alternatives exist, the scientific rationale is compelling, and the general public is unknowingly at risk (1). HPV vaccine does not meet these criteria, and HPV is not spread through casual contact.

How can doctors respond to adolescents and parents who refuse HPV vaccination? When disagreements arise in other clinical situations, physicians are encouraged to understand the perspective of patients (in this case, parents) and to respond to their concerns. Such a patient-centered approach might also be useful regarding HPV vaccination (20).

Some parents question the need for vaccination because they believe their daughters are not sexually active. Physicians should acknowledge that HPV vaccine is not needed until just before sexual activity starts. It is also not unreasonable to delay vaccination because of uncertainty about long-term effectiveness and rare adverse effects that may not have been identified. Doctors need to help parents consider a different perspective: Their child may become more sexually active than they would like or approve. By age 14 to 15, 28% of US girls are sexually active. Other parents might fear that the HPV vaccine will encourage sexual activity. It is understandable that parents fear that children grow up too quickly in the 21st century. Once parents have their underlying concerns acknowledged, they might be more willing to accept that evidence indicates that the vaccine is unlikely to increase sexual activity.

Some adolescents might want to be vaccinated against HPV even though their parents object, and they might not want to discuss their sexuality candidly with their parents. Adolescents who know they are likely to become sexually active should have the opportunity to benefit from the HPV vaccine. Most states allow adolescents to obtain care for sexually transmitted infections, contraception, and pregnancy care without parental consent (*see* Chapter 37). The ethical rationale is that reducing serious harms to adolescents and respecting their emerging independence outweigh parental interests in control over their children in these situations. Similarly, adolescents should be permitted to receive HPV vaccination without parental permission.

SUMMARY

1. In public health emergencies, time for physicians to deliberate about a particular case may be limited.
2. Before a crisis occurs, physicians should think through in advance how they would respond to foreseeable dilemmas arising when patients disagree with public health recommendations or requirements.

REFERENCES

1. Gostin LO. *Public Health Law: Power, Duty, Restraint.* 2nd ed. Berkeley, CA: University of California Press; 2008:287–330.
2. Childress JF, Faden RR, Gaare RD, et al. Public health ethics: mapping the terrain. *J Law Med Ethics.* 2002;30:170–178.
3. Gostin LO, Bayer R, Fairchild AL. Ethical and legal challenges posed by severe acute respiratory syndrome: implications for the control of severe infectious disease threats. *JAMA.* 2003;290:3229–3237.
4. Knobler S, Mahmoud M, Lemon S, et al., eds. *Learning from SARS: Preparing for the Next Disease Outbreak.* Washington, DC: National Academies Press; 2004.
5. Markel H, Gostin LO, Fidler DP. Extensively drug-resistant tuberculosis: an isolation order, public health powers, and a global crisis. *JAMA.* 2007;298:83–86.
6. Fidler DP, Gostin LO, Markel H. Through the quarantine looking glass: drug-resistant tuberculosis and public health governance, law, and ethics. *J Law Med Ethics.* 2007;35:616–628, 512.
7. Centers for Disease Control and Prevention. *Community Containment Measures, Including Isolation and Quarantine.* 2004. http://www.cdc.gov/ncidod/sars/quarantine.htm. Accessed May 5, 2008.
8. Lo B, Katz MH. Clinical decision making during public health emergencies: ethical considerations. *Ann Intern Med.* 2005;143:493–498.
9. U.S. Department of Health and Human Services. *NVAC/ACIP Recommendations on Use of Vaccines and NVAC Recommendations on Pandemic Antiviral Drug Use.* 2005. http://www.hhs.gov/pandemicflu/plan/appendixd.html. Accessed June 2, 2008.
10. White DB, Katz MH, Luce JM, et al. Who should receive life support during a public health emergency? Using ethical principles to improve allocation decisions. *Ann Intern Med.* 2009;150:132–138.
11. Emanuel EJ, Wertheimer A. Public health. Who should get influenza vaccine when not all can? *Science.* 2006;312:854–855.
12. Altevogt B, Stroud C, Hanson SL, et al. *Guidance for Establishing Crisis Standards of Care for Use in Disaster Situations.* Washington, DC: The National Academies press; 2009. http://www.nap.edu/catalog.php?record_id=12749&m=0003000740. Accessed December 9, 2011.
13. Godlee F, Smith J, Marcovitch H. Wakefield's article linking MMR vaccine and autism was fraudulent. *BMJ.* 2011;342:c7452.

14. Omer SB, Salmon DA, Orenstein WA, et al. Vaccine refusal, mandatory immunization, and the risks of vaccine-preventable diseases. *N Engl J Med.* 2009;360:1981–1988.
15. Healy CM, Pickering LK. How to communicate with vaccine-hesitant parents. *Pediatrics.* 2011;127 (suppl 1):S127–S133.
16. Lo B. HPV vaccine and adolescents' sexual activity. *BMJ.* 2006;332:1106–1107.
17. Charo RA. Politics, parents, and prophylaxis—mandating HPV vaccination in the United States. *N Engl J Med.* 2007;356:1905–1908.
18. Gostin LO, DeAngelis CD. Mandatory HPV vaccination: public health vs private wealth. *JAMA.* 2007;297: 1921–1923.
19. Colgrove J, Abiola S, Mello MM. HPV vaccination mandates—lawmaking amid political and scientific controversy. *N Engl J Med.* 2010;363:785–791.
20. Lo B. Human papilloma virus vaccination programmes. *BMJ.* 2007;335:357–358.

ANNOTATED BIBLIOGRAPHY

1. Childress JF, Faden RR, Gaare RD, et al. Public health ethics: mapping the terrain. *J Law Med Ethics.* 2002;30:170–178.
Presents an ethical framework for public health policies.
2. Gostin LO. *Public Health Law: Power, Duty, Restraint.* 2nd ed. Berkeley, CA: University of California Press; 2008.
Comprehensive treatise on public health law and policy.
3. Altevogt B, Stroud C, Hanson SL, et al., eds. *Guidance for Establishing Crisis Standards of Care for Use in Disaster Situations.* Washington, DC: The National Academies Press; 2009. http://www.nap.edu/catalog.php?record_id=12749&m=0003000740. Accessed December 9, 2011.
Consensus recommendations for modifying legal standards of care in disasters where the need for care overwhelms available resources.
4. Lo B, Katz MH. Clinical decision-making during public health emergencies: ethical considerations. *Ann Intern Med.* 2005;143:493–498.
Analyzes ethical dilemmas that frontline clinicians face during public health emergencies.
5. Emanuel EJ, Wertheimer A. Who should get influenza vaccine when not all can? *Science.* 2006;312:854–855.
Analyzes ethical principles for the allocation of scarce resources during an influenza pandemic and argues for a life-cycle approach.
6. White DB, Katz MH, Luce JM, et al. Who should receive life support during a public health emergency? Using ethical principles to improve allocation decisions. *Ann Intern Med.* 2009;150:132–138.
Analyzes the allocation of scarce ICU beds during an influenza pandemic, highlighting the changes from ordinary clinical care.

44

Ethical Issues in Cross-Cultural Care

T he cultural backgrounds of US patients are becoming increasingly diverse. By 2050, non-Hispanic Caucasians will no longer be a majority of the population. Furthermore, immigrants are settling in new areas of the country. Thus, physicians across the country will care for patients from many cultural heritages, which will change over their careers.

Previous chapters discussed specific ethical dilemmas in which culture influences patients' values and medical decisions, including the disclosure of a serious diagnosis (*see* Chapter 6), surrogate decision making (*see* Chapter 12), and insistence on life-sustaining interventions (*see* Chapter 14). Those chapters focused on how to resolve the specific ethical issue. In this chapter, we address two cross-cutting questions: First, what can physicians be expected to know about the cultural issues that are salient in an ethical dilemma? Second, how can physicians respond to these cultural issues in an ethically appropriate manner?

THE IMPACT OF CULTURE ON CLINICAL CARE

Physicians need to appreciate how a patient's cultural background impacts on how he or she views ethical dilemmas and how they should be resolved.

UNDERSTAND HOW CULTURE INFLUENCES PATIENTS

Culture molds a patient's values, beliefs, and expectations about health, medical care, the doctor–patient relationship, and decision-making style (1). It shapes what concerns patients express to physicians and how they describe their symptoms. Patients draw upon cultural values when they weigh risks and benefits and make health care decisions. In many cultures, individual patient autonomy is less important than protecting patients from distress and fulfilling obligations to family members.

Physicians should be familiar with cultures to which many of their patients belong and how these cultures view common ethical dilemmas. Doctors, however, cannot be expected to have in-depth knowledge of every culture. To obtain more information, physicians need to consult the literature and knowledgeable colleagues and cultural interpreters, such as religious leaders. As with other aspects of medicine, training cannot provide physicians all the information they will need during their career.

AVOID CULTURAL STEREOTYPING

Physicians must not make assumptions about a patient's values based on her cultural heritage (1–3). Culture is not homogeneous or monolithic. Individuals and subgroups within a culture vary in their attitudes and values. In addition to culture, education, socioeconomic status, and many other factors also shape preferences for decision making and care. Furthermore, cultures change over time, and immigrants typically acculturate to the United States.

ELICIT INFORMATION ABOUT A PATIENT'S CULTURE

To respect the patient's values and preferences, physicians need to understand how an individual patient is shaped by his culture. Open-ended questions help the doctor to do this, regardless of the patient's background (2).

DISCLOSURE OF A SERIOUS DIAGNOSIS TO THE PATIENT

| CASE 44.1 | Family requests not to tell the patient he has cancer |

Mr. Z, a 70-year-old Spanish-speaking man with a change in bowel habits and weight loss, is found to have colon cancer. His daughter and son ask the physician not to tell their father he has cancer. Mr. Z lived in Mexico most of his life, where people in his generation are not told they have cancer. His children fear if Mr. Z is told, he will lose hope.

WHAT SHOULD A PHYSICIAN KNOW ABOUT CULTURAL ISSUES?

In many cultures, patients traditionally are not told of a diagnosis of cancer or other serious illness. In one study, 87% of European American patients and 89% of African American patients wanted to be told if they have cancer, compared with 65% of Mexican Americans and 47% of Korean Americans (4). In some cultures, disclosure of a grave diagnosis is believed to cause patients to suffer, while withholding the diagnosis allows serenity, security, and hope (5). Communicating the diagnosis directly and explicitly might be considered insensitive and cruel. Families might try to protect the patient by communicating the diagnosis nonverbally or indirectly or by taking on decision-making responsibility (6, 7). They may mistrust or get angry at physicians who tell the patient of his diagnosis.

Supporting for disclosing the diagnosis of cancer is growing. In traditional cultures the percentage of people who want to be told of a diagnosis of cancer is increasing (8). Immigrants tend to acculturate to the United States.

HOW SHOULD PHYSICIANS RESPOND TO CULTURAL ISSUES?

Regardless of the percentage of persons in a culture who do not want to be told they have cancer, the key ethical issue for doctors is whether the individual patient wants to know the diagnosis (9).

| CASE 44.1 | *Continued* |

Physicians should routinely ask each patient whether he wants to be told of his test results and diagnosis or whether he wants someone else to receive the information. Such individualized assessment is particularly important with patients from cultures that traditionally do not disclose serious diagnoses. Physicians, however, should also ask patients of Northern European heritage, because some of them may not want to know that they have cancer. Because patients and their families might hold different views, it is important to ask the patient directly and not rely on what the family believes the patient would want.

Chapter 6 gives more specific suggestions regarding how to disclose a grave diagnosis to patients (9,10). It may be appropriate to disclose the diagnosis indirectly and to determine the degree of disclosure the patient desires (10).

END-OF-LIFE DECISION MAKING

CASE 44.2   Family insistence that everything be done (11)

Bishop P is a 60-year-old African American man with diabetes, quadriplegia, and refractory infections. He was hospitalized with urosepsis from Enterobacter cloacae complicated by hypotension, respiratory failure, renal failure, stroke, and seizures. He required mechanical ventilation and dialysis. Despite multiple courses of antibiotics, his blood cultures remained positive for E. cloacae, resistant to all antibiotics. A drug reaction caused a total body rash, and his skin sheared away around his bandages and electrocardiographic leads. The physicians believed that further interventions would be inhumane and disfiguring, that he would not survive the hospitalization, and that attempts at CPR would be futile.

Bishop P's Pentecostalist church emphasizes faith healing. Bishop P was obtunded and could not state his preferences for care. His family insisted that everything be done because he believed that all life was sacred.

WHAT SHOULD A PHYSICIAN KNOW ABOUT CULTURAL ISSUES?

African Americans complete advance directives and forego life support less frequently than other patients (12, 13). Physicians need to understand how these decisions are based on cultural values and religious beliefs. For many African Americans, spiritual beliefs provide comfort and a way to cope with illness (12). Many African Americans believe that God is ultimately responsible for health, that the physician is God's instrument, and that prayer can promote healing. Because only God has power to decide life and death, human beings must preserve life until God determines its end. Many African Americans also believe in divine intervention and miracles (14). They may also view illness as something to endure or as a test of their faith. All these beliefs tend to make African American patients desire life support (12).

Inequalities and discrimination in health care have shaped beliefs of African American patients about end-of-life decisions (3). Many African Americans worry that a Do Not Attempt Resuscitation (DNAR) order or an advance directive might lead to withholding of needed care.

HOW SHOULD PHYSICIANS RESPOND TO CULTURAL ISSUES?

Whenever the physician disagrees with a patient or family over care, it is crucial to understand their concerns and values and to identify cultural or religious values that influence their decisions (Table 44-1). Open-ended questions are particularly helpful, no matter what the patient's culture.

Empirical studies suggest how doctor–patient communication affects patient trust. African American patients and patients whose race differs from their physician receive less information from

TABLE 44-1   Caring for patients from different cultures

Understand the concerns and values of the patient and family.

    Use open-ended questions.

    Show you understand their perspective through empathic comments.

    Summarize what the patient or family has said, and check that it is correct.

Seek help from cultural and religious leaders or cultural interpreters, including caregivers who has experienced caring for similar patients.

Find common ground, such as providing the best care possible and forging an ongoing partnership.

physicians and play a less active role in decisions. There might be a vicious cycle in which such patients do not prompt doctors to provide more information and doctors, in turn, provide less information (15). Furthermore, African American patients perceive their physicians as less informative, less partnering, and less supportive than Caucasian patients consider their physicians, and these perceptions are associated with lower trust in physicians (16).

CASE 44.2 | *Continued*

Knowing that religion is important to Bishop P, the physicians can ask open-ended questions to better understand how religious beliefs impact on his and his family's medical decisions. "How does religion or spirituality play a role in your life?" (10, 17, 18). "In your religion or culture, is there anything that should be done now?"

With an African American family, the physician might also ask open-ended questions focused on mistrust of the medical system. "Many African-Americans are concerned that they will not receive the care they need. I wonder what stories you might have heard?" Asking the question with regard to "stories" rather than a patient's personal experience might be useful because people may be deeply influenced by stories about people like them (19). After listening to a family's concerns, physicians should acknowledge that mistrust is an understandable reaction. The physician might say, "I've heard stories like that too." Or "I think it would be hard for me to trust doctors and hospitals if I heard stories like that." Physicians should not try to reassure the family immediately that they will provide all appropriate care (20). Premature reassurance might be ineffective or counterproductive, deterring patients from disclosing their concerns and emotions in enough detail that they feel understood (21).

The physician should try to find common ground, for example, by acknowledging that religion is an important source of comfort for patients and their families.

Chapter 14 gives more specific suggestions regarding resolving disagreements over life-sustaining interventions.

ADVANCE CARE PLANNING

Although federal policies encourage patients to provide advance directives, in some cultures advance directives are viewed with skepticism (10).

CASE 44.3 | **Reluctance to provide an advance directive**

Mrs. W is a 73-year-old woman with congestive heart failure who was hospitalized a month ago for a severe exacerbation of CHF, which almost required intubation and mechanical ventilation. Mrs. W emigrated from China 30 years ago and speaks Cantonese at home. To try to ascertain her preferences for life support if she suffered another severe exacerbation, the physician tries to raise the topic of advance directives. Mrs. W smiles politely and says simply, "Thank you." When pressed further, she says, "My children will know what to do." Similar attempts to engage in advance planning have also been unproductive in the past.

WHAT SHOULD A PHYSICIAN KNOW ABOUT CULTURAL ISSUES?

Because posthospitalization visits provide an opportunity to discuss advance planning with patients with congestive heart failure (22), Mrs. W's physician feels frustrated. Physicians need to understand that there may be strong cultural reasons why some patients are reluctant to consider advance directives.

In traditional Chinese culture, advance care planning is viewed as impractical and unnecessary (23). Many patients would prefer to consider the issues only when an actual decision needs to be made. Imagining a hypothetical situation may seem futile. The culture encourages people to avoid topics that make them feel negative and protect themselves against unnecessary worry. Finally, the patient may prefer to rely on family responsibilities to care for relatives who are ill and to make decisions. Giving explicit directives or designating one person as surrogate might imply that the family cannot be trusted to make the right decisions and might cause the patient and family to lose face. In addition, children's filial responsibility and respect for parents might lead them to insist on maximal life-sustaining interventions to prolong her life.

HOW SHOULD PHYSICIANS RESPOND TO CULTURAL ISSUES?

Physicians need to respect the family's sense of responsibility, while ascertaining whether limiting some life-sustaining interventions is consistent with that responsibility. Once the family realizes that the doctor understands their values, they may be more willing to consider limiting life-sustaining interventions. Conversely, physicians who understand the family's perspective may be more flexible regarding life-sustaining interventions.

Physicians also need to pay attention to ethical issues surrounding the decision to use a professional translator rather than a bilingual health care worker or a family member (24). The decision to call a professional interpreter should depend on the clinical situation, degree of language gap, available resources, and patient preference. Different options for interpretation have advantages and disadvantages. Although bilingual staff may be convenient and available, their language skills are usually not tested and might be inadequate. Having family members serve as interpreters may be congruent with patient preferences and cultural expectations. Relatives may also serve as patient advocates and participate in decisions regarding a patient's care. Family members, however, often have inadequate language skills and may also interpret selectively to fit their own beliefs. Physicians should inform patients with low English proficiency of the available resources for language assistance and offer a professional interpreter at each major stage of an encounter. Many patients may not appreciate that they have the right to translation services, without charge. Physicians should ensure that patients understand the advantages of professional interpreters and not assume that patients prefer to have family members interpret. Informed patients should decide the type of interpreter.

CASE 44.3   *Continued*

With any patient, it is useful for the physician to summarize what the patient has said and check that it is accurate. "I want to make sure I understand what you want. You want your children to make medical decisions for you if you were too sick to talk to me directly. But rather than talk with them about what kinds of care you want or not want, you trust them to make decisions. Have I understood you correctly?"

Children, who often are more acculturated to the United States, may be more willing to consider decisions in advance. If the physician infers that the children's sense of responsibility to parents is important, then she could ask more focused questions that still are open-ended: "Some Chinese Americans feel that to respect their parents, they must have all life-sustaining interventions done. How do you feel about that?"

ACCOMMODATING CULTURAL PREFERENCES ABOUT CARE

Some patients have culturally based preferences regarding who may provide medical care (24).

CASE 44.4 **Request for a Muslim physician**

Mrs. K is a 62-year-old woman who presented to the emergency department (ED) the day after a fall on her back. She has dull low back pain and shooting pains down her right leg, as well as an inability to urinate. An hour ago, she developed substernal chest pain and short-ness of breath. Mrs. K was born in Pakistan and has lived in the United States for 15 years. She is a devout Muslim. The ED physician assigned to her care is male.

Mrs. K refuses a physical examination, but is eventually persuaded to allow her heart and lungs to be examined. She refuses a back examination. After coaxing, she allows the physi-cian to examine her spinal column with gloves on. There is spinal tenderness. She adamantly refuses a rectal examination. Because of her chest pain, Mrs. K is placed on a cardiac monitor and bed rest. She becomes agitated and refuses a bedpan and bedside commode. Later, a nurse allows Mrs. K to walk to the bathroom, where she has a large bowel movement.

Her workup is negative for spinal or cardiac disease. The following morning her symp-toms have greatly improved, and she is discharged.

WHAT SHOULD A PHYSICIAN KNOW ABOUT CULTURAL ISSUES?

In Case 44.4, Mrs. K had strong preferences regarding caregivers, which complicated her care. Many Muslims prefer a Muslim physician of the same gender, or at least a non-Muslim physician of the same gender (25). In Muslim culture, separation of genders is important (26). With a male clinician, Muslim women might object to making direct eye contact, answering direct questions, undressing for examinations, being touched, or removing their headscarves (26). Care from a male physician is not strictly banned, because medical necessity allows "things that are ordinarily forbidden to be permissible" (25). Theologic debates, however, are not appropriate or constructive at the bedside. Mrs. K refused a bedpan and commode because of her modesty and privacy, which are highly valued in Muslim culture (25). Standards of modesty and privacy vary across cultures (27). In a patient with possible cardiac ischemia, both the exertion of going to the bathroom and the stress of not having a bowel movement might be dangerous. In this case, given Mrs. K's distress, overriding the routine ED procedures to allow her to walk with assistance to the bathroom was appropriate.

HOW SHOULD PHYSICIANS RESPOND TO CULTURAL ISSUES?

There are good reasons to accommodate a patient's preferences regarding the type of physician. The doctor–patient relationship is highly personal, and trust is important. Since 9/11, many Muslims report they have faced stereotyping, stigma, and discrimination (26). Trying to meet Mrs. K's prefer-ences respects her cultural heritage and her as a person.

The legal concept of reasonable accommodation provides a helpful conceptual framework. Physicians should take reasonable steps to accommodate Mrs. K's preferences regarding a female physician, even if standard hospital procedures need to be modified.

The suggestions in Table 44-1 can help physicians understand the patient's concerns and develop practical plans to address them.

CASE 44.4 *Continued*

Physicians who have little experience with Muslim patients might not anticipate Mrs. K's preferences for a female Muslim physician or the importance of bathroom privacy. After seeing that she is refusing routine medical procedures, the physician should try to elicit the reasons for her refusal through open-ended questions: "I want to try to take care of your medical problems. Is there anything I need to know to give you the best care we can?" Open-ended questions to elicit the patient's expectations and concerns are an effective communication technique, regardless of the patient's cultural background.

After learning of Mrs. K's strong preference for a female physician, the doctors can try to accommodate them. If there is a female physician working in the ED that shift, she could take over Mrs. K's care with little burden on the ED and its staff. If a female physician is not available, then the treating physician should explain the situation and ask the patient and family how the patient would like to proceed. The physician might also ask permission to talk with the patient's imam for suggestions. Such joint problem-solving helps build a partnership to care for the patient. The patient or family may offer suggestions, such as having the physician wear gloves or placing her behind a drape during an examination. These measures to accommodate Mrs. K's preferences place only small burdens on the ED staff. There are limits, however, on what physicians or a hospital could reasonably be asked to do. The ED is not required to call in a female physician from home or disrupt the care of other patients in ways that place them at serious risk or inconvenience

ETHICALLY PROBLEMATIC CULTURAL REQUESTS

Some requests for a specific type of health care worker may be ethically problematical, as in the following case.

CASE 44.5   Racist cultural requests

Mr. D is a 52-year-old Caucasian man who came to the ED because of crushing substernal chest pain and is found to have ST elevation in the lateral leads. He will be admitted to the cardiac care unit (CCU). The CCU physician, an African American woman, comes to the ED to admit him. He refuses to allow her to care for him, calling her names that are racially and sexually offensive and loudly declaring his white supremacist beliefs.

Patients have health care needs that physicians and hospitals are in a unique position to address. Because patients depend on them, the professional ideal is that physicians should place the patient's best interests foremost. For example, in wartime, military physicians are expected to attend to the medical needs of enemy combatants, even those who espouse and articulate offensive ideologies. Respect for the patient's culture, however, has limits. Physicians and other health care workers should

CASE 44.5   *Continued*

The CCU and ED physician are ethically justified in setting limits on Mr. D's actions. A patient who expects his beliefs to be respected and to have his health needs addressed needs to respect health care workers and other patients. A hospital or health care worker is ethically justified in expecting patients to refrain from discrimination and abusive behavior as a condition of receiving care. Patients should not insult or disparage health care workers. It is ethically permissible to set limits on patient behaviors even though beliefs should not be regulated. Patients may think whatever they want, but they should not say things or act in ways that offend, demean, or harm others.

The CCU doctor might say, "I am the doctor on call tonight in the CCU. You may be having a heart attack and you need treatment. If you want to be treated in this hospital tonight, I have to ask you not to use that kind of language. I can try to transfer you to another heart doctor tomorrow if you wish. If you want to leave this hospital and seek care elsewhere, you are free to do so, but delaying care would put you at serious medical risk." The ED physician should reinforce these conditions, particularly if he is Caucasian or male. If Mr. D agrees to receiving treatment, the physicians should strive to provide high-quality and compassionate care (28).

not be subjected to verbal or physical abuse (*see* Chapter 34). Race, religion, and national origin are protected under the US Constitution, and people should not be discriminated against because of these characteristics.

Many physicians would seek to accommodate Mrs. K, the Muslim patient in Case 44.4, but not Mr. D, the white supremacist patient in Case 44.5. Can these cases be logically distinguished? Physicians should not try to judge the validity of cultural beliefs or determine if some beliefs are more deserving of respect. Physicians should focus on actions and words, rather than beliefs. Mrs. K does not insult or disparage non-Muslim physicians. Had she framed her refusal of care in terms of a hatred of infidels and used racial insults to staff, the situation would be similar to Case 44.5.

FEMALE GENITAL CUTTING

Ritual genital cutting of female minors (a more neutral term than female genital mutilation) is widely practiced in Africa and the Middle East (29). Parents believe that it will integrate their daughter's into their culture, protect her virginity and family honor, and make her a wife. The term refers to a range of procedures, including excision of the clitoris and labia minora and infibulation, in which labial surfaces are stitched together to cover the urethra and vaginal introitus. Serious complications include infection, dysmenorrhea, painful intercourse, infertility, and childbirth complications. In the United States, some parents ask physicians to perform female genital cutting using sterile conditions and anesthesia. Otherwise, they might have the procedure done in their home country or by someone without medical training.

These procedures violate the ethical principle of "do no harm" and the rights of children to health and well-being. Some physicians consider a ritual nick as a possible compromise to avoid greater harm. Under United States federal law, however, all types of female genital cutting on minors are criminal offenses. In declining these procedures, physicians should express respect for parents and their cultural, religious, and ethnic traditions. Cessation of this practice will require community educational programs led by immigrant women (30).

SUMMARY

1. Physicians should be sensitive to how culture may influence a patient's values and decisions.
2. Physicians can use open-ended questions to elicit from patients how their cultural backgrounds influence their expectations and values regarding ethical dilemmas.
3. Doctors can then address cultural differences in a respectful manner.

REFERENCES

1. Kleinman A, Benson P. Anthropology in the clinic: the problem of cultural competency and how to fix it. *PLoS Med.* 2006;3:e294.
2. Betancourt JR. Cultural competence and medical education: many names, many perspectives, one goal. *Acad Med.* 2006;81:499–501.
3. Crawley LM, Marshall PA, Lo B, et al. Strategies for culturally effective end-of-life care. *Ann Intern Med.* 2002;136:673–679.
4. Blackhall LJ, Murphy ST, Frank G, et al. Ethnicity and attitudes toward patient autonomy. *JAMA.* 1995;274:820–825.
5. Gordon DB, Paci E. Disclosure practices and cultural narratives: understanding concealment and silence around cancer in Tuscany, Italy. *Soc Sci Med.* 1997;44:1433–1452.
6. Surbone A. Truth telling to the patient. *JAMA.* 1992;268:1661–1662.
7. Surbone A. Telling the truth to patients with cancer: what is the truth? *Lancet Oncol.* 2006;7:944–950.
8. Jiang Y, Liu C, Li JY, et al. Different attitudes of Chinese patients and their families toward truth telling of different stages of cancer. *Psychooncology.* 2007;16:928–936.
9. Kagawa-Singer M, Blackhall LJ. Negotiating cross-cultural issues at the end of life: "you got to go where he lives". *JAMA.* 2001;286:2993–3001.

10. Barclay JS, Blackhall LJ, Tulsky JA. Communication strategies and cultural issues in the delivery of bad news. *J Palliat Med.* 2007;10:958–977.
11. Alpers A, Lo B. Avoiding family feuds: responding to surrogates' demands for life-sustaining treatment. *J Law Med Ethics.* 1999;27:74–80.
12. Johnson KS, Elbert-Avila KI, Tulsky JA. The influence of spiritual beliefs and practices on the treatment preferences of African Americans: a review of the literature. *J Am Geriatr Soc.* 2005;53:711–719.
13. Raghavan M, Smith AK, Arnold RM. African Americans and end-of-life care #204. *J Palliat Med.* 2010;13:1382–1383.
14. Widera EW, Rosenfeld KE, Fromme EK, et al. Approaching patients and family members who hope for a miracle. *J Pain Symptom Manage.* 2011;42:119–125.
15. Gordon HS, Street RL Jr, Sharf BF, et al. Racial differences in doctors' information-giving and patients' participation. *Cancer.* 2006;107:1313–1320.
16. Gordon HS, Street RL Jr, Sharf BF, et al. Racial differences in trust and lung cancer patients' perceptions of physician communication. *J Clin Oncol.* 2006;24:904–909.
17. Lo B, Ruston D, Kates LW, et al. Discussing religious and spiritual issues at the end of life: a practical guide for physicians. *JAMA.* 2002;287:749–754.
18. Lo B, Kates LW, Ruston D, et al. Responding to requests regarding prayer and religious ceremonies by patients near the end of life and their families. *J Palliat Med.* 2003;6:409–415.
19. Holloway KFC. *Passed On: African American Mourning Stories.* Durham, NC: Duke University Press; 2003.
20. Lo B, Quill T, Tulsky J. Discussing palliative care with patients. *Ann Intern Med.* 1999;130:744–749.
21. Maguire P, Faulkner A, Booth K, et al. Helping cancer patients disclose their concerns. *Euro J Cancer.* 1996;32A:78–81.
22. Selman L, Harding R, Beynon T, et al. Improving end-of-life care for patients with chronic heart failure: "let's hope it'll get better, when I know in my heart of hearts it won't". *Heart.* 2007;93:963–967.
23. Bowman KW, Singer PA. Chinese seniors' perspective on end-of-life decisions. *Soc Sci Med.* 2001;53:455–464.
24. Schenker Y, Lo B, Ettinger KM, et al. Navigating language barriers under difficult circumstances: a conceptual and practical approach for clinicians. *Ann Int Med.* 2008;149:264–269.
25. Padela AI. Can you take care of my mother? Reflections on cultural competency and clinical accommodation. *Acad Emerg Med.* 2007;14:275–277.
26. Inhorn MC, Serour GI. Islam, medicine, and Arab-Muslim refugee health in America after 9/11. *Lancet.* 2011;378:935–943.
27. Fiester A. What "patient-centered care" requires in serious cultural conflict. *Acad Med.* 2012;87:20–24.
28. Tweedy DS. A case of racism and reconciliation. *Ann Intern Med.* 2012;156:246–247.
29. American Academy of Pediatrics Board of Directors. Ritual genital cutting of female minors. *Pediatrics.* 2010;126:191.
30. Appiah KA. *The Honor Code: How Moral Revolutions Happen.* New York, NY: W.W. Norton; 2010.

ANNOTATED BIBLIOGRAPHY

1. Fiester A. What "patient-centered care" requires in serious cultural conflict. *Acad Med.* 2012;87:20–24.
   Physicians need to learn skills to provide quality care to patients from anywhere, no matter what differences in cultural background might exist.
2. Kagawa-Singer M, Blackhall LJ. Negotiating cross-cultural issues at the end of life: "you got to go where he lives." *JAMA.* 2001;286:2993–3001.
   Analyzes issues of truth-telling, life-sustaining interventions, and decision-making styles, which are salient in cross-cultural care at the end of life. Practical suggestions for how to address these issues.
3. Inhorn MC, Serour GI. Islam, medicine, and Arab-Muslim refugee health in America after 9/11. *Lancet.* 2011;378:935–943.
   American Academy of Pediatrics Board of Directors. Ritual genital cutting of female minors. *Pediatrics.* 2010;126:191.
   Thoughtful articles, illustrating the value of search for articles in the medical literature on specific ethical dilemmas in cross-cultural care.
4. Barclay JS, Blackhall LJ, Tulsky JA. Communication strategies and cultural issues in the delivery of bad news. *J Palliat Med.* 2007;10:958–977.
   Thorough review of cultural aspects of delivering bad news and discussing end-of-life care.
5. Schenker Y, Lo B, Ettinger KM, et al. Navigating language barriers under difficult circumstances: a conceptual and practical approach for clinicians. *Ann Int Med.* 2008;149:264–269.
   Analyzes ethical and practical dilemmas regarding when to call for a professional translator, rely on other health care workers, or rely on relatives of the patient.

45

Ethical Issues in Digital Health Information

Digital communication through e-mail, the Internet, and social media are becoming increasingly common in medicine, as in other areas of life. In addition, the US government is urging the adopting of electronic health records (EHRs). These digital technologies present the promise of more efficient and higher quality health care. However, digital health information presents risks and burdens as well as benefits and may have unintended adverse effects on the doctor–patient relationship.

E-MAIL WITH PATIENTS

E-mail allows patients and physicians to communicate asynchronously outside of clinic hours without being frustrated by "telephone tag." Patients can ask questions, report their condition, and request appointments, referrals, and refills of medications. Doctors can communicate with patients without interrupting their workflow, write orders, and route messages to other staff. If the e-mail platform is linked to an EHR, doctors can easily document their actions. However, e-mail communication with patients also presents risks and challenges, as the following case illustrates.

CASE 27.1	New chest pain

A 63-year-old woman e-mailed her physician, "I was awakened this morning with persistent discomfort in the middle of my chest (which I had once a few years ago). It has since gone away. Given the fact that my brother had to get five stents last year, I wonder if I should be evaluated. I am hoping to be seen today." The message was not opened until 2 hours after it was sent.

ETHICAL ISSUES WITH E-MAILS

In responding to e-mails, physicians should follow the same ethical guidelines that they follow in face-to-face visits, taking into account the peculiarities of the medium.

First, physicians should respect patients by ascertaining their concerns and needs, educating them, forming a mutually acceptable plan of care, and protecting their privacy and confidentiality.

Second, doctors should act in the patient's best interests. Some clinical situations require real-time conversation and attention to the patient's emotions and are better handled through phone calls or face-to-face conversations than e-mail. An example is telling a patient that an imaging study shows probable cancer. In conversations, nonverbal communication such as the tone and loudness of voice, pauses, and interruptions can transmit valuable information. In face-to-face meetings, facial expression, eye contact, body position, head nods, and physical contact convey meaning and emotion.

CASE 27.1   *Continued*

Because this patient may have new-onset coronary artery disease, she needs triage to a possible paramedic call, emergency department visit, or same-day clinic visit. When her e-mail was not answered promptly, the patient phoned the clinic and was connected with the nurse, who determined that she could be scheduled for an appointment for that afternoon. At that visit, the physician determined that the pain was not typical of angina, confirmed that the EKG was normal, and ordered an urgent treadmill test.

The clinic realized it needed to set up procedures to screen e-mails in real time, identify urgent messages, and respond to them promptly. Also, it began to send automated e-mail responses to patients telling them when to expect a reply and explaining how to communicate urgent concerns.

HEALTH INFORMATION ON THE INTERNET

About one quarter of adults use the Internet for information related to issues they are discussing with their physicians (1). Physicians need to keep in mind the benefits and risks of such information (2).

PROSPECTIVE BENEFITS

Improved Access to Health Information

The Internet offers more health information to the public than conventional media and makes it searchable and accessible at any time.

Enhanced Patient Role in Decision-Making

The Internet may help patients play a more active role in their care. Bringing information from the Internet to a physician is associated with patients feeling more in control during the physician visit, more willingness to ask questions, and greater confidence in their perceived ability to manage disease (3).

Psychosocial Benefits

Social networking sites organized around specific conditions may provide psychosocial support to patients and help them learn how to cope with their illness.

RISKS AND BURDENS

Inaccurate or Misleading Information

Medical information and advice on the Internet is not screened, edited, or rated for accuracy. It is difficult for patients to judge the quality of medical websites or the information presented (4). Furthermore, patients may have difficulty putting information into the context of their specific clinical situation. Personal narratives and dramatic cases may lead patients to overestimate the frequency of rare events.

Medical risks

Some physicians fear that Internet information will lead patients to request medical interventions that are not indicated. However, in one study 71% of patients who brought information from the Internet to physicians did so simply to obtain the physician's opinion, not to obtain a test, medication, or referral (3). Whether or not patients received the requested intervention did not affect their rating of the doctor–patient relationship (3). Thus, at the point of clinical services, most patients accept the physician's recommendations.

Some interactive Internet sites offer advice from physicians to individual users. The qualification of these physicians and the quality of such advice is not known. Furthermore, it is not clear whether sound medical advice for complicated problems can be given without a face-to-face discussion and physical examination.

Psychosocial Risks

Patients may suffer psychosocial harms if they directly access on the Internet test results that reveal a serious diagnosis such as cancer, rather than learning the diagnosis through a physician (5).

The Doctor–Patient Relationship

Patients report that bringing information from the Internet to the physician generally has a positive impact on the doctor–patient relationship, provided that the physician had adequate communication skills and did not appear challenged (3). Other data confirm the importance of the physician's response to patients bringing information from the Internet. Physicians who perceived that the patient was challenging their authority were more likely to believe the doctor–patient relationship had deteriorated (6). Thus, certain responses by the physician might worsen the doctor–patient relationship.

WHAT PHYSICIANS SHOULD DO

Doctors should promote the benefits of these information innovations and minimize their risks and burdens (2).

Promote Informed Decision-Making by Patients

Physicians and health care organizations should encourage patients to seek information about their condition, help them with the quality of medical information on the Internet, and recommend websites that contain reliable information.

Recognize and Minimize Counterproductive Reactions

Doctors need to recognize that they might feel threatened when patients bring in health information from the Internet. Physicians should not let their own emotions compromise patient care. In other situations, doctors learn not to overreact and to form alliances with patients rather than polarize the situation (*see* Chapter 14). If a patient requests a medically inappropriate intervention because of information from the Internet, the physician should explain why it is not appropriate and negotiate a plan of care that is mutually acceptable.

ELECTRONIC HEALTH RECORDS

EHRs can improve care by making comprehensive information immediately available to physicians and enabling quality of care initiatives. The 2009 Health Information Technology for Economic and Clinical Health (HITECH) Act offers incentives to adopt EHRs (7). Currently, there are financial incentives, and in 2015 there will be lower reimbursements for physicians who do not use EHRs. To qualify for these financial incentives, EHRs must provide electronic prescribing, decision support, and data for quality-of-care indicators (7). These capabilities will enhance the quality and efficiency of care.

CONCERNS ABOUT EHRs

Affordability of EHRs

For small practices, which include the majority of physicians, EHRs are very expensive despite the financial incentives under HITECH. Some EHR vendors have business plans to provide the EHR to physicians for free or at a deep discount, in exchange for receiving de-identified patient data for data mining. In addition, vendors may send pop-up banners with advertisements. Physicians are already familiar with pop-up ads, for example when accessing medical journals or medical websites online. However, pop-up advertisements raise ethical concerns, as discussed later (2).

Fair Reimbursement

Physicians commonly have pay-for-performance incentives linked to quality-of-care indicators. EHRs allow efficient collection of data on a wide variety of indicators. Inaccurate reporting of quality data, however, may lead to unfair reimbursement. Justified exceptions to clinical practice guidelines occur in around 5% of cases. Complex, sick patients may be exceptions to practice guidelines because they cannot tolerate the intervention, decline it, or have medical contraindications. Hence, justified exceptions will be higher in practices that see many such patients. Automated reporting of quality indicators may be inaccurate because current EHRs do not document if a recommended intervention was declined or is contraindicated.

Privacy of EHRs

Many patients want control over their personal health information (*see* Chapter 5). They may regard some information as highly sensitive or not relevant to the current problem, for example, an abortion or marijuana use many years ago. Furthermore, patients may worry that data in an EHR may be disclosed to the government or to companies who mine large data sets for profit. Once information is entered into the EHR, patients might lose control over who has access to it. Thus, some patients choose to withhold some information from the EHR.

Security of EHRs

Large security breaches have been reported at health care organizations, other businesses, and Internet servers. Compared with paper medical records, a breach of security in EHRs typically involves information about a large number of patients.

New federal regulations stiffen penalties for breaches of privacy, increase enforcement, and provide incentives for encryption of patient information (7). Data that have been encrypted according to federal standards is presumed to be unreadable, unusable, and undecipherable. To provide incentives for encryption, the regulations require patients be notified of breaches of security of unsecured personal health information. For breaches involving more than 500 patients, local news media also need to be notified. There are financial incentives to adopt EHRs that meet federal encryption standards. These security measures are intended to increase patient trust in EHRs and willingness to allow information in EHRs to be shared with other providers and used for other purposes, such as research and quality improvement.

SHARING PATIENT INFORMATION AMONG PROVIDERS

Different doctors and hospitals caring for a patient need to share information in order to coordinate care and reduce redundant care.

Models for Sharing Electronic Health Information

Health information exchanges (HIEs) are agreements among health care providers to exchange health care information electronically. Spurred by federal financial incentives, a number of local and regional hospitals and health care systems have agreed to exchange information (8). HIEs lower costs because electronic exchange of information is less expensive than photocopying, faxing, or mailing medical records. Currently, the goal of HIEs is to improve patient care. However, the HIEs might also be used for quality improvement, research, or public health. HIEs vary in whether patients consent to exchange information for different purposes (9).

National networks for sharing health information are envisaged. Serious adverse events identified after the drug was approved for market led the FDA to withdraw approval of rofecoxib and restrict the use of rosiglitazone. The FDA also created the Sentinel program to use data from medical records to investigate postmarketing adverse events (10). Rather than collecting patient-specific data, Sentinel will use a distributed data network. Hospitals, health care plans, insurers, and other organizations will respond to specific data queries by analyzing their data and submitting their de-identified results. No patient consent is needed for Sentinel because HIPAA allows a health care organization to carry out quality improvement without patient authorization.

Ethical Guidelines Regarding Sharing Electronic Health Information

Patients may want to restrict access to personal health information that they consider very sensitive or not relevant to the problem at hand, for example, information regarding alcohol or substance use, mental health, a history of marijuana use, or abortion. Alternatively, they may disclose information to a physician orally but ask them not to place it in the medical record. Respect for patient freedom and autonomy requires following patient preferences regarding who will have access to their health information. However, there also are countervailing ethical guidelines.

To act in the best interests of the patient, physicians need to know the patient's medications or previous test results. Failure to have such information may result in suboptimal care, including delays or errors in diagnosis, unnecessary repetition of tests, and trials of therapies that have already failed. Knowing a patient's psychiatric medicines will help physicians evaluate common complaints such as palpitations, fatigue, or gastrointestinal distress. Not duplicating previous imaging studies avoids the risks of contrast media or radiation exposure.

The principle of justice requires the equitable distribution of health benefits and the promotion of the health of the community. The FDA Sentinel program uses electronic medical records for postmarketing surveillance of adverse drug effects. Incomplete information in medical records could bias the results of such postmarketing studies, potentially placing other patients at unnecessary risk.

Legal Issues

HIPAA allows the use and disclosure of personal health information for the purposes of treatment, billing, and administration (11). When a doctor or hospital shares information about a patient with another treatment provider, although patient permission is commonly requested as a matter of respect, it is not required. This provision favors benefiting the patient over respecting patient preferences not to disclose information.

HIPAA gives patients the right to request that physicians and health care organizations restrict the use and disclosure of their personal health information for treatment, payment, or billing. However, health care institutions and physicians are not required to honor those requests, except when the patient requests that their insurer not be notified of care that they paid for out of the pocket.

When patients request that information not be shared with other providers, the physician should explain that this might compromise care. The doctor should also explain confidentiality protections that are in place, for example, to restrict access to health care workers who have a need to know a patient's personal health information. Usually, the patient then agrees to share his or her information.

If patients decide not to place some information in the record, they assume the risk of substandard care. Because health care is increasingly a team endeavor, it is important that other health care workers caring for the patient—including specialists and nurses—know that there is incomplete information. Thus, the attending physician should place in the note a comment that there is additional information, together with her pager or phone number.

PERSONAL HEALTH RECORDS

Personal health records (PHRs) are controlled by the patient rather than by the physician, clinic, or hospital. They are also known as patient-controlled health records. In its full-fledged format, patients assemble their health information from the physicians, clinics, and hospitals that have cared for them, add patient-measured outcomes (such as home blood pressure and glucose measurements, functional status, and quality of life), and determine what information they wish to share with various providers. EHRs controlled by health care providers may incorporate some of these functions.

PHRs have several potential advantages (2). They are more comprehensive than the information held by a single health care provider. They enhance patient autonomy by giving patients more information, responsibility, and control over their health care. By including patient-generated data, PHRs focus physicians on patient-centered outcomes. Some PHRs have links to medical information and practice guidelines or offer social networking with other patients with the condition.

PHRs also present ethical challenges. They may complicate the problem of patients withholding pertinent information from treating physicians. As discussed later, PHRs also raise issues regarding privacy, confidentiality, and equitable access.

PHYSICIAN USE OF SOCIAL MEDIA

Physicians post information on social media, including blogs, websites, and social networks at similar rates as the general population. Medical students and residents use social media more than older physicians. Some materials that physicians post are problematic (12, 13). Postings that contain sufficient detail to identify a patient violate confidentiality. Physicians might express frustration or anger over incidents at work. Some posts contain offensive or discriminatory language, disparage patients or colleagues, or picture the physician intoxicated, using illegal drugs, or in sexually suggestive poses. Even if such photos are not on the physician's own site, persons in photos can be readily identified. Physicians commonly fail to use strict privacy settings on sites. Furthermore, physicians might use online dating sites where they reveal highly personal information. Such communications would be considered inappropriate in face-to-face or telephone encounters. On social media, however, people may be less inhibited and formal.

Physicians should keep in mind the following guidelines (14–16). First, postings on the Internet and social networking sites are accessible to the public and patients unless physicians consistently use highly restrictive privacy settings. Professional websites, social networking accounts, and blogs should be separate from personal ones. Physicians should expect some patients to Google them and forward information to others. Once posted, materials may be permanent. Second, behaviors and words that are inappropriate in face-to-face encounters should also be avoided on the Internet. Patients and potential patients who view problematic materials might question the physician's judgment, common sense, or trustworthiness.

OVERARCHING ETHICAL CONCERNS

As mentioned previously, several ethical concerns apply to all these digital information technologies.

Privacy and confidentiality. Risks to confidentiality may be greater because digital breaches usually involve more patients and larger amounts of personal information than breaches of paper records. The HIPAA Health Privacy Rule protections do not apply to companies that do not provide medical care but present themselves as sites for social networking, information, "recreational" genomic testing, or PHRs (7).

The rich personal information that consumers reveal to health websites and in electronic health records presents opportunities for targeted advertisements for drugs or other health products. PHR vendors also might sell such information to data mining companies. Such advertising raises several concerns (2). Patients may not appreciate that such ads might be possible and might have no meaningful ability to opt out of agreements between health care institutions and EHR vendors. Visitors to websites and purchasers of Internet services typically agree to a company's privacy policies using a click-through button as a condition of using the application or website.

Point of ordering advertisements that appear on an EMR when a physician is about to order a test or medication raise particular ethical concerns. Because these ads are salient when a physician is about to make a patient care decision, they may be particularly persuasive. Businesses that carry out such marketing seek to increase sales of their product; unlike physicians, they are not bound by professional standards to give advice that is consistent with scientific evidence or to act in the best interests of patients. The ethical issue is whether companies should be allowed to insert point of ordering advertisements that are inconsistent with evidence-based practice guidelines or FDA labeling. Alternatively, evidence-based advertising at the point of ordering to support evidence-based prescribing might be encouraged, for example, through government incentives or programs (17).

Just distribution of benefits and risks. Disadvantaged populations use digital health information technologies less frequently (18). They are less likely to be offered such secure patient portals and EHRs by their physicians. Even if offered, they are less likely to become regular users. This "digital divide" has multiple causes, including poor Internet access, health literacy, and English proficiency. Outreach to disadvantaged populations may be needed to ensure that the benefits of digital information technologies are fairly distributed and existing health disparities do not worsen (19).

SUMMARY

1. Digital information technologies not only offer unprecedented opportunities to improve the quality and efficiency of medical care but also pose novel ethical concerns, particularly regarding confidentiality and justice, that need to be addressed.

REFERENCES

1. Couper MP, Singer E, Levin CA, et al. Use of the internet and ratings of information sources for medical decisions: results from the DECISIONS survey. *Med Decis Making.* 2010;30:106S–114S.
2. Lo B, Parham L. The impact of web 2.0 on the doctor–patient relationship. *J Law Med Ethics.* 2010;38:17–26.
3. Murray E, Lo B, Pollack L, et al. The impact of health information on the internet on the physician–patient relationship: patient perceptions. *Arch Intern Med.* 2003;163:1727–1734.
4. Wald HS, Dube CE, Anthony DC. Untangling the Web—The impact of internet use on health care and the physician–patient relationship. *Patient Educ Couns.* 2007;68:218–224.
5. Halamka JD, Mandl KD, Tang PC. Early experiences with personal health records. *J Am Med Inform Assoc.* 2008;15:1–7.
6. Murray E, Lo B, Pollack L, et al. The impact of health information on the internet on health care and the physician–patient relationship: national U.S. survey among 1.050 U.S. physicians. *J Med Internet Res.* 2003;5:e17.
7. Blumenthal D. Wiring the health system—origins and provisions of a new federal program. *N Engl J Med.* 2011;365:2323–2329.
8. Office of the National Coordinator for Health Information Technology. *Get the Facts about the State Health Information Exchange Program.* http://healthit.hhs.gov/portal/server.pt?open=512&mode=2&objID=1834. Accessed December 28, 2011.
9. Goldstein MM. Health information technology and the idea of informed consent. *J Law Med Ethics.* 2010;38:27–35.
10. Behrman RE, Benner JS, Brown JS, et al. Developing the Sentinel System—a national resource for evidence development. *N Engl J Med.* 2011;364:498–499.
11. Lo B, Dornbrand L, Dubler NN. HIPAA and patient care: the role for professional judgment. *JAMA.* 2005;293:1766–1771.
12. Chretien KC, Greysen SR, Chretien JP, et al. Online posting of unprofessional content by medical students. *JAMA.* 2009;302:1309–1315.
13. Chretien KC, Azar J, Kind T. Physicians on Twitter. *JAMA.* 2011;305:566–568.
14. American Medical Association. *Professionalism in the Use of Social Media.* 2010. http://www.ama-assn.org/ama/pub/physician-resources/medical-ethics/code-medical-ethics/opinion9124.page. Accessed December 28, 2011.
15. Greysen SR, Kind T, Chretien KC. Online professionalism and the mirror of social media. *J Gen Intern Med.* 2010;25:1227–1229.
16. Mostaghimi A, Crotty BH. Professionalism in the digital age. *Ann Intern Med.* 2011;154:560–562.
17. The Prescription Project. *Academic Detailed: Evidence-based Prescribing Information.* 2008. http://www.prescriptionproject.org/tools/solutions_factsheets/files/0007.pdf. Accessed March 9, 2009.
18. Sequist TD. Health information technology and disparities in quality of care. *J Gen Intern Med.* 2011;26:1084–1085.
19. Kahn JS, Hilton JF, Van Nunnery T, et al. Personal health records in a public hospital: experience at the HIV/AIDS clinic at San Francisco General Hospital. *J Am Med Inform Assoc.* 2010;17:224–228.

ANNOTATED BIBLIOGRAPHY

1. Lo B, Parham L. The impact of web 2.0 on the doctor–patient relationship. *J Law Med Ethics.* 2010;38:17–26.
   Overview of the impact of new digital communication technologies on the doctor–patient relationship.
2. Greysen SR, Kind T, Chretien KC. Online professionalism and the mirror of social media. *J Gen Intern Med.* 2010;25:1227–1229.
   Recommendations on physician use of social media.

CASES FOR DISCUSSION

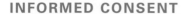

INFORMED CONSENT

CASE 1 **Choosing among therapeutic options for breast cancer**

An asymptomatic 52-year-old computer programmer is diagnosed with stage T1 localized breast cancer. Options for treatment include total mastectomy or lumpectomy plus radiation therapy. Suppose that you are the attending surgeon.

QUESTIONS FOR DISCUSSION

1. You are hosting a visiting physician from China, who says he does not understand why Americans regard informed consent as so important: "I can understand that in your country, you tell patients they have cancer. But why don't you then just do what is the best treatment for them, rather than going through what you call informed consent?" How would you explain (a) the purposes of informed consent and (b) the ethical reasons for informed consent?

2. An intern asks you how to determine what information about surgery he needs to discuss with the patient. "I just read a chapter in a surgery textbook, and I'm not sure how much information I should tell her before asking her to sign the consent form," he says. "There's no way I can tell her everything! What do I need to discuss with her?" How would you answer the intern's question?

3. Suppose, on the basis of your critical reading of the published evidence, you believe that breast-conserving surgery plus radiation therapy offers the best outcome for this patient. How do you incorporate this judgment in your discussions with the patient?

4. One resident has read articles reporting that patients do not understand basic information that physicians discuss with them and says, "Why do we bother with the informed consent? Patients don't understand what we tell them and don't remember any of it." How do you respond to the resident's objections?

5. A student asks if patients need to be told of the role that students and residents play during surgery and in postoperative care. One of the residents says, "We don't need to tell the patient about that. They have given implied consent to have residents and students participate in their care by choosing to come to a teaching hospital." Do you agree or disagree? Give the ethical considerations for your position. How have the courts used the term *implied consent*?

REFUSAL OF CARE

CASE 2 **Refusal of treatment by a patient with inoperable cancer**

A 64-year-old man has inoperable pancreatic cancer and obstructive jaundice. He had an internal drainage tube placed in the common duct in an attempt to decompress his biliary tree; however, he developed cholangitis, which was treated with antibiotics. He entered hospice care, and over the next 2 weeks he had progressive jaundice, abdominal pain, nausea, pruritis, anorexia, and weight loss. He is unlikely to live more then a few weeks. His drainage tube obstructs and he is admitted with another episode of biliary sepsis. As his physician, you discuss with him plans for care. He is lucid and shows no sign of mental impairment during your conversation.

QUESTIONS FOR DISCUSSION

1. The patient says he does not want cardiopulmonary resuscitation (CPR) attempted if he suffers a cardiac arrest. Would you write a Do Not Attempt Resuscitation (DNAR) order? What are the ethical reasons for your decision?
2. What would you do if his wife or family disagrees with his refusal of CPR? What is the ethical rationale for your response?
3. The patient also refuses antibiotics for biliary sepsis, saying, "There isn't any point in going through this again only to have another infection next week or the week after." The intern exclaims, "How can we not give him antibiotics? He'll die without them, and we have an ethical duty to save lives." Do you agree to withhold antibiotics? What is the ethical rationale for your position?

CASE 3	Refusal of blood transfusions by a Jehovah's Witness

A 34-year-old grade school teacher is hospitalized after an automobile accident that ruptures his spleen. A devout Jehovah's Witness, he refuses transfusion. He does agree to a splenectomy and states emphatically, "I wish to live, but with no blood transfusions." He also refuses blood components and court-ordered transfusions. He declares, "It is between me and God, not the courts. I'm willing to take my chances. My faith is that strong." He is lucid throughout the conversation.

QUESTIONS FOR DISCUSSION

1. His hematocrit drops to 14.1%. One of the residents says, "How can we just stand by and let him bleed to death when we could bring him back to full health with transfusions? Aren't doctors supposed to act for the good of the patient? How can it be good for a young, healthy man to die needlessly?" Do you agree with the resident? What is the ethical rationale for your position?
2. The patient's wife was a Jehovah's Witness but left the faith. "I know that he says he doesn't want a blood transfusion, but I also know he loves his children and his work," she says. "He could never agree to a transfusion, but he couldn't bear to leave us either. Can't you just give him blood without telling him when he's in surgery? Then he would get the care he needs." How do you respond to the wife? Explain the ethical rationale for your approach.
3. The surgeon is reluctant to operate without transfusion support. "What's the point of taking someone to the operating room to have him die on the table?" he says. "If he wants to refuse transfusions and die in the emergency room, then that's his right. But he can't force me to operate and be responsible for his death." Do you agree or disagree with the surgeon? What is the ethical rationale for your position?

CASE 4	No clear reason for refusal of medically effective treatment

A 45-year-old sales clerk has a 1/2-cm breast mass that is found to be malignant on needle aspiration. With either mastectomy or lumpectomy plus radiation, she has an excellent chance of being cured of her cancer. She refuses any form of therapy, saying that she wants to try natural healing through herbal remedies, megavitamin therapy, spiritual healing, and relaxation techniques.

QUESTIONS FOR DISCUSSION

1. One resident objects, "How do we just stand by when she would most likely be cured of her cancer with surgery? Aren't we supposed to act in the patient's best interests? How can it be in

the patient's best interests to lose the chance to cure her cancer?" Another resident says, "Wait a minute, we're supposed to respect patient autonomy. It's her body and her life, and it's her decision." How do you respond to these viewpoints? What is the ethical rationale for your position? How would you carry out your views in practice?

CONFIDENTIALITY

CASE 5	Reporting a patient with syncope to the Department of Motor Vehicles

A 76-year-old retired teacher with a history of coronary artery disease is hospitalized after a syncopal episode. He is found to have ventricular tachycardia. He had two previous syncopal episodes during the past 3 years. An automatic implantable cardioverter defibrillator (AICD) is implanted. During the first year after implantation, about 10% of patients experience syncope or near-syncope because of defibrillation.

QUESTIONS FOR DISCUSSION

1. A nurse in a clinic asks if the patient needs to be reported to the Department of Motor Vehicles. How do you respond? What ethical considerations support your position?
2. Suppose that your patient is a 47-year-old bus driver instead of a retiree. The patient tells you that he is willing to try anything, even take temporary leave from work, as long as you don't report him to the Department of Motor Vehicles. "Doc, if you take my license away, I can't support my family," he pleads. "I need this job." How do you respond? What ethical considerations support your position?

CASE 6	Use of anabolic steroids by an athlete

A colleague asks your advice on a difficult case. A 19-year-old college swimmer reveals that she has started to take anabolic steroids, which she obtains through friends at the gym where she lifts weights. She says that she is aware of the long-term side effects but plans to use the drugs only while she is competing in intercollegiate athletics. She doesn't want to lose her scholarship. Because many of her competitors are using steroids, she believes there is no other way for her to be competitive.

QUESTIONS FOR DISCUSSION

1. Your colleague asks whether she should tell the swim coach about the patient's steroid use, saying, "Maybe the coach can discourage her from taking these drugs. It's so dangerous for her, and her health can't be worth winning a few races. We need to act in her best interests." How do you respond? What ethical considerations support your position?
2. Another colleague, joining your discussion, suggests, "She should be reported to the intercollegiate athletic officials. It isn't fair to other swimmers for her to have an advantage. If she wants to risk her health, then that's her business, but let's keep the pool lanes fair." How would you respond? What ethical considerations support your position?
3. A third colleague says, "If you tell anyone, it should be her parents. If I were her mother, I'd certainly want to know." What is your view on talking to her parents? What ethical considerations support your position?

| CASE 7 | Disclosure of genetic illness to relatives |

A 40-year-old auto mechanic is found to have a localized breast cancer, which is treated with lumpectomy and radiation. Because of a family history of both ovarian and breast cancer in several first-degree relatives, she is tested for BRCA-1 and is found to be positive for a muta-tion that confers a greatly increased risk for these cancers. As her physician, you discuss the implications of this autosomal recessive condition for her 34-year-old and 36-year-old sisters and urge her to disclose her test results to them so they also can be tested for BRCA-1. A relative who has the same mutation has a lifetime 85% risk of breast cancer and a 50% risk of ovarian cancer. An affected relative will probably want to begin screening mammog-raphy earlier than is usually recommended and also may want to consider interventions such as bilateral mastectomy, tamoxifen, and experimental therapies. Your patient refuses to disclose her results to her sisters or to allow you to do so. "We had a major falling out when mom died," she tells you. "They did some things that I don't think I can ever forgive. I just don't want to get involved with them at this point in my life."

QUESTIONS FOR DISCUSSION

1. A nurse is outraged at the patient's refusal to inform her sisters that they might be at high risk for cancer. "We should pick up the phone and call them," she says. "This is more serious than tuber-culosis and we notify contacts of TB patients. What if her sisters years later present with inoperable cancer?" How do you respond to the nurse? What ethical considerations support your position?

DECISION-MAKING CAPACITY

| CASE 8 | Refusal of colonoscopy |

A 72-year-old retired lawyer comes into the hospital with lower abdominal pain. He is found to have guaiac positive stools and anemia. You plan to do a colonoscopy, but the patient refuses. During your conversation, you learn that the patient spends all day inside his house where the electricity has been turned off due to outstanding bills.

One intern says that it is appropriate to seek a court order, saying, "This guy can't even pay his bills, how can we expect him to make decisions about his health care?" Another intern responds, "Look, I have trouble paying my bills on time. I hope that no court would override my medical decisions."

The patient's only relative is a niece who lives in a distant state. She says that he is somewhat cantankerous and has always been independent and stubborn. She is unable to persuade him over the phone to have the colonoscopy. She tells the doctors, "If you believe that he's not able to make decisions for himself, then I would certainly give permission for you to do the tests and treatments he needs. I want the best care for him."

QUESTIONS FOR DISCUSSION

1. What will happen if it is determined that the patient is competent to make medical decisions? What if he is determined to lack decision-making capacity?
2. What questions would you ask this patient to better evaluate whether he is competent to make decisions about his care?
3. The intern says, "I was told that we have to get a psychiatry consultation to declare a patient incompetent." Do you agree or disagree? What ethical considerations support your position?

DECISIONS FOR INCOMPETENT PATIENTS

CASE 9	Mechanical ventilation in end-stage lung disease

Mrs. O, a 64-year-old retired grocery store owner with end-stage interstitial lung disease, presents to the emergency department (ED) for shortness of breath that began several days ago. On room air, she is breathing at a rate of 36 and has an O_2 saturation of 54%. She is cyanotic and using her accessory muscles. On examination, she is afebrile and has no signs of consolidation. She is unable to have a coherent conversation. Her chest x-ray shows no acute infiltrates. At baseline, her FEV1 is 0.8 L, and her room air blood gas is PH 7.38, pO_2 51 mm Hg, pCO_2 55 mm Hg. She has shortness of breath walking around her house. She lives with her daughter and two grandchildren, her closest relatives. Mrs. O pulls off both nasal cannulae and a mask delivering oxygen. Her daughter is unable to get her to keep the supplemental O_2 on.

Mrs. O has never completed a durable power of attorney for health care, and there is no Do Not Intubate (DNI) order in the computerized record system. You are unable to get the ambulatory records, and the on-call physician does not know the patient.

QUESTIONS FOR DISCUSSION

1. The daughter says that her mother knows that she has end-stage lung disease and has told her primary physician several times that she does not want to be intubated. The patient has also told the daughter that she would not want intubation. Her daughter reports, "She knows what intubation is. She had it several years ago when she had pneumonia. But she knows that her lungs have just gotten worse and worse. She's ready to die when the time comes, but she wants to die with dignity, without machines or tubes." Your resident says doctors must provide treatment for potentially reversible conditions, saying, "This may be aspiration pneumonia, from which she could recover. Without a written advance directive or DNI order, we have to intubate her." Do you agree? What are the ethical justifications for your position?
2. One intern says, "We have to intubate her. All we know is what the daughter is telling us. How can we be sure that she is saying what her mother wants? You cannot always trust family members; maybe she is trying to get an inheritance. Whenever there is any doubt, we have to err on the side of preserving life." The other intern responds, "But that means we would never trust a family to make decisions for an incompetent patient, except when patients complete a health care proxy. That doesn't seem right." Do you agree with either intern? What are the ethical justifications for your position? How might the first intern's concerns be addressed in emergency situations?

CASE 10	Stroke and aspiration pneumonia

Mr. S, a 74-year-old retired gas station owner with Alzheimer disease and coronary artery disease, is admitted with a stroke. An ECG also shows an acute myocardial infarction with many premature ventricular contractions. He develops an aspiration pneumonia that is treated with antibiotics. Three days after admission, he has a dense hemiplegia, is unable to speak coherently, and has difficulty swallowing. At his baseline, he often does not recognize family members and needs help with all activities of daily living. He has not given any written advance directives.

QUESTIONS FOR DISCUSSION

1. According to his wife and daughter, he had said many times that becoming demented and living in a nursing home would be a fate worse than death. He had helped care for an uncle with Alzheimer disease and had said that not being able to recognize people and take care of himself would be intolerable. The wife and daughter request that he be transferred out of the intensive care unit (ICU) and allowed to die. They want a DNAR order, no intubation, no feeding tube, and no antibiotics for infections. "Just keep him comfortable and let him die in peace," they say. In the emergency room, they agreed to active treatments because they were told that his stroke might be reversible and that he might return home; however, he has not improved after 3 days. They are unable to care for him at home because of his wife's medical problems and his daughter's job. They also cannot afford to hire full-time help. The nurses comment that they seem devoted to him. Do you agree with the DNAR and DNI orders? What are the ethical justifications for your position?
2. How would the ethical and legal analysis be different if the patient had completed an advance directive appointing his wife as proxy?

| CASE 11 | Stroke and aspiration pneumonia |

Assume the same medical facts as in Case 10, but Mr. S has made no statements about his preferences for care. His wife and daughter believe that he would not want to receive continued intensive care after failing to improve from his stroke. "He never really talked about what he would want in this situation for himself," his wife explains. "But he was a man who prided himself on his independence and dignity. He never wanted anyone to help him when he was injured or sick. He was always immaculately dressed. He would never even go out to pick up the newspaper in the morning before getting dressed because he didn't want anyone to see him in his robe or pajamas. It's hard enough for him to have us help him. He would be mortified to have strangers help him with his bathing and dressing. We've been married over 50 years, and I know in my heart he wouldn't want to live like this."

QUESTIONS FOR DISCUSSION

1. The intern says that without some indication of the patient's own preferences, either written or oral, it is inappropriate to discontinue antibiotics or write DNAR and DNI orders. "What the family is saying is pure speculation," the intern points out. "Also he may still improve from his stroke." Do you agree with the intern? What are the ethical justifications for your position?

| CASE 12 | Stroke and aspiration pneumonia |

Assume the same medical facts as in Case 10, but Mr. S has made no statements about his preferences for care and has no family members. He has lived in a nursing home for several years and has no friends who visit him regularly. The nurses did not know him before he became demented.

QUESTIONS FOR DISCUSSION

1. One of the interns says, "We have to continue ICU care because we don't know what the patient would want in this situation. Without any surrogate, we have to give maximal treatment. How can we say that it's better for him to be dead than to live like this, when we don't know him?" Do you agree with the intern? What are the ethical justifications for your position?

CONFUSING ETHICAL DISTINCTIONS

> ### CASE 13   Withdrawal of mechanical ventilation
>
> *Assume that Mrs. O, the 64-year-old retired grocery store owner with end-stage interstitial lung disease from Case 9, was intubated in the ED. The next morning you obtain old records, which document extensive discussions with her primary physician that she does not want to be intubated or have resuscitation attempted. You also speak with the primary physician, who confirms that the patient did not want to be intubated and says, "This is exactly what she most feared—being on a ventilator with nothing readily reversible."*

QUESTIONS FOR DISCUSSION

1. An ICU nurse says, "I would have no problem if we hadn't intubated her in the first place. But we can't just turn off the ventilator or extubate her. She would die in a couple of minutes. That would be killing her, pure and simple, just as if we injected potassium." Do you agree with the nurse? What are the ethical justifications for your position?
2. Because the patient will be dyspneic, you want to administer morphine and also provide sedation. An intern objects, saying that it could reduce her respirations or lower her blood pressure, which would kill her: "That would be active euthanasia, and that's wrong." Do you agree? What are the ethical justifications for your position?

> ### CASE 14   Withdrawal of antibiotics and withholding tube feedings
>
> *Assume that Mrs. O, the 64-year-old retired grocery store owner with end-stage interstitial lung disease from Case 9, is transferred out of the ICU with DNAR and DNI orders, based on the family reports of her previous statements.*

QUESTIONS FOR DISCUSSION

1. The neurology consultant exclaims, "I have no problem with the DNAR and DNI orders. But feeding her and giving her antibiotics are basic, ordinary care. It would be inhumane to withhold them." Do you agree? What are the ethical justifications for your position?

DNAR ORDERS

> ### CASE 15   DNAR orders during endoscopy
>
> *A 58-year-old woman with dysphagia is found to have inoperable carcinoma of the esophagus. She realizes her poor prognosis and opts for palliation. With the concurrence of her family, she agrees to a DNAR and DNI order. Because she has difficulty maintaining adequate oral intake, she agrees to endoscopic placement of an intraluminal esophageal stent.*

QUESTIONS FOR DISCUSSION

1. The gastroenterologist who performs the procedure insists that the DNAR order be lifted during the procedure, saying, "I understand that she has chosen palliative care, and I respect that. But if she has a cardiac arrest during the endoscopy, it is due to the medications that we give for

conscious sedation. Our ability to resuscitate patients in this situation, even those with inoperable cancer, is close to 100%. The situation is completely different from a cardiopulmonary arrest that occurs spontaneously in the course of illness." Do you agree with the gastroenterologist that the DNAR order should be suspended during the procedure? What are the ethical justifications for your position?

CASE 16   Pneumonia and Alzheimer disease

A 74-year-old man with severe Alzheimer disease is transferred from a nursing home for treatment for pneumonia. Except for mild hypercholesterolemia and osteoarthritis of the knees and hips, he has no active medical problems and takes no medications regularly. He has no living relatives or friends, and before becoming demented he had not indicated what he would want done in such a situation. His baseline state in the nursing home is that he requires assistance with all activities of daily living, including eating. He usually does not recognize nursing home staff, but he does smile when watching television. The nursing home physician says that he does not know what the patient would want, but that it seems reasonable to administer antibiotics but not to provide interventions, such as mechanical ventilation.

QUESTIONS FOR DISCUSSION

1. The resident on the team says, "He should be DNAR. It doesn't make any sense to resuscitate someone with such a terrible quality of life. It would be futile." Do you agree with the resident's view? What are the ethical justifications for your position?

FUTILE INTERVENTIONS

CASE 17   Multiorgan failure

Mr. D is a 72-year-old homebound man with multisystem failure admitted to a community hospital for pneumonia, a myeloproliferative disorder, and failure to thrive. He develops stupor and adult respiratory distress syndrome (ARDS), for which he requires mechanical ventilation. He is transferred to a referral center, where he develops renal failure requiring dialysis and recurrent episodes of hypotension and sepsis. No primary site of infection has been identified.

His major problem now is abdominal pain and distention, which requires opioids. A CT scan shows dilated extrahepatic bile ducts but no intrahepatic dilatation or other abnormalities. His liver function tests are only mildly and occasionally elevated. The patient's daughter believes that an operation on his biliary tract would cure his abdominal problem and that relief of his abdominal distention would allow him to be weaned off the ventilator. The surgical service believes that there is no abdominal problem that surgery would improve and that general anesthesia would be extremely high risk. Two attempts at endoscopic retrograde cholangio-pancreatography (ERCP) were unable to visualize the ampulla of Vater. Interventional radiology is unwilling to attempt percutaneous biliary drainage because there is no intrahepatic duct dilatation.

Mr. D has given no advance directives. The patient's wife tends to defer to the daughter in discussions and agrees with her. His family believes that if he had widespread cancer or were in a permanent coma, he would not want life-prolonging treatment, but they point out that this is not currently the case. They refuse to agree to a DNAR order or limitation of medical interventions.

QUESTIONS FOR DISCUSSION

1. The surgical chief resident says that it would be "crazy" to operate on Mr. D and remarks, "He's not a surgical candidate. There is no reason to operate. It would be futile. We won't take him to the operating room, no matter what the family wants." Do you believe that exploratory laparotomy would be futile and that the surgery team may refuse to do the procedure? What are the ethical justifications for your position?

2. The gastrointestinal (GI) service declines to make another attempt at ERCP. The GI fellow says, "We've already tried the procedure twice. There's no point in trying again. The family can't force us to do something that's futile." Do you believe that ERCP would be futile and that the GI team may refuse to do the procedure? What are the ethical justifications for your position?

3. The nephrology service believes that continuing dialysis is futile, saying, "What's the point of dialyzing him? That's not going to allow him to leave the ICU." Do you believe that continued dialysis would be futile and that the nephrology team may refuse to do the procedure? What are the ethical justifications for your position?

4. When you sign out the patient to the night float resident, she notes that the last time she covered, the patient suffered an episode of hypotension, which she treated with fluids, vasopressors, and antibiotics. "What if that happens again, but he doesn't respond and develops progressive hypotension despite maximal therapy?" she asks. "Do you still want me to do CPR if he suffers a cardiac arrest? Why don't you write a medical DNAR order? CPR would be futile." In that situation, would it be appropriate to withhold CPR despite the family's wishes? What are the ethical justifications for your position?

PHYSICIAN-ASSISTED SUICIDE AND ACTIVE EUTHANASIA

CASE 18　　Head and neck cancer

Mrs. M is 57-year-old machinist who has recurrent head and neck cancer that has progressed despite radiation and chemotherapy. She cannot swallow foods and secretions and has to sit upright at night to spit out her secretions. She asks her physician for a prescription for a lethal dose of sleeping pills and says, "It's barbaric that the medical system does not allow me to retain the last shreds of my dignity. Why can't I have the same humane, compassionate treatment that we give our pets at the end of their lives? I do not want to wait for pneumonia or starvation to deliver me. I want to end my life freely and rationally. I am not depressed, but it is inhumane to ask me to live this way. Don't force me to shoot myself to get relief." Her husband and children agree with her decision.

QUESTIONS FOR DISCUSSION

1. What actions should a physician who supports physician-assisted suicide take before deciding that it is appropriate to write a prescription for a lethal dose of medication in this case?

2. What actions should a physician who opposes physician-assisted suicide take in addition to refusing the patient's request?

3. Does the moral responsibility of the physician differ when writing a lethal prescription compared to injecting a lethal dose of medication, such as potassium?

CASE 19	Failed suicide attempt

Mrs. M, the patient with head and neck cancer in Case 18, is found at home by her husband after a suicide attempt. She has ingested a combination of tricyclic antidepressants, barbiturates, and alcohol and has left a long explanatory note. She had held a good-bye party for her friends and then ingested the medications while he played her favorite music. As they agreed, they left her alone for 3 hours. When he returned with a friend, they were shocked to find her grunting for breath but not conscious. Horrified that she was suffering, they called 911.

In the field, she is found to have an O_2 saturation of 70% and is intubated. In the ED, she is placed on mechanical ventilation and given intravenous fluids and vasopressors. The patient's primary physician confirms her progressive cancer, her recent deterioration, and the absence of depression or other psychiatric illness, saying, "She didn't want to be a burden on her family or spend her last days waiting for an infection. I personally wouldn't do what she did, but I respect her choice. There is no question that she thought about this long and hard."

QUESTIONS FOR DISCUSSION

1. Would you continue mechanical ventilation, fluids, and vasopressors? One ED resident says, "If we withdraw support, we'll be abetting a suicide. That's illegal and morally wrong. My conscience won't let me do that. What message does it send to other patients if the emergency room helps people kill themselves?" Do you agree with this position? What are the ethical justifications for your position?

2. While the medical and nursing staff are discussing the case, the patient begins to awaken. She is weaned off vasopressors, and 2 hours later she is extubated. As per ED protocol, a psychiatrist talks with her. She says, "Of course, I'll do this again as soon as I get home and can figure out how to do it right. We'll have to get on the Internet and find out. Don't you understand that waiting for some medical catastrophe to occur is an inhumane way to die? Wouldn't you do the same thing? Do you expect me to lie about my intentions to make you all feel less guilty?" As the psychiatrist, do you place her on an involuntary hold because she is actively suicidal? What are the ethical justifications for your position?

CASE 20	Withdrawal of mechanical ventilation

Mrs. O, the 64-year-old retired grocery store owner with end-stage interstitial lung disease from Case 9, has mechanical ventilation withdrawn based on evidence that she would not want such treatment. She is placed on oxygen via nasal cannulae and morphine and diazepam drips to palliate her dyspnea and anxiety. On 10 mg morphine per hour and 2 mg diazepam per hour, the patient appears comfortable, without any tachypnea, use of accessory muscles, tachycardia, or restlessness. Her respiratory rate is 12 per minute. She does not respond when called or when an intravenous line is restarted.

QUESTIONS FOR DISCUSSION

1. The patient's family requests that you increase the dose of medications: "She said many times she didn't want to linger or to have a prolonged death." Do you agree with the family's request? What are the ethical justifications for your position?

REFUSAL TO CARE FOR PATIENTS

CASE 21	Caring for a patient with AIDS

A 34-year-old unemployed homeless man with AIDS (CD4 level 47) is admitted to your service with Pneumocystis carinii *pneumonia. His IV has infiltrated, and you are asked to restart it.*

QUESTIONS FOR DISCUSSION

1. How would you feel if you suffered a needlestick injury while caring for an HIV-infected patient?
2. One of the interns on the admitting team refuses to take care of this patient. What are the ethical considerations if each of the following holds true?
   a. The intern says he is inexperienced at starting IVs and thinks that a more experienced physician should care for the patient.
   b. The intern is a deeply religious person who believes that homosexuality is a sin. Because the patient is gay, the intern does not want to care for him. The intern says, "I couldn't live with myself if I helped him live in sin."
   c. The patient is an injection drug user. An injection drug user at the hospital had earlier mugged the intern in his internship. The intern is still experiencing flashbacks about that earlier incident and does not want to be subjected to more stress.

ETHICAL DILEMMAS FACING STUDENTS AND HOUSE STAFF: LEARNING ON PATIENTS

CASE 22	Outcomes of coronary artery bypass and graft

Suppose your favorite uncle has been recommended to have coronary artery bypass and graft (CABAG) by his primary care physician and cardiologist in New York. From your clinical epidemiology course you recall that the mortality rates for this operation vary from less than 1% to more than 8% and that New York State publishes mortality rates for hospitals and for individual surgeons.

QUESTION FOR DISCUSSION

1. Do you want to know the outcomes experience for the hospital or for the surgeon who would operate on your uncle? What are your reasons?

CASE 23	Carrying out an invasive procedure

Recall the first time you did a lumbar puncture (LP) (or central line, major suturing, or other major procedure).

QUESTIONS FOR DISCUSSION

1. How did you feel before doing your first invasive procedure?
2. One of your classmates says that by coming to a teaching hospital, patients have given implied consent to having students and residents do procedures. Thus, there is no need to tell the patient that a student will be performing a procedure. Do you agree, and why?

3. What would you do if before your first LP, the resident calls to say go ahead and do it yourself, because he and the interns are in the emergency room with critically ill new patients? The LP needs to be done today. How would you respond?

CASE 24   Unethical behavior of an attending physician

On a clerkship, you observe what you consider unethical behavior by one of your attending physicians. On several occasions, his speech is slurred and you smell alcohol on his breath. He also fails to round on his patients for days at a time, without having anyone cover for him, and does not return your pages or those of your resident.

QUESTIONS FOR DISCUSSION

1. What are the ethical reasons for reporting the situation to an appropriate senior physician?
2. What are some of the risks to you if you report the situation?
3. In practical terms, how might you proceed?

DISCLOSING ERRORS

CASE 25   Muscle weakness due to inadequate potassium replacement

A 42-year-old man is admitted to you with diabetic ketoacidosis. After treatment with intravenous fluids and an insulin drip, the patient's glucose declines from 745 to 289 mg per dL after 4 hours. However, the patient develops progressive weakness and difficulty breathing and requires transfer to the ICU for mechanical ventilation. In reviewing the case, you check the computer for lab results and realize that the patient had a potassium of 2.3 mmol per L. No potassium replacement had been given during the treatment of the ketoacidosis.

The patient's family asks what happened and whether he had a stroke. They say that the patient has been hospitalized several times for ketoacidosis but has never required mechanical ventilation.

QUESTIONS FOR DISCUSSION

1. If you were the subintern on the case, what would your feelings be?
2. In your experience, how have colleagues reacted to mistakes?
3. What would your concerns be about telling the attending physician about this mistake?
4. Would you tell the attending physician about the episode?
5. A nurse asks you what she should tell the patient and family, saying that they are very concerned about what happened. How do you respond? What are the ethical reasons for your response?

ETHICAL ISSUES IN PEDIATRICS

CASE 26   Treating adolescents without parental consent

A 15-year-old high-school student comes to the physician because of dysuria and a discharge from his penis after intercourse without a condom. He wants to be tested and treated but does not want his parents to know about his problems. "They would completely freak out if they knew I was having sex," he says.

QUESTIONS FOR DISCUSSION

1. You ask a colleague whether you can treat the patient without his parents' authorization. She says that you may do so, provided that he is capable of giving informed consent to treatment. Do you agree with her advice? What are the ethical justifications for your position?

2. The patient is so concerned about his parents' finding out that he asks you to write on the encounter form that the visit is for shoulder pain. "I don't want them getting a bill that tells them why I came in." How do you respond to his request? Give the ethical considerations for your decision.

CASE 27	Treating children despite refusals

A 10-year-old boy is taken to the ED with vomiting and right lower quadrant abdominal pain and is found to have appendicitis.

QUESTIONS FOR DISCUSSION

1. The patient says that he does not want surgery, saying that the pain is getting better and he does not want to have a scar the rest of his life. His parents are willing to authorize surgery for him. The resident on the team says, "We're not going to operate on a patient who is screaming that he doesn't want surgery. That's assaulting the patient." Do you agree with the resident? What are the ethical reasons supporting your position?

2. Suppose instead that the parents refuse surgery after an aunt who was baby-sitting brought the child to the ED. The parents are devout Christian Scientists who believe that their child will recover with prayer therapy. The intern says that parents are not permitted to make irrational decisions, so the surgery should proceed as recommended. Do you agree with the intern? What are the ethical reasons supporting your position?

INDEX

Note: Page numbers followed by *f* indicate figures; those followed by *t* indicate tables respectively.

Abandonment, patient, 187
Abortion(s)
    cases, 281
    as ethical issue in obstetrics/gynecology, 281
    ethical issues associated with, 281
    family planning and, 279
    objections of, 184
    performance of, 182
    rights, 278
Abuse(s). *See also* Domestic violence
    active euthanasia and physician-assisted suicide,
            151–152
    of children, 48–49, 282–283
    of elderly, 49
    substance, 247, 265, 282–283
Accountability, maintaining, 56
Accreditation Council for Continuing Medical
            Education, 237
Active euthanasia
    abuses and, 151–152
    case of alleged, 126
    declining, 156
    definitions of, 149
    justified, 156
    medical interventions and, 150
    in Netherlands, 154
    opioids or sedatives and, 150
    in Oregon, 152–153
    physician-assisted suicide and, 347–348
    practice of, 153–154
    procedural and proposed safeguards associated with, 154
    reasons against, 150–152
    reasons in favor of, 150–151
    requests for, 151, 153
    responding to requests for, 155–156, 155*t*
    summary on, 157
    survivors of patients who underwent, 154
    unintended consequences of, 154
    U.S. policy options for, 154–155
    withdrawal of requests for, 154
Active injection drug use, 299
ADHD. *See* Attention deficit/hyperactivity disorder
Adolescent(s). *See also* Children
    confidentiality of, 266–267
    minors as
        emancipated, 265
        mature, 265
        parental requests for treatment of, 266
        treatment of specified conditions with, 265

patients, 265–266
    reproductive health for, 279–280
Advance care planning, 94
    cultural issues and, 326–327
Advance directives
    cases, 91, 97, 100, 101
    conflict with patients' best interests, 93
    definition of, 90
    discussions of
        improvement of, 95–96, 95*t*
        initiation of, 95, 95*t*
        problems with, 94
        rationale for, 94
    interpretations of, 93
    limitations of, 92–93
    oral
        cases, 93
        statements to physicians, 91
    summary on, 101
    types of, 91–92
    written documents of, 96
        health care proxies as, 92, 95*t*
        living wills as, 91
        physician orders for life-sustaining treatment
                (POLST), 92
African Americans, 111, 112, 178, 300, 314, 324, 325
AIDS (autoimmune deficiency syndrome), 90.
            See also HIV
    patient, caring, 349
Alcohol, use of, 36, 200, 248
Alcoholism, 299
Allocation. *See also* Microallocation; Rationing
    definition of, 216
    interventions and resource, 38
    public health guidelines for triage and, 316–317
    of various organs, 300
Alzheimer disease, 247
    pneumonia and, 346
AMA. *See* American Medical Association
American College of Physicians, 237
American Medical Association (AMA), 237
    on patients' best interests, 217
    on sexual contact, 195, 197, 198
Americans with Disabilities Act, 182
Anabolic steroids, use of, 341
Anesthesia, 124
    for surgery and invasive procedures, 140
Anthrax
    inhalational, 314
    outbreaks, 316
Antibiotic(s), 130, 256, 316
    administration of, 3
    courses of, 111, 121

Antibiotic(s) (*continued*)
   development of, 182
   for infections, 161
   new, 205
   not active against organism cases, 71
   prophylactic, 314
   refusal of, 98, 267
   sulfonamide, 242
   treatments, 132
   withdrawal of, 345
Antidepressants, 38
Antiretroviral therapy, 47
Aortic stenosis, 32
Aortic valve replacement, 36
Aristotle, 16
ARTs. *See* Assisted reproductive technologies
Assisted reproductive technologies (ARTs), 278, 283
Attending physician, unethical behavior of, 350
Attention deficit/hyperactivity disorder (ADHD), 268
Autoimmune deficiency syndrome. *See* AIDS
Autonomy, 8
   of caregivers, 115
   of children, 263
   concept of, 12
   deception and, 53
   definition of, 12
   individual liberty and, 315–316
   nondisclosure and, 53
   patient
      impairment of, 286
      respect for, 85, 150–151

Baby Doe Regulations, 269
Battery, malpractice and, 25
Bedside rationing, of health care, 216–221.
      See also Microallocation
   arguments against, 217
   arguments in favor of, 217–219, 217*t*
   on basis of costs, 219–221
   cases
      blood product shortage as, 218
      expensive care as, 219
      limited physician's time as, 218
   limited CCU beds as, 216, 218
   resources for, 221
   second opinion on, 221
   suggestions for, 221, 221*t*
   summary on, 221
   tiered formulary benefits of, 220–221
Behavior(s)
   impact of genes on, 304–305
   unethical, conflicts of interest and, 213
Beneficence, 8. *See also* Best interests of patients
   guideline of, 13, 231
   principle of, 202
   recipients of organ transplantation and, 299
Best interests of patient(s), 69*f*, 74, 271. *See also*
      Beneficence
   agreement on, 39, 39*t*
   AMA's recommendations on, 217

cases, refusal of surgery as, 32
   conflict with advance directives and, 93
   contradictions/decisions by, 25
   doing no/lack of harm as, 33, 194, 242
   fiduciary nature of, 33
   guidelines, 13–14
   intervention requests and, 36–39
   as not absolute duty, 217
   paramount, 214–215
   problems associated with, 34–36
   promotion of, 32–39
   substituted judgments and
      assessing, 99–100
      determination of, 99
   summary on, 39
Bioethics
   definition of, 4
   training programs, 132
Bioterrorism, 314
BiPAP. *See* Noninvasive ventilation (NIV)
Birth control, 279
Blackmun, Harry, 169
"Blame-free" culture, 241
Blood
   product shortage of, 218
   transfusions
      Jehovah's Witness and legal issues
         associated with, 86
      suggestions on, 86–87
Born-Alive Infants Protection Act (2002), 269
Brain death, 296
   definitions of, 164
   higher, 165
   legal status of, 165
   practical suggestions on, 166
   summary on, 166
   whole-, 164
Breast cancer, therapeutic options for, 339
Brennan, William, 169
Bronchodilators, 121
Bronchoscopy, 62
Bundled payments, 228
Bush, Jeb, 171

Calcium, 256
California, proxy guidelines in, 105
California law, 254
California Supreme Court, rulings of, 22
Cancer, head and neck, 347
Cardiac arrest, 72
Cardiac care unit (CCU), 329
   beds, 216, 218
Cardiac transplantation, 164
Cardiopulmonary criteria, for death, 163–164
Cardiopulmonary resuscitation (CPR), 27, 74, 161
   attempt at, 72
   cases
      desire for mechanical ventilation, 110, 113
      no response to, 72
   characteristics of, 92

DNAR and
  discussions on, 136–138, 139*t*
  effectiveness of, 135
  family request case for, 136
  implementation of, 139–140
  interpretation of, 139–140
  justifications for, 136
  special settings for, 140
  summary on, 140–141
  writing, 139
 misunderstandings about, 137
 recommendations about, 138
 refusal of, 136
 show or slow codes in, 139–140
Care. *See also* Cross-cultural care; Health care; Patient care;
        Refusal to care
 beneficial, 228
 for contagious patients, refusal to, 319
 continuance of, 186
 crisis standards of, 319
 emergency, 187
 extraordinary or heroic, 122
 life-sustaining intervention cases and, 3, 110
   desire for CPR/mechanical ventilation, 110, 113
   withdrawal of mechanical ventilation,
           114, 115, 121, 126
 life-sustaining interventions and
   clinical considerations with, 110–111
   ethical considerations on, 111–112
   family insistence on everything be done cases,
           111, 113
   physician insistence on, 114–116, 115*t*
   recommendations for, 112–114, 112*t*
   summary on, 116
 managed, 227
 medical
   termination of, 197
   time since last, 197–198
 ongoing, 114, 138
 palliative, 155
 persistent disagreements over, 110–116
 psychiatric, 286–287
 refusal of, 339–341
   for patients, 349
 substandard, 258
 summary on, 116
 transference of, 116
Caregiver(s)
 autonomy of, 115
 on interventions
   arguments for, 115
   objections to, 115–116, 115*t*
 on suffering, 112
Carrier screening, 304
Casuistry, 16
Catholicism, 123, 168, 182
CCU. *See* Cardiac care unit
CDC. *See* Centers for Disease Control
        and Prevention
Centers for Disease Control and Prevention
        (CDC), 281

Cesarean sections
 elective, 280
 forced, 280
CF. *See* Cystic fibrosis
Chemotherapy, 21
Chest pain, 332, 333
Childhood immunizations, 320
Children, 279, 326
 abuse of, 48–49, 282–283
 advocates of, 263
 autonomy of, 263
 best interests of, 263–264
 confidentiality of, 266–267
 disclosure of information to, 266
 emergencies and, 265
 feelings/emotions of, 131
 genetic testing, informed consent and, 309
 morality of, 5
 parent's interests and, 264
 preferences of, 264
 refusal of medical interventions for, 267–268
 relationships of physician and parents with, 266–267
 standards for making decisions for, 263–264
 treatment of specified conditions and, 265
 truth and, 52
Chinese, 327
Christian Science, 267
Chromosomal abnormalities, screening for, 281–282
Cigarettes, 36
Ciprofloxacin, 316
Citizenship, 300
Clinical contexts, of decision-making capacity, 80
Clinical ethic(s). *See also* Ethical dilemmas
 approaches to, 3–10
 definition of, 4
 difference between law and, 4–5
 fundamentals of, 1
 medical facts and, 8
 moral guidance sources for, 5–6
 physicians and, 6–7
 professional *v.*, 4
 summary on, 10
Clinical interventions. *See* Interventions
Clinical judgment, impairment of, 191
Clinical research
 benefits and risks with, 203
 cases
   dementia, 205
   finder's fee, 205, 206
   osteoporosis trials, 203
 conflicts of interests with, 205–206
 ethical principles for, 202–205, 204*t*
 misconceptions about, 204
 nature of, 204
 overview of, 203
 participants in, 205
 procedures of, 204
 summary on, 206
 voluntary participation in, 204
Clinical situations, decision-making capacity in
        specific, 82–83

Clinical skills, basic, 253
Clinical standards, for decision-making capacity, 79–80, 79*t*
Clinician-investigators, 206
CME. *See* Continuing medical education
Coercion, 23
Colonoscopy, refusal of, 342
Colostomy, 275
Competence
    informed patients, 12, 28–29, 70
        refusal of renal dialysis by, 87
        refusal of treatment by, 85–88
        respecting patient refusals and, 85
        restrictions on refusal and, 87–88
        scope of refusal by, 85–87
        summary on, 88
    legal standards for, 78–79
Computed tomography (CT), 224, 240, 242, 273
Concierge medicine, 178
Confidentiality, 286–287, 341–342
    of adolescents, 266–267
    cases
        HIV transmission risks as, 45
        information omission as, 44
        relatives as, 43–44
    of children, 266–267
    countervailing, 43
    difficulties maintaining, 42
    disclosure and
        of information on public figures, 44
        of patients' conditions, 43–44
    ethical dilemma guidelines and, 12–13
    exceptions to, 41, 41*t*, 266
    federal regulations on, 43
    of genomic results, 309–311
    HIV and, 3, 5, 15
        cases of transmission risks and, 45
        infections and, 46–47
        partner notification and, 47
    importance of, 41*t*, 42–43
    information omission from medical records and, 44
    overriding
        impaired drivers and, 47
        justification for, 46, 46*t*
        to protect patients, 41*t*, 48–49
        reporting to public officials and, 46–47, 46*t*
        third parties and, 45–48
    patient, 3, 9
    reasons for, 42
    of recipient/donors, 298
    summary on, 50
    waivers of, 42
Conflicts of interest(s), 209, 295
    addressing, 214–215
    apparent or perceived, 213
    cases, for a judge, 212
    with clinical research, 205–206
    conflicting *v.* competing, 213
    definition of, 212
    disclosure of, 215
    financial, 214

in nonmedical situations, 211–212
    overview of, 211–215
    physicians and, 14
    situations with no, 214
    summary on, 215
    among surrogates, 106–107
    unethical behavior and, 213
Conscience, claims of, 6
Consensus panel, 164
Consent. *See also* Informed consent
    doctrine of implied, 27
    of donors, 297
    forms, 26
    presumed, 296
Consequentialist theories, 15
Consultation(s)
    ethics
        family and health care disagreement case on, 130
        goals of, 130–132, 131*t*
        potential problems with, 132, 132*t*
        procedures for, 132–133
        stakeholders and, 131–132, 131*t*
        summary on, 133
    of psychiatrists, 82
Contact, renewal of, 198
Contact tracing, 47
Continuing medical education (CME)
    conferences as drug company gifts, 234
    programs, 236
    sponsorship of, 215
Contraception, 184
Contraceptives, oral, 306
Coronary artery bypass and graft, outcomes of, 349
Counterproductive reactions, recognize and minimize, 334
CPR. *See* Cardiopulmonary resuscitation
Cross-cultural care. *See also* Cultures
    ethical issues in
        advance care planning, 326–327
        cases, 324, 325
        disclosure of serious diagnosis as, 324
        impact of, 323–324
        summary on, 330
Cruzan, Nancy, 159, 169–170
Cruzan case
    court rulings on, 169
    death and, 170
    implications of, 170
CT. *See* Computed tomography
Culture(s)
    expectations within, 190
    influences of, 323
    issues and advance care planning, 326–327
    issues associated with, 324
    preferences within, 328
    racial request case and, 329
    stereotyping of, 323
    in United States, 53
Cystic fibrosis (CF), 304

"Dead donor rule," 164
Death(s), 150. *See also* Euthanasia; Suicides; Uniform
        Determination of Death Act
    brain, 296
        criteria for, 164–165
        definitions of, 164
        higher, 165
        legal status of, 165
        practical suggestions on, 166
        summary on, 166
        whole-, 164
    cardiopulmonary criteria for, 163–164
Deception, 13. *See also* Nondisclosure
    in administration of medications
        reasons against, 54
        reasons for, 54–55
    autonomy and, 53
    avoidance of, 52–60
    cases
        cancellation of travel plans, 59
        covert administration of medications, 54–55, 56
        excuse from work, 57–58, 59
        family request to withhold diagnoses from patient,
                52, 56, 59, 324
        insurance coverage, 57
    with colleagues, 59–60
    as culturally appropriate, 53
    definition of, 52
    dilemmas regarding, 55–56, 55*t*
    minimizing the amount/consequences of, 56
    to patient, 53–56, 55*t*
    summary on, 60
    surrogates' authorization of, 55
    to third parties
        reasons against, 58, 58*t*
        reasons for, 57–58
        resolving dilemmas regarding, 58–59, 58*t*
    trainees and, 59
    withholding bad news from patients as
        reasons against, 54
        reasons for, 53
Decision(s)
    for children, standards for making, 263–264
    delusions and patients', 80
    during disasters, 127
    during Hurricane Katrina, 127
    informed, 8, 138
    microallocation, 217–218
    patients'
        control over treatment, 155
        delusions and, 80
        to future reactions, 25
        made by, 13
        reluctance to make, 24
    physicians' unilateral, 74
    prudent, 15
    reluctance to make, 24
Decision making, 212. *See also* Advance directives;
        Competence; Informed consent; Substituted
        judgments
    end-of-life, 325–326

    enhanced patient role in, 333
    by family, 105, 264–266
    by parents, 264–266
    shared, 20–21, 67, 177–178
        informed consent and, 27–29, 28*t*
        promotion of, 28*t*
    styles, 178
    surrogate, 8, 10
        case of, 104
Decision-making capacity, 13, 70, 342. *See also*
        Competence
    assessment of, 80, 81*t*
    clinical contexts of, 80
    clinical standards for, 79–80, 79*t*
    emergencies and, 83
    ethical implications of, 78
    lack of, 27, 205
        advance directives, 91–97, 95*t*
        standards for decisions on, 90–101
        substituted judgment and, 97–99
    legal standards for, 78–79
    mental illness impairing, 82
    of patients, 13, 70
    patients lacking, 78, 83
    refusal to explain decision case on, 77
    in specific clinical situations, 82–83
    summary on, 83
Delusions, patients' decisions and, 80
Dementia. *See also* Intravenous feedings; Tube feedings
    clinical research case of, 205
    severe, 72, 145
        cases, 143, 160
Deontologic theories, 15–16
Depression, 45, 53, 153, 195, 195*t*, 247
Diabetes, 87
Dialysis, 219
Digital communication, 332
Digital health information, ethical issues in
    benefits and risks, distribution of, 338
    digital communication, 332
    electronic health records (EHRs), 334–337
    internet, health information on, 333–334
    patients, e-mail with, 332
    privacy and confidentiality, 337
    social media, physician use of, 337
    summary, 338
Digoxin, 247, 250
Disabilities Act, 45
Disability certification, requests for, 190
Disaster(s). *See also* Hurricane Katrina
    decisions during, 127
    plan for, 127
Discernment, 15
Disclosure(s), 200. *See also* Nondisclosure
    of abnormal results case and genomics, 310
    of approaches/experiences/outcomes in surgery,
            272–273
    benefits of, 54
    confidentiality and
        of information on public figures, 44
        of patients' conditions, 43–44

Disclosure(s) (*continued*)
  of conflicts of interests, 215
  deception and non, 13
  of errors
    cases, 239, 242
    communication of physicians in, 241
    controversial, 242–243
    by other health care workers, 244–245
    to patients/surrogates, 240–241, 244
    responsibility for, 241
    summary on, 245
    by trainees, 243–244
  of genomic results, 310
  of gifts, 236–237
  of information to children, 266
  options with health care costs, 230–231
  of patients' conditions and confidentiality, 43–44
  professional, 25–26
  of prognostic information cases, 22
  to schools, 266
  of secret information about patients, 200
  of serious diagnosis in cross-cultural care, 324
  standards for, 25–26
  of surgical innovation, 272
Discrimination, 305
  genetic
    employers and, 308
    insurers and, 308
    laws against, 308
Discussion(s)
  of advance directives
    improvement of, 95–96, 95t
    initiation of, 95, 95t
    problems with, 94
    rationale for, 94
  on CPR and DNAR, 136–138, 139t
  of documents in medical records, 97
  with patients and surrogates, futility
    of, 74–75
Disease(s)
  communicable, 87
  infectious
    reporting of, 46, 46t
    warnings of, 48
DNA
  -based genetic testing, 304
    genomics and, 305–307
  mitochondrial, 307
  screening, 306
  testing, types of, 304
DNAR. *See* Do Not Attempt Resuscitation
DNR. *See* Do Not Resuscitate
Do Not Attempt Resuscitation (DNAR), 72
  CPR and
    discussions on, 136–138, 139t
    effectiveness of, 135
    family request case for, 136
    implementation of, 139–140
    interpretation of, 139–140
    justifications for, 136
    special settings for, 140

  summary on, 140–141
  writing, 139
  limited or partial, 139
  orders, 95, 113, 345–346
  written, 73
Do Not Resuscitate (DNR), 70, 126
Doctor–patient relationship(s), 175, 334
  cases, disruptive and uncooperative, 185
  changes in, 190–191
  conscientious objections with, 184–185
  context of
    definitions of, 182
    ethical obligations regarding patient
      care as, 181–182
  difficult, 185–187, 185t
  fiduciary nature of, 33
  nature of, 197
  occupational risks associated with, 182–184
    responses to, 183–184
  overview of
    different, 177–179
    models of, 177–178
    preferences, 178
  power within, 196
  summary on, 187
  taking advantage of, 195–196, 195t
  termination of, 186–187
Doctors. *See* Physicians
Doctrine of double effect, 123–124, 171
Document(s)
  advance directives in written, 96
    health care proxies as, 92, 95, 95t
    living wills as, 91
    physician orders for life-sustaining treatment
      (POLST), 92
  discussions in medical records, 97
  recommendations, 133
Domestic violence, 49
Donation(s). *See also* Transplantations
  of cadaveric organs, current system for, 295–296
  live
    consent from, 297
    current system for, 298
    harm to, 297
    motives of, 297
    payment to, 297–298
  of organs from living donors, 296–298
  to strangers, 301
Donation after circulatory determination of death
      (DCDD), 296
Donor(s)
  cards, 296
  confidentiality of recipient, 298
  consent of, 297
  "Good Samaritan," 296
  harm to, 297
  motives of, 297
  paired, 298
  payment to, 297–298
  reimbursement for, 298
Down syndrome, 269, 281

Drinking, 247
  cessation, 144–145
  voluntary stopping of, 125
Drivers, impaired, 47
Drug(s), 203. *See also* Medications
  addictions, 87
  companies, 215
  detailing, 235
  generic, 229
  monitoring side effects of performance-enhancing, 36
  nonpreferred, 220, 229
  pain and request for controlled, 37
  preferred, 220
  psychotropic, 291
  resistant tuberculosis, 314–315
Drug companies, gifts from
  CME and conferences as, 234
  expectations of reciprocity with, 236
  health care costs and, 236
  hospitality and meals as, 234
  objections to accepting, 235–236, 235*t*
  objectivity and, 236
  practices regarding, 237
  reasons, 235
    for accepting, 235
    for offering, 235
  recommendations regarding, 236–237
  summary on, 237
  types of, 234–235
Drug Enforcement Agency, 37
Duties
  absolute, 217
  definition of, 16
  of ethical guidelines, 15–16
  in prevention of harm, 289
Dying. *See also* Euthanasia; Suicides
  aid in, 152–153
  process of, 91
  withholding tube feedings to only prolong, 144

E-mail, 332
Eating, voluntary stopping of, 125
EEG. *See* Electroencephalogram
Elderly
  abuse of, 49
  patients, 95, 178, 189
Electrocardiogram (ECG), 216
Electroencephalogram (EEG), 164
Electroencephalography (EEG) technique, 160
Electronic health information, sharing
  ethical guidelines regarding, 336
  models for, 335
Electronic health records (EHRs)
  concerns about, 334–335
  patient information, sharing, 335–336
  personal health records (PHRs), 336–337
Elevation, 329
Emergency(ies). *See also* Public health emergencies
  care, 187, 319
  children and, 265

  decision-making capacity and, 83
  informed consent and, 26–27
  medical service, 140
  obstetric, 280
  surgeries, 274, 275
Emergency Medical Treatment and Labor
      Act (EMTLA), 187
Emotion(s)
  feelings of children, 131
  needs
    of patients, 113
    reactions to, 125–126
    of surrogates, 113
  support for, 131–132
Employers, 308
EMTLA. *See* Emergency Medical Treatment and
      Labor Act
End-of-life
  decision making, 325–326
  treatments during, 98
End-stage lung disease, mechanical ventilation in, 343
Endoscopy, DNAR orders during, 345
Error(s), disclosure of
  cases, 239, 242
  communication of physicians' in, 241, 243–244
  controversial, 242–243
  by other health care workers, 244–245
  to patients/surrogates, 240–241, 244
  responsibility for, 241
  summary on, 245
  by trainees, 244
Ethic(s). *See also* Bioethics; Clinical ethics
  of caring, 17
  case-based, 16
  code of, 4
  consultations
    family and health care disagreement case on, 130
    goals of, 130–131, 131*t*
    potential problems with, 132, 132*t*
    procedures for, 132–133
    stakeholders and, 131–132, 131*t*
    summary on, 133
  definition of, 4
  morality and, 5
  professional *v.* clinical, 4
  virtue, 17
Ethical consensus, areas of, 7
Ethical dilemma(s). *See also* Clinical ethics
  approaches to
    in clinical dilemmas, 7–8, 7*t*
    in patient care, 3–10
  associated with secret information about patients, 200
  cases
    HIV confidentiality as, 3, 5, 15
    life-sustaining interventions as, 3, 110
    physician certification of eligibility as, 3
  in clinical medicine, 7–8, 7*t*
  guidelines during, 9, 43
    confidentiality as, 12–13
    deception and nondisclosure as, 13
    definition of, 14, 15

Ethical dilemma(s) (*continued*)
  different and conflicting, 15
  duties, principles and rules of, 15–16
  exceptions to, 14–15
  keeping promises as, 13, 64–65
  other approaches to, 16–17
  patients' best interests as, 13–14
  prima facie, 15
  respect for persons as, 12–13, 240
  specific cases and interpretation of, 14
  summary on, 17
  usage of, 14–15
  learning on patients
    dead or unconscious, 254–255
    students and, 252–255
  moral guidance sources for, 5–6
  practical considerations of, 9–10
  psychosocial issues within, 9
  for students
    cases, 255, 256, 257
    clinical responsibility as, 255
    colleague relationships as, 256
    learning on patients and, 252–255
    on professionalism, 257
    summary on, 259
    unethical care as, 257–258
    work hours as, 255–256
  summary on, 10
Ethical distinctions
  confusing, 345
  during Hurricane Katrina, 126
  within life-sustaining interventions
    doctrine of double effect and, 123–124, 171
    emotional reactions to, 125–126
    extraordinary or heroic care and, 122
    relief of symptoms with opioids/sedatives and, 123
    summary on, 128
    unprecedented cases for, 126–128
    withdrawal and withholding of, 121–122
Ethical guidelines, 9, 43
  confidentiality as, 12–13
  conflicts and uncertainty over, 131
  deception and nondisclosure as, 13
  definition of, 14, 15
  different and conflicting, 15
  duties, principles and rules of, 15–16
  exceptions to, 14–15
  for keeping promises, 13, 64–65
  other approaches to, 16–17
  patients' best interests as, 13–14
  prima facie, 15
  respect for persons as, 12–13, 240
  specific cases and interpretation of, 14
  summary on, 17
  usage of, 14–15
Ethical issues, 261
  in cross-cultural care
    advance care planning, 326–327
    cases, 324, 325
    disclosure of serious diagnosis as, 324
    impact of, 323–324

    summary on, 330
    framing of, 8–9
  in gynecology/obstetrics
    abortion as, 281
    assisted reproductive technologies as, 283
    differences with, 278–279
    informed consent in, 279–281
    maternal-fetal medicine as, 281–283
    summary on, 283
  identification of, 7
  in organ transplantations
    case, 301
    donation of cadaveric organs as, 295–296
    donation of organs from living donors as, 296–298
    selection of recipients as, 298–301
    summary on, 301–302
  in pediatrics
    differences in, 263
    handicapped infants and, 268–269
    interventions, 268
    refusal of medical interventions and, 267–268
    relationships of physician–child–parent within, 266–267
    standards for, 263–264
    summary on, 269
  in psychiatry
    dangerous patients as, 289–290
    differences with, 286–287
    involuntary commitment as, 287–288
    refusal of treatment as, 290
    suicides as, 288–289
  in surgery
    cases, 273, 274, 275
    differences with, 271
    informed consent as, 271–273
    risks associated with, 274–276
    summary on, 276
Ethnic backgrounds, 300
Europeans, 306, 324
Euthanasia. *See also* Active euthanasia
  case of alleged active, 126
  definitions of, 149–150
  involuntary, 149
  nonvoluntary, 149
  passive, 150
  voluntary, 149
Extracorporeal membrane oxygenation (ECMO), 164

Face-to-face meetings, 332
Factor V Leiden, 306
Fair reimbursement, 334–335
False-negative tests, 306
Family, 305
  decision making by, 105, 264–266
  definition of, 105
  health care disagreement case, 130
  members
    disagreement between, 104
    no, 106
    as surrogates, 105

planning, 184
  abortion and, 279
presence during resuscitation, 140
requests
  case for CPR/DNAR, 136
  to withhold diagnoses from patient, 52, 56, 59, 324
Federal law, 330
Federal regulations, 335
Fee-for-service reimbursement, 214, 223, 231
Female genital cutting, 330
Fetal DNA fragments, genomic sequencing of, 282
Fetus
  concepts of, 279
  during pregnancy, interests of women, 279
Fiduciary
  definition of, 33
  nature
    of doctor–patient relationships, 33
    of patients' best interests, 33
  relationships, 33
  roles of physicians, 228
Financial incentives, 214
  to patients, 229–230
  to physicians, 228–229
Florida Legislature, 171
Florida Supreme Court, 171
Food(s), 145
  covert administration of medications in, 54
Functional magnetic resonance imaging (fMRI), 159–160
Functional status, 135
Futile interventions, 346–347
Futility
  cases of
    antibiotics not active against organism, 71
    no response to CPR, 72
    progressive septic shock, 71
    recurrent aspiration pneumonia and severe
      dementia, 72
  definitions of, 71–72, 71t
  discussions with patients and surrogates, 74–75
  failed interventions and, 72
  guidelines and procedures on, 75
  judgments, 73–74
  no pathophysiologic rationale for, 71, 71t
  physicians on, 74
  practical problems with, 73–74
  problematic appeals to, 136
  safeguards during, 74–75
  summary on, 75

Gene(s)
  abnormalities, 281
  BRCA1, 306
  BRCA2, 306
  impact of, 304–305
  mutations of, 306
Genetic discrimination
  employers and, 308
  insurers and, 308
  laws against, 308

Genetic enhancement, 311
Genetic illness to relatives, disclosure of, 342
Genetic Information Nondiscrimination Act, 308
Genetic testing
  ancestry, 307
  DNA-based, 305–307
  informed consent and
    challenges of, 308–309
    children and, 309
    importance of, 308–309
    nondirective counseling and, 309
    recommendations for, 309
Genomic(s)
  ancestry testing and, 307
  blueprint/future diary of, 304
  differences with, 304–305
  disclosure of abnormal results case and, 310
  discrimination and, 307–308
  DNA-based genetic testing and, 305–307
  enhancement in, 311
  information, 305
  informed consent and, 308–309
  knowledge, 305
  results
    confidentiality of, 309–311
    disclosure of, 310
    recommendations for, 310–311
  summary on, 311
  testing, 305
    over Internet, 307
Gift(s)
  advice about, 192
  appropriate, 191–192
  cases
    disability certification requests, 190
    elderly patient, 189
    opera tickets, 192
  declining, 192
  disclosure of, 236–237
  from drug companies
    CME and conferences as, 234
    expectations of reciprocity with, 236
    health care costs and, 236
    hospitality and meals as, 234
    objections to accepting, 235–236, 235t
    objectivity and, 236
    practices regarding, 237
    reasons for, 235
    reasons for accepting, 235
    reasons for offering, 235
    recommendations regarding, 236–237
    summary on, 237
    types of, 234–235
  from patients to physicians
    problems with, 190–191
    reasons for, 189–190
    summary on, 193
    how to respond to, 191–192
  solicitation of, 191
Global Initiative for Chronic Obstructive
      Lung Disease, 7

Global payments, 228
Gonorrhea, 46, 46*t*
Gynecology, ethical issues in obstetrics
    abortion as, 281
    assisted reproductive technologies as, 283
    differences with, 278–279
    informed consent in, 279–281
    maternal-fetal medicine as, 281–283
    summary on, 283

Harm
    best interests of patients and doing no/lack
        of, 33, 194, 242
    to donors, 297
    to patients, 248, 286
    prevention of
        duty in, 289
        steps in, 289–290
Health. *See also* Public health; Public health emergencies
    mental, 266
    plans, 229
    policy, definition of, 4
    reproductive
        for adolescents, 279–280
        philosophic quandaries regarding, 278
        third parties and, 278
Health care, 240
    access to, 179
    bedside rationing cases
        blood product shortage as, 218
        expensive care as, 219
        limited physician's time as, 218
    bedside rationing of, 216–221
        arguments against, 217
        arguments in favor of, 217–219, 217*t*
        on basis of costs, 219–221
        limited CCU beds as, 216, 218
        resources for, 221
        second opinion on, 221
        suggestions for, 221, 221*t*
        summary on, 221
        tiered formulary benefits of, 220–221
    costs
        cases, 227, 230, 231–232
        controlling, 227–232
        disclosures and options with, 230–231
        economic incentives and, 230
        financial incentives to patients, 229–230
        financial incentives to physicians, 228–229
        gifts and, 236
        physicians' responses to incentives to decrease
            services and, 230–232, 230*t*
        requests for inappropriate medical interventions
            and, 230*t*
        summary on, 232
    providers, reactions of, 86
    proxies and advance directives, 92, 95, 95*t*
    quality improvement act, 249
    in United States, 227
    workers, 55, 108

    disclosure of errors by, 244–245
    occupational risks associated with, 183–184
Health care proxy(ies)
    advance directives and, 92, 95, 95*t*
    choice of, 95
    guidelines in California, 105
    statements by, 98
Health information exchanges (HIEs), 335
Health Information Technology for Economic
        and Clinical Health (HITECH) Act
        2009, 334
Health Insurance Portability and Accountability Act.
        See HIPAA
Health maintenance organizations (HMOs), 182, 229
Health promotion, incentives for, 229–230
Heart, transplants of, 299
Hemlock Society, 149
Hemochromatosis, 306
Hepatitis B infections, 298
Hereditary nonpolyposis colorectal cancer
        (HNPCC), 306
HIPAA (Health Insurance Portability and Accountability
        Act), 43, 48, 307, 336
HIPAA Health Privacy Rule, 337
Hippocratic Oath, 42, 194
Hispanic-Americans, 178
HIV (human immunodeficiency virus), 274, 298.
        See also AIDS
    confidentiality, 3, 5, 15
        cases of transmission risks and, 45
        infections and, 46–47
        partner notification and, 47
    occupational risks associated with, 183
    surgery case, 181
HLAs. *See* Human leukocyte antigens
HMOs. *See* Health maintenance organizations
HNPCC. *See* Hereditary nonpolyposis colorectal
        cancer
Home birth, 283
"Homeostasis," 8
Hospital-specific/surgeon-specific outcomes,
        dissemination of, 272
Hospitals, 132, 182, 205, 272
House staff, ethical dilemmas of
    cases, 255, 256, 257
    clinical responsibility as, 255
    colleague relationships as, 256
    learning on patients and, 252–255, 349
    on professionalism, 257
    summary on, 259
    unethical care as, 257–258
    work hours as, 255–256
HPV. *See* Human papilloma virus
Human leukocyte antigens (HLAs), 296, 300
Human papilloma virus (HPV) vaccine, 320–321
Hurricane Katrina
    alleged active euthanasia case during, 126
    decisions during, 126
    ethical distinctions during, 126
Hypotension, 72, 111
Hypoxemia, progressive refractory, 72

IBS. *See* Irritable bowel syndrome
ICDs. *See* Implantable cardiac defibrillators
ICU. *See* Intensive care unit
Illness(es), 150
  impairment of decision-making capacity and
      mental, 82
    medical, 247
    psychiatric, 82, 247, 286
    terminal, 170
Immunizations, 320
Impaired physician(s)
  cases, 247, 250
  dealing with, 250–251, 250*t*
  legal issues regarding, 249
  reasons
    for intervention with, 247–248, 248*t*
    not to intervene with, 248–249
  whistle-blowers and, 249
Impairment, causes of, 247, 248*t*
Implantable cardiac defibrillators (ICDs), 122
Implied consent, doctrine of, 27
Inaccurate/misleading information, on internet, 333
Inadequate potassium replacement, muscle weakness due
      to, 350
Incompetence, 78
Incompetent patients, decisions for, 343–344
Infants, handicapped, 268–269
Infection(s)
  antibiotics for, 161
  confidentiality, HIV and, 46–47
  hepatitis B, 298
Infectious diseases
  reporting of, 46, 46*t*
  warnings of, 48
Influenza pandemic, vaccines during, 316
Informal arrangements, 265
Information
  cases of disclosure of prognostic, 22
  comprehensible, 28
  patients' understanding of medical/pertinent, 24, 28,
      79–80
Informed choice, 177
Informed consent, 37, 81, 271, 339
  cases
    disclosure of prognostic information, 22
    lumpectomy or mastectomy, 19, 22, 28
    reluctance to make decisions as, 24
  decision making and, 27–29, 28*t*
    promotion of, 28*t*
    shared, 20–21
  definition of, 19–20
  emergencies and, 26–27
  as ethical issue in surgery, 271–273
  as ethical issues in obstetrics/gynecology, 279–281
  exceptions to, 26–27
  genetic testing and
    challenges of, 308–309
    children and, 309
    importance of, 308–309
    nondirective counseling and, 309
    recommendations for, 309

legal issues regarding, 25–26
  problems with, 24–25
  reasons for, 20–21
  requirements for, 21–24, 21*t*
  for sterilization, 257, 280–281
  summary on, 30
  for surgery, 271–273
  voluntary, 203–204, 204*t*
Informed decision-making by patients,
      promoting, 334
Informed dissent, 20
Inoperable cancer, refusal of treatment by patient
      with, 339
Insistence on treatment(s)
  everything be done cases by family, 111, 113
  life-sustaining interventions and physicians,
      114–116, 115*t*
Institute of Medicine, 240
Institutional review boards (IRBs), 202
Insulin, overdose of, 239
Insurance, coverage deception cases, 57
Insurers, 308
Intensive care unit (ICU), 73
  cases, 110
  full, 218
Internet, 172, 307
  health information on, 333–334
Intervention(s). *See also* Medical interventions
  alternatives, 21
  assent to, 83
  benefits, consequences and risks of, 21, 21*t*
  cases
    expensive, low-yield test requests as, 38
    monitoring side effects of performance-enhancing
        drug, 36
    request for controlled drug for pain, 37
  causing suffering, 112
  clinical, 69–70, 69*f*
    flowchart for, 69*f*
  effective
    with few side effects, 267–268
    with side effects, 267–268
  futile
    definitions of, 71–72, 71*t*
    discussions with patients and surrogates, 74–75
    failed interventions and, 72
    judgments, 73–74
    no pathophysiologic rationale for, 71, 71*t*
    practical problems with, 73–74
    safeguards during, 74–75
    summary on, 75
  futile, cases of
    antibiotics not active against organism, 71
    no response to CPR, 72
    progressive septic shock, 71
    recurrent aspiration pneumonia and severe
        dementia, 72
  imposition of medical, 85
  nature of, 21
  patient refusal of beneficial, 32
  public health emergencies and

Intervention(s) (*continued*)
    non-recommended, 316–318
    refusal of, 318–319
  requests and patients' best interests, 36–39
  resource allocation and, 38
  right to refuse, 20
  suicide, 288–289
Intimate examinations, learning, 253–254
Intravenous feedings
  benefits and burdens of, 145
  clinical recommendations for, 146
  legal issues associated with, 146
  reasons to provide
    considered ordinary care, 144
    starvation as, 144
  reasons to withhold
    not considered ordinary care as, 144–145
    not suffering as, 144
    only prolong dying as, 144
  reversible causes of, 143
  severe dementia case, 143
  summary on, 147
Invasive procedures
  anesthesia for surgery and, 140
  complications associated with, 243
  learning, 254
  performing, 252
Involuntary court-ordered interventions, 286
Involuntary psychiatric commitment
  adverse consequences with, 288
  ethical issues in, 287–288
  outpatient commitment and involuntary
     treatment, 287–288
  procedures for, 287
  rationale for, 287
  standards for, 287
Involuntary treatment, 287–288
IRBs. *See* Institutional review boards
Irritable bowel syndrome (IBS), 38
Isolation, 315

Jehovah's Witness, 274
  health care providers and, 86
  refusal of blood transfusions by, 340
    legal issues associated with, 86
    suggestions on, 86–87
Joint Commission, 240, 249
Judges, conflicts of interest case, 212
Judgment(s). *See also* Substituted judgments
  detrimental outcomes or compromised, 212–213
  futility, 73–74
  impairment of clinical, 191
  of physicians, 48, 212
  QOL, 35
Justice
  definition of, 14
  principle of, 203
  recipients of organ transplantation
    and, 299–300

Kidneys, transplants of, 300
Korean-Americans, 324

Law(s), 282
  criminal, 5
  difference between clinical ethics and, 4–5
  eugenic, 305
  against genetic discrimination, 307–308
  reporting of, 249
  Texas, 75
Legal issue(s), 70
  associated with intravenous/tube feedings, 146
  associated with refusal of blood transfusions by
     Jehovah's Witness, 86
  associated with sexual contact between patients and
     physicians, 196
  constraints of physicians as, 10
  regarding informed consent, 25–26
  requirements of physicians as, 21
Legal ruling(s)
  abortion cases, 281
  Cruzan case
    court rulings on, 169
    death and, 170
    implications of, 170
  on life-sustaining interventions, 168–172
  physician-assisted cases
    court rulings on, 170–171
    implications of, 171
  Planned Parenthood v. Casey, 281
  Quinlan case
    court ruling on, 168
    implications of, 168–169
  Roe v. Wade, 281
  Schiavo case
    court rulings on, 171
    implications of, 171–172
  summary on, 172
  Tarasoff case, 289
Legal standard(s)
  for competence, 78–79
  for decision-making capacity, 78–79
Legal status, of brain deaths, 165
Life, sanctity of, 151
Life-sustaining intervention(s)
  care and, 3, 110
    clinical considerations with, 110–111
    ethical considerations on, 111–112
    family insistence on everything be done cases,
      111, 113
    physician insistence on, 114–116, 115*t*
    recommendations for, 112–114, 112*t*
    summary on, 116
  cases, 3, 110
    desire for CPR/mechanical ventilation, 110, 113
    family insistence on everything be done, 111, 113
    withdrawal of mechanical ventilation, 114, 115,
      121, 126
  ethical distinctions within

doctrine of double effect and, 123–124, 171
emotional reactions to, 125–126
extraordinary or heroic care and, 122
during Hurricane Katrina, 126
relief of symptoms with opioids/sedatives and, 123
summary on, 128
unprecedented cases for, 126–128
withdrawal and withholding of, 121–122
legal rulings on, 168–172
Live donors. *See* Transplantations
Liver, transplants of, 299
Living wills, 91
Locked-in syndrome, 160
Long-term improvement, 160
Louisiana, 126
Lumpectomy, case, 19, 22
Lying
definition of, 52
equivocating on rounds, 256
objections to, 53

Magnetic resonance imaging (MRI), 38, 57,
    224, 227, 231
Malpractice
battery and, 25
negligence and, 25
Managed care, 227
Manipulation, 23
Marshall, Thurgood, 169
Mastectomy cases, 19, 22, 28
Maternal-fetal medicine, 281–283
Maternal serum, prenatal screening using fetal
    DNA in, 282
MCS. *See* Minimally conscious state
Mechanical ventilation, cases
desire for CPR, 110, 113
withdrawal of, 114, 115, 121, 126
Mechanical ventilation, withdrawal of, 345, 348
Medicaid, 300
reimbursements, 223
services, 216
Medical decision(s)
issues and, 244
Medical information, patients' understanding of,
    24, 28, 79–80
Medical intervention(s), 69
euthanasia and, 150
health care costs and requests for
    inappropriate, 230*t*
physician-assisted suicides and, 150
for PVS, 161
unwanted, 185
Medical paternalism. *See* Paternalism
Medical record(s)
confidentiality and information omission from, 44
document discussions in, 97
Medical treatments, refusal of, 291
Medically effective treatment, refusal of, 340
Medicare, 223, 300

Medication(s), 185, 282. *See also* Drugs
case on covert administration of, 54–55, 56
deception and administration of
reasons against, 55
reasons for, 54–55
effectiveness of, 290
pain, 144
psychiatric, 290
psychoactive, 291
MELD. *See* Model for End-Stage Liver Disease
Mental illness, impairment of decision-making capacity
    and, 82
Mental status testing, role of, 81–82, 81*t*
Mercy killings, 149
Methicillin-Resistant-Staphylococcus aureus (MRSA), 71
Mexican-Americans, 324
Microallocation
decisions, 217–218
definition of, 216
Mini Mental Status Exam, 81
Minimally conscious state (MCS), 160
Minors. *See also* Adolescent(s); Children
emancipated, 265
mature, 265
parental requests for treatment of, 266
treatment of specified conditions with, 265
Misrepresentation, 12
definition of, 52
dilemmas regarding, 55–56, 55*t*
Missouri Supreme Court, 169
Mistakes. *See* Errors, disclosure of
Model for End-Stage Liver Disease (MELD), 299
Morality, 305
of children, 5
ethics and, 5
personal, 5–6
of physicians, 5–6
Morphine syringes, 126
MRI. *See* Magnetic resonance imaging
MRSA. *See* Methicillin-Resistant-Staphylococcus aureus
Multiorgan failure, 346
Muslim, 328, 330

National Practitioner Data Bank, 249
Native Americans, 307
Negative rights, 115–116
Negligence, malpractice and, 25
Neonatal intensive care unit (NICU), 268
Netherlands, physician-assisted suicides and active
    euthanasia in, 154
New Jersey Supreme Court, right to privacy rulings
    by, 168
New Orleans, 126
New York, 170, 272
NICU. *See* Neonatal intensive care unit
Nondisclosure, 13. *See also* Deception
in administration of medications
reasons against, 54
reasons for, 54–55

Nondisclosure (*continued*)
  autonomy and, 53
  avoidance of, 52–60
  cases
    cancellation of travel plans, 59
    covert administration of medicine, 54–55, 56
    excuse from work, 57–58, 59
    family request to withhold diagnoses from patient,
        52, 56, 59, 324
    insurance coverage, 57
  with colleagues, 59–60
  as culturally appropriate, 53
  definition of, 52
  dilemmas regarding, 55–56, 55*t*
  minimizing the amount/consequences of, 56
  to patient, 53–56, 55*t*
  summary on, 60
  to third parties
    reasons against, 58, 58*t*
    reasons for, 57–58
    resolving dilemmas regarding, 58–59, 58*t*
  withholding bad news from patients as
    reasons against, 54
    reasons for, 53
Noninvasive positive pressure ventilation.
        See Noninvasive ventilation (NIV)
Noninvasive ventilation (NIV), 139
Nonmaleficence, guidelines of, 13
Nonverbal communication, 332
Nonvoluntary eugenic sterilization, 280
NPPV. *See* Non-positive-pressure ventilation
Nursing homes, 143, 145

Observed behaviors, 34
Obstetric(s)
  emergencies, 280
  ethical issues in gynecology
    abortion as, 281
    assisted reproductive technologies as, 283
    differences with, 278–279
    informed consent in, 279–281
    maternal-fetal medicine as, 281–283
    summary on, 283
Opioid(s)
  active euthanasia/physician-assisted suicides, sedatives
        and, 150
  doses of, 123, 125
  prescription for, 37
  relief of symptoms with sedatives, 123
Oregon, physician-assisted suicides and active euthanasia
        in, 152–153
Organ(s). *See also* Donations; Transplantations
  allocation of various, 301
  cadaveric donor
    current system for donation of, 295–296
    donation after circulatory determination of death
        (DCDD), 296
    ethical issues associated with, 295–296
    proposals to increase, 296
    respect for, 295

    donation, 301
  transplantations, ethical issues in
    case, 301
    donation of cadaveric organs as, 295–296
    donation of organs from living donors as,
        296–298
    selection of recipients as, 298–301
    summary on, 301–302
Orthopedics operations, 181
Outpatient commitment, 287–288
Oxycodone (Oxycontin), 37
Oxycontin. *See* Oxycodone
Oxygen, home, 3, 5

Paired donation, 298
Paired kidney donations, 298
Palliative sedation
  case and refractory suffering, 126–127
  refractory suffering and, 124–125, 126–127
Parent(s)
  decision making by, 105, 264–266
  interests and children, 263–264
  relationships of physician–child with, 266–267
  requests for treatment of adolescent minors, 265
Parental consent, treating adolescents without, 350
Parental permission, 265
Paternalism, 177
  critics of, 35
  definition of, 35
  medical, 35–36
    problems associated with, 35–36
Patient(s), 236, 258. *See also* Informed consent;
        Refusal to care
  abandonment of, 187
  adolescent, 265–266
  advances by, 198
  advocate, 231
  agreements, 23, 127
  autonomy
    impairment of, 286
    respect for, 85, 150–151
  choices of, 20, 79
  confidentiality, 3, 9
    protection of, 41*t*, 48–49
  cost sharing, 229
  decision-making capacity of, 13, 70
  decisions
    control over treatment, 155
    delusions and, 80
    to future reactions, 25
    made by, 13
    reluctance to make, 24
  disclosure of errors to, 240–241, 244
  "dumping," 255
  elderly, 95, 178
  emotions and needs of, 113
  family request to withhold diagnoses from,
        52, 56, 59, 324
  gifts from, 189–192
  goals/values of, 80, 95, 156

harm to, 248, 286
incompetent, 169
individual, 26
informed, competent, 12, 28–29, 70
laws restricting physician discussions with, 26
learning on, 349–350
    dead or unconscious, 254–255
    students and, 252–255
notification of, 116, 221
out-, 287–288
participation, 132
perspectives of, 112–113, 186
persuasion of, 23, 83
physicians' therapeutic privilege and, 27
preferences and values of, 8, 56, 95–96, 99
promote informed decision-making by, 334
protection of, 215
reasonable, 26
recommendations to, 29
refusal
    of beneficial interventions, 32
    of surgery, 32
rejection of, 192
relatives of, 200
respect for, 12–13, 240
    self-determination of, 20–21
risks for, 248
roles of
    active, 28
    partnership, 28
    perspective, 28
secret information about
    approaches to, 200–201
    disclosure of, 200
    ethical dilemmas associated with, 200
    revealing, 200–201
    summary on, 201
    types of, 200
special treatments for, 192
treatment plans for, 23
understanding of medical/pertinent information by, 24, 28, 79–80
use of reasoning by, 80
values of, inconsistencies with, 106
violence by psychiatric, 48
vulnerability of, 196
waiver by, 27
well-being of, 21
Patient care. *See also* Doctor–patient relationships
    approaches to ethical dilemmas in, 3–10
    compromising of, 196
    options and diagnosis, 54
    refusal to provide, 181–187
Patient-controlled health records. *See* Personal health records (PHRs)
Patient Protection and Affordable Care Act 2010, 179, 227
Patient Self-Determination Act, 90, 170
Patients, best interests of. *See* Best interests of patients
Patient's cancer tissue, DNA profiling of, 304
Pay for performance. *See* Quality incentives

Pediatric(s), ethical issues in, 350–351
    differences in, 263
    handicapped infants and, 268–269
    interventions, 268
    refusal of medical interventions and, 267–268
    relationships of physician–child–parent within, 266–267
    standards for, 263–264
    summary on, 269
Pediatric intensive care unit (PICU), 121
Pelvic examinations, 254
Persistent vegetative state (PVS), 73, 91, 144
    appropriate treatments for, 160–161
    cases, 168
    clinical features of, 159–160
    definition of, 159–160
    MCS and, 160
    medical interventions for, 161
    prognosis of, 160
    summary on, 161
Personal health records (PHRs), 336–337
Persuasion, of patients, 23, 83
Pharmaceutical Manufacturers Association, 237
Physician(s), 243–244, 263, 286. *See also* Doctor–patient relationships
    -assisted suicide cases
        court rulings on, 170–171
        implications of, 171
    -assisted suicides and active euthanasia, 347–348
        abuse and, 151–152
        declining, 156
        justified, 156
        medical interventions and, 150
        in Netherlands, 154
        opioids or sedatives and, 150
        in Oregon, 152–153
        practice of, 153–154
        procedural and proposed safeguards associated with, 154
        reasons against, 150–152
        reasons in favor of, 150–151
        requests for, 151, 153
        responding to requests for, 155–156, 155t
        summary on, 157
        survivors of patients who underwent, 154
        unintended consequences of, 154
        U.S. policy options for, 154–155
        withdrawal of requests for, 154
    as advocates, 263
    assistance by, 10
    certification of eligibility as cases of, 3
    clinical ethics and, 6–7
    concerns, preferences and values of, 8–10
    conflicts of interests and, 14
    core values for, 34
    disagreements between parents and, 267
    disclosure of errors by/to, 241, 243–244
    dying and
        aid in, 152–153
        process of, 91
        withholding tube feedings to only prolong, 144

Physician(s) (*continued*)
  emotions of, 154
  entrepreneurism and, 178
  expertise of, 33
  fiduciary nature of relationships between
      patients and, 33
  fiduciary roles of, 228
  on futility, 74
  impaired
    cases, 247
    dealing with, 250–251, 250*t*
    legal issues regarding, 249
    reasons for intervention with, 247–248, 248*t*
    reasons not to intervene with, 248–249
    whistle-blowers and, 249
  in-office services of, 225
  incentives for
    to increase services, 223–225
    nonfinancial, 225
    problems with, 223
    self-referral as, 223–225
    summary on, 225
  joint ventures of, 224
  judgments of, 48, 212
  lack of social opportunities for, 194
  legal constraints of, 10
  legal issues associated with sexual contact between
      patients and, 196
  legal requirements of, 21
  licensed, 235
  morality of, 5–6
  primary interests of, 212
  promise-keeping suggestions for, 63–65
  recommendations, 19–20, 29
  responses to incentives to decrease services and health
      care costs, 230–232, 230*t*
  roles of, 316
  suggestions for, 221, 221*t*
  supervising, 243
  therapeutic privilege of, 27
  time of, 218
  unilateral decisions by, 74
  warnings by, 48
  wellness programs, 249
Physician orders for life-sustaining treatment (POLST), 92
Physician Payment Sunshine Act, 236
Physician–child–parent, relationships of, 266–267
PICU. *See* Pediatric intensive care unit
Placebo, uses of, 203
Planned Parenthood v. Casey, 281
Pneumonia
  and Alzheimer disease, 346
  recurrent aspiration. *See* Recurrent aspiration
      pneumonia
  stroke and aspiration, 343, 344
Poddar, Prosenjit, 289
Point of service (POS), 229
POS. *See* Point of service
Positron emission tomography (PET), 224
PPOs. *See* Preferred provider organizations
Preferred provider organizations (PPOs), 229

Pregnancy, 87, 266
  interests of women and fetus during, 279
  with other medical problems, 282
Prenatal genetic testing, 304
Prenatal testing, 281
Prescription(s)
  incorrect, 242
  for opioids, 37
Prescription Drug Monitoring Programs, 37
Principle(s)
  definition of, 16
  of ethical guidelines, 15–16
Principle of justice, 203, 336
Privacy, 41
  concept of, 42
  federal regulations on, 43
  respect for, 194
Professionalism, 4, 34, 236
  comparisons of, 196
  disclosure and, 25–26
  ethical dilemmas of students on, 257
  self-regulation and, 248
Professions, definition of, 257
Progressive septic shock, 71
Prolife advocacy groups, 172
Promise-keeping
  cases
    not to inform patient about cancer diagnosis, 62
    to schedule tests, 62–63, 64
  ethical guidelines for, 13, 64–65
  problems with, 63
  significance of, 63
  suggestions for physicians regarding, 63–65
Proportionate palliative sedation, 124
Proxy(ies)
  advance directives and health care, 92, 95, 95*t*
  choice of, 95
  guidelines in California, 105
  statements by, 98
Psychiatric care, 286–287
Psychiatric illnesses, 82, 247, 286
Psychiatric medications, 290
Psychiatric patients, violence by, 48
Psychiatric therapies, 286
Psychiatrists, consultation of, 82
Psychiatry. *See also* Involuntary psychiatric commitment
  ethical issues in
    cases, 289
    dangerous patients as, 289–290
    differences with, 286–287
    involuntary commitment as, 287–288
    refusal of treatments as, 290
    suicides as, 288–289
Psychosocial benefits, to patients through internet, 333
Psychosocial risks, to patients through internet, 334
Public health
  emergencies, ethical issues in
    differences in, 315–316
    non-recommended interventions during, 316–318
    recent, 314–315
    refusal of interventions during, 318–319

refusal to care for contagious patients as, 319
summary on, 321
vaccinations, controversies over, 320–321
guidelines for allocation and triage, 316
policies, 320
protection of, 316
Public officials, 46–47
confidentiality and reporting to, 46–47, 46t
partner notification by, 47
PVS. See Persistent vegetative state

QOL. See Quality of life
Quality incentives, 228
Quality of life (QOL)
case assessment of, 35
factors, 34
judgments by others, 35
unacceptable, 73
Quantitative information, 22
Quarantine, 315
Quinlan case
court ruling on, 168
implications of, 168–169
Quinlan, Karen Ann, 159, 161, 168–169

Racism, 329
Radiation therapy, 19, 22
Rationing
bedside cases of
blood product shortage as, 218
expensive care as, 219
limited physician's time as, 218
definition of, 216
of health care, bedside, 216–221
arguments against, 217
arguments in favor of, 217–219, 217t
on basis of costs, 219–221
limited CCU beds as, 216, 218
resources for, 221
second opinion on, 221
suggestions for, 221, 221t
summary on, 221
tiered formulary benefits of, 220–221
Recipient(s), of organ transplantation
beneficence and, 299
confidentiality of, 298
historical background of, 298–299
justice and, 299–300
selection of, 298–301
Recurrent aspiration pneumonia, 72
Refusal of treatment(s)
by competence/informed patients, 85–88
medical, 291
psychiatry, 290
Refusal to care, for patients, 181–187
antibiotics and, 88, 98, 267
beneficial interventions for patients and, 32
children and medical interventions, 267–268
by competence/informed patients, 12, 70

renal dialysis and, 87
respecting, 85
restrictions on, 87–88
scope of, 85–87
summary on, 88
for contagious patients, 319
CPR and, 136
by Jehovah's Witness
legal issues associated with blood transfusions
and, 86
suggestions on blood transfusions, 86–87
patient's best interests, surgery and, 32
public health emergencies/interventions and, 318–319
rights, 115
surgery and patient's, 32
Reimbursement, for donors, 298
Reimbursement incentive(s)
to increase services, 223–225
Medicaid, 224
nonfinancial, 225
problems with, 223
self-referral as, 223–225
summary on, 225
Religious beliefs
Christian, 115
on interventions, 112
sensitivity to, 113
in United States, 83
Renal dialysis, refusal of, 87
Reporting
abuse of children, 48–49, 282–283
of domestic violence, 49
of elder abuse, 49
of impaired colleagues/physicians, 249–251
of infectious diseases, 46–47, 46t
of laws, 249
to public officials and overriding confidentiality,
46–47, 46t
of unethical care by senior physicians, 257–258
Research ethic(s)
benefits and risks with, 203
cases
dementia, 205
finder's fee, 205, 206
osteoporosis trials, 203
conflicts of interests with, 205–206
ethical principles for, 202–205, 204t
misconceptions about, 204
nature of, 204
overview of, 203
participants in, 205
procedures of, 203
summary on, 206
Resource(s)
allocation and interventions, 38
for bedside rationing, of health care, 221
Respect
for patient, 12–13, 240
autonomy, 85, 150–151
refusals, 85
self-determination, 20–21

Respect (*continued*)
  for persons
    as ethical dilemma, 12–13
    principle of, 202
  for privacy, 194
Right(s)
  abortion, 278
  affirmative or positive, 115
  claims of, 6
  to die rulings by U.S. Supreme Court, 169
  negative, 115–116
  to privacy rulings by New Jersey Supreme Court, 168
  of refusal, 115
  to refuse interventions, 20
Roe v. Wade, 281
Rule(s)
  definition of, 16
  of ethical guidelines, 15–16

SARS. *See* Severe acute respiratory syndrome
Schiavo, Theresa, 159, 171–172
Schiavo case
  court rulings on, 171
  implications of, 171–172
Second opinions, 74
Sedation, palliative
  case and refractory suffering, 126–127
  refractory suffering and, 124–125, 126–127
Sedative(s)
  active euthanasia/physician-assisted suicides,
        opioids and, 150
  doses of, 123, 125
  relief of symptoms with opioids, 123
  uses of, 124
Seizures, 47
Selective serotonin reuptake inhibitors (SSRIs), 291
Sentinel program, 335, 336
Serotonin reuptake, 38
Serum potassium, 9
Severe acute respiratory syndrome (SARS),
        181, 183, 315, 319
Sexual contact
  cases
    current patient receiving active therapy as, 195
    former patient with no ongoing relationship, 197
    recent surgical patient, 197
  justifications for, 194
  between patients and physicians, 194–198
  with patients
    current, objections to, 195–196, 195*t*
    former, objections to, 196–198
    suggestions for, 198
  summary on, 198
Shared decision making, 20
Slow codes, 139–140
Smoking, 200
Social media, physician use of, 337
South Carolina, 283
Specificity, importance of, 8–9
Spiritual beliefs. *See* Religious beliefs

SSRIs. *See* Selective serotonin reuptake inhibitors
Sterilization, informed consent for, 257, 280–281
Steroids, oral anabolic, 36
Student(s)
  ethical dilemmas of
    cases, 255, 256, 257
    clinical responsibility as, 255
    colleague relationships as, 256
    learning on patients and, 252–255
    on professionalism, 257
    summary on, 259
    unethical care as, 257–258
    work hours as, 255–256
  introduction of, 252
Substituted judgment(s)
  case of disagreements over, 98
  inaccuracy with, 98
  inconsistency with, 98
  patients' best interests and
    assessing, 99–100
    determination of, 99
  problems with, 98–99
  questionable considerations with, 98
  summary on, 101
  unavoidable speculation and, 98
Suffering
  caregivers on, 112
  compassion for, 151
  interventions causing, 112
  refractory
    aspects of, 124
    emotional reactions to, 125–126
    palliative sedation and, 124–125, 126–127
    palliative sedation case and, 126, 128
    responses to, 124–125
    summary on, 128
    unprecedented cases for, 125
    voluntary stopping of drinking/eating and, 125
  relief of, 151
  withholding intravenous/tube feedings due to not, 144
Suicide(s), 53. *See also* Euthanasia
  definitions of, 149–150
  as ethical issue in psychiatry, 288–289
  interventions, 288–289
  physician-assisted
    abuse and, 151–152
    declining, 156
    justified, 156
    medical interventions and, 150
    in Netherlands, 154
    opioids or sedatives and, 150
    in Oregon, 152–153
    practice of, 153–154
    procedural and proposed safeguards associated
          with, 154
    reasons against, 150–152
    reasons in favor of, 150–151
    requests for, 151, 153
    responding to requests for, 155–156, 155*t*
    summary on, 157
    survivors of patients who underwent, 154

unintended consequences of, 154
U.S. policy options for, 154–155
withdrawal of requests for, 154
Sulfonamide antibiotics, 242
SUPPORT study, 110, 123
Surgeon(s)
decline to operate by, 273–274
experience of, 23
individual, 271
lumpectomy or mastectomy cases of, 19, 22, 28
outcomes of, 271
Surgery
anesthesia for invasive procedures and, 140
consent for, 254
disclosure of approaches/experiences/outcomes in, 272–273
ethical issues in
cases, 273, 274, 275
differences with, 271
informed consent as, 271–273
risks associated with, 274–276
summary on, 276
exploratory, 38
HIV and, 181
patient refusal of, 32
recent patient case undergoing, 197
trainees' role during, 22
Surgical innovation, disclosure of, 272
Surrogate(s), 69f, 90, 93, 94, 98
agreement of, 127
authorization of deception, 55
conflicts of interests among, 106–107
decision making, 8, 10
case of, 104
improvement of, 107–108, 107t
disclosure of errors to, 240–241, 244
emotions and needs of, 113
futile intervention discussions with, 74–75
interests and needs of, 99
notification of, 221
perspectives of, 112–113
potential
court-appointed guardians as, 104–105
disagreements among, 107
family members as, 105
no family members as, 106
selection of, 105
summary on, 108
Sweden, 145
Syndrome(s), 6

Tarasoff, Tatiana, 289
Tarasoff case, 289
Teaching styles, 256
Terminal sedation. See Palliative sedation
Terri's Law, 171, 172
Texas laws, 75
Therapeutic portal-systemic shunt (TIPS), 218
Therapeutic privilege, of physicians, 27
Therapies, 69

Third parties
deception and nondisclosure to
reasons against, 58, 58t
reasons for, 57–58
resolving dilemmas regarding, 58–59, 58t
overriding confidentiality and, 45–48
reproductive health and, 278
Time, use of, 113
TIPS. See Therapeutic portal-systemic shunt
Toss-ups, 29
Trainee(s), 254. See also Students
cognitive and procedural skills of, 271
deception and, 59
disclosure of errors by, 243–244
emotional distress of, 244
responses, 243–244
suggestions for, 258
surgery and role of, 22
Transparency, maintaining, 56
Transplantation(s)
anticipated benefit of, 300
cadaveric donor organs and
current system for donation of, 295–296
donation after circulatory determination of death (DCDD), 296
ethical issues associated with, 295–296
proposals to increase, 296
respect for, 295
ethical issues in organ
cadaveric donor organs as, 295–296
case, 301
donation of organs from living donors as, 296–298
selection of recipients as, 298–301
summary on, 301–302
heart and liver, 299
kidney, 300
living donors, donation of organs and, 296–298
previous, 300
Trust, 93
issues, 56, 196
loss of, 53
public, 191, 236
undermining of, 58
Truth telling, 52. See also Deception
Tube feedings
benefits and burdens of, 145
clinical recommendations for, 146
legal issues associated with, 146
reasons to provide
considered ordinary care, 144
starvation as, 144
reasons to withhold
not considered ordinary care as, 144–145
not suffering as, 144
only prolong dying as, 144
reversible causes of, 143
severe dementia case, 143
summary on, 147
withholding, 345
Tuberculosis, 46, 46t, 314–315

Unconscious patients, learning on, 254–255
Unethical care, by other physicians, 257–258
Uniform Anatomical Gift Act, 295
Uniform Determination of Death Act, 165
Unilateral DNAR orders, 136
United Kingdom, 145
United Network for Organ Sharing (UNOS), 300
United States (U.S.), 164, 298, 300, 308, 314
    cultures in, 53
    health care in, 227
    policy options for euthanasia and suicides in, 154–155
    policy policies, 220
    religious beliefs in, 83
UNOS. *See* United Network for Organ Sharing
Unprofessional actions, patterns of, 34
U.S. *See* United States
U.S. Congress, 249
U.S. Constitution, 85
U.S. Food and Drug Administration, 145
U.S. Ninth Circuit Court, 170
U.S. Supreme Court
    right to die rulings by, 169

rulings of, 85, 123, 149, 281
Utilitarianism, 15

Vaccine(s)
    case, 317–318
    development of, 182
    during influenza pandemic, 317
Vasopressors, 71, 72, 125
Vegetative state. *See* Persistent vegetative state
Venous thromboembolism, 306
Violence, by psychiatric patients, 48

Washington, 170
Whistle-blowers, 258
Whole-genome sequencing, 306–307
Wisdom, practical, 15, 16
Women, fetus, pregnancy and, 279
Work
    excuse from, 57–58, 59
    hours, 255–256